Scientific and Technical Publication No. 631

UNHAPPY HOURS:
alcohol and partner aggression in the Americas

Editors: Kathryn Graham, Sharon Bernards, Myriam Munné, and Sharon C. Wilsnack

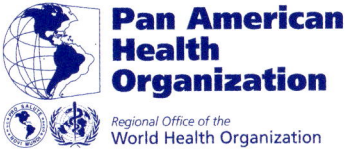

UNHAPPY HOURS:

To be published in Spanish (2009) as:
El brindis infeliz: el consumo de alcohol y la agresión entre parejas en las Américas
ISBN 978-92-75-31631-3

PAHO HQ Library Cataloguing-in- Publication Data

Pan American Health Organization
Unhappy Hours: Alcohol and Partner Aggression in the Americas
Washington, D.C.: PAHO, © 2008
(Scientific and Technical Publication No. 631)

ISBN 978-92-75-11631-9

I. Title   II (Series)

1. ALCOHOL DRINKING – adverse effects
2. AGGRESSION –psychology
3. DOMESTIC VIOLENCE – legislation and jurisprudence
4. ALCOHOL-RELATED DISORDERS – psychology
5. BATTERED WOMEN
6. SPOUSE ABUSE
7. AMERICAS

NLM WM274

The Pan American Health Organization welcomes requests for permission to reproduce or translate its publications, in part or in full. Applications and inquiries should be addressed to the Scientific and Technical Publication Project, Knowledge Management and Communications Area, Pan American Health Organization, 525 23rd Streets, N.W., Washington, DC, USA, which will be glad to provide the latest information on any changes made to the text, plans for new editions, and reprints and translations already available.

©Pan American Health Organization, 2008

Publications of the Pan American Health Organization enjoy copyright protection in accordance with the provisions of Protocol 2 of the Universal Copyright Convention. All rights are reserved.

The designations employed and the presentation of the material in this publication do not imply the expression of any opinion whatsoever on the part of the Secretariat of the Pan American Health Organization concerning the status of any country, territory, city or area or of its authorities, or concerning the delimitation of its frontiers or boundaries.

The mention of specific companies or of certain manufacturers' products does not imply that they are endorsed or recommended by the Pan American Health Organization in preference to others of a similar nature that are not mentioned. Errors and omissions excepted, the names of proprietary products are distinguished by initial capital letters.

Table of Contents

Preface v
Foreword vii
Introduction ix

Gender, Alcohol, and Culture: An International Study (GENACIS)—A Brief History, Present Work, and Future Initiatives
Benjamin Taylor, Sharon Wilsnack, and Jürgen Rehm 1

General Issues in Research on Intimate Partner Violence: An Overview
Sharon Wilsnack and Richard Wilsnack 7

Common Survey Methods and Analyses Conducted for Each Country Chapter
Sharon Bernards and Kathryn Graham 25

Argentina: Alcohol and Partner Physical Aggression in Buenos Aires Province and City
Myriam Munné 35

Belize: Alcohol and Partner Physical Aggression
Claudina Ellington Cayetano and Kathryn Graham 55

Brazil: Alcohol and Partner Physical Aggression in Metropolitan São Paulo
Florence Kerr-Corrêa, Janaina Barbosa de Oliveira, Maria Cristina Pereira Lima, Adriana Marcassa Tucci, Maria Odete Simão, Mariana Braga Cavariani, and Miriam Malacize Fantazia 73

Canada: Alcohol and Partner Physical Aggression in the 10 Provinces
Kathryn Graham and Sharon Bernards 91

Costa Rica: Alcohol and Partner Physical Aggression in the Greater Metropolitan Area of San José
Julio Bejarano 111

Mexico: Alcohol and Partner Physical Aggression in Ciudad Juárez, Monterrey, Querétaro, and Tijuana
Martha Romero Mendoza, María Elena Medina-Mora, Jorge Villatoro Velázquez, Clara Fleiz, Leticia Casanova, and Francisco Juárez 129

Nicaragua: Alcohol and Partner Physical Aggression in Bluefields, Estelí, Juigalpa, León, and Rivas
José Trinidad Caldera Aburto, Sharon Bernards, and Myriam Munné 147

Peru: Alcohol and Partner Physical Aggression in Lima and Ayacucho
Marina Piazza 163

United States: Alcohol and Partner Physical Aggression—Findings from a National Sample of Women
Sharon C. Wilsnack, Richard W. Wilsnack, and Arlinda F. Kristjanson 187

Uruguay: Alcohol and Partner Physical Aggression in Various Cities
Raquel Magri, Hector Suárez, and Laurita Regueira 207

Comparison of Partner Physical Aggression across Ten Countries
Kathryn Graham and Sharon Bernards 221

Acknowledgments 249

UNHAPPY HOURS:

Preface

For many years we have known and been concerned about the damage that partner violence has inflicted on women, children, and even men in our Region. We have also known that alcohol is one of the leading risk factors for the burden of disease in the Americas—in 2002 alone, alcohol was responsible for more than 323,000 deaths and more than 14 million years of healthy life lost to premature death and disability.

For as many years, PAHO has steadfastly worked to combat gender-based violence, promote gender equality, and construct more just societies with health for all. The publication of *Unhappy Hours: Alcohol and Partner Aggression in the Americas* is the latest contribution to a better understanding of partner violence and, in so doing, find more effective interventions to right this wrong.

I am proud to introduce this book, which for the first time explores the relationship between alcohol consumption and partner violence. It brings to light evidence of alcohol's impact on partner aggression from 10 of the Region's countries, and represents an unprecedented effort to collect and analyze information from the general population that can be compared across countries. The book reminds us how alcohol consumption can contribute to violence, distort gender relations, and erode the dream of attaining health for all women, men, and children in the Americas.

Finally, the book's message is clear: effective policies to decrease excessive, harmful alcohol consumption in a population will have a beneficial impact on the rates of violence against women. Let this publication begin to chart the way to putting in place a comprehensive strategy to reduce alcohol-related problems and harmful drinking, and so address gender inequity and many of the health conditions reducing the lives and quality of life of the people living in the Region.

Mirta Roses Periago
Director

Foreword

This is a brave and important study. It explores an element of partner violence that has long been taboo among feminist activists and researchers: the role of alcohol in contributing to the frequency and severity of violence in intimate relationships.

I began researching the issue of violence against women in the early 1980s. At that time, the problem of partner violence—especially on an international scale—was still deeply hidden. Victims suffered in silence and few global institutions acknowledged, let alone tackled, the issue.

Women's groups were beginning to organize in countries outside of the United States and Europe. But they still saw the problem of partner violence as an aberration—a problem unique to their culture. It was not until the late 1990s that advocates began to join forces across national boundaries and frame intimate partner violence as a global issue, first as an abuse of women's human rights at the United Nations World Conference on Human Rights in Vienna in 1993 and later as a global health issue.

Research helped consolidate this realization—both by collecting women's stories and by generating numbers to communicate the frequency and breadth of these experiences. Certain things became clear: physical and sexual violence by an intimate partner was a common occurrence in women's lives and, to a lesser extent, in the lives of men. The health consequences of violence are serious and can persist long after the violence has stopped.

I was privileged to be involved in helping to launch the first global study of violence against women and its health consequences. Sponsored by the World Health Organization, this study was the first to provide comparable data across 15 sites in 10 nations. Our understanding of violence takes a major step forward with the publication of the present study on partner aggression and alcohol.

The GENACIS study—Gender, Alcohol, and Culture: An International Study—explores how gender and culture combine to affect alcohol consumption and alcohol-related problems. The PAHO Multicentric Study is an arm of this initiative that specifically examines these issues in 10 countries of the Americas and explores the relationship between alcohol consumption and partner violence. Not only does the PAHO study address an under-attended aspect of the violence dilemma, it advances research methodology by collecting detailed information on how women and men experience the event: "How severe was it? What was your level of fear? How upset were you just after the incident happened?"

If you talk to women about their experiences of violence, they frequently link drinking and abuse, especially drinking by their male partners. Women have long suspected what this study now confirms: the risk of violence goes up when men drink heavily.

This will come as no surprise to many victims of partner violence, but it is a truth that the anti-violence movement has been loath to embrace. The fear has always been that drunkenness will be used as an excuse to explain away violence—that fingering alcohol will deflect attention away from the power and gender dimensions of abuse.

If we are to deal with the problem of partner aggression, however, we must acknowledge its hydra-like nature. It is a problem with many interlocking antecedents that operate at multiple levels: biological proclivities and personal history, relationship factors and immediate triggers, social and neighborhood contexts, and macro dimensions such as gender hierarchies and social norms around conflict resolution and violence.

Alcohol is most certainly a part of this complex puzzle. And it is one of the factors most open to intervention and change. The challenge now is how to use this knowledge to help make relationships safer and reduce the chances of partner violence. This will require new collaborations between the substance abuse practitioners and researchers and the anti-violence movement.

PAHO is in an excellent position to take leadership in this arena, charting a course that other regions can follow. In the 1990s, PAHO spearheaded a unique project to strengthen community and health sector response to partner violence in Latin America. And it has long worked to study and respond to both substance abuse and community violence. I look forward to helping to actualize a new set of interventions that can mobilize the combined wisdom of these multiple fields, to make relationships safer for women, men, and their children.

Lori Heise

Research Fellow,
Gender Violence and Health Centre, London School of Hygiene and Tropical Medicine

Core Research Team Member
WHO Multi-Country Study on Women's Health and Domestic Violence against Women

Director, Global Campaign for Microbicides, PATH

Introduction

Alcohol consumption ranked first among 26 risk factors for ill-health in the Americas in 2000, ranking higher than tobacco, overweight, or lack of sanitation (Rehm and Monteiro, 2005), based on statistics compiled for the World Health Organization comparative risk assessment study (Rehm et al, 2004). The pattern of alcohol consumption in many countries in the Region is among the most harmful to health in the world, according to WHO estimates, as the way people typically drink is to consume excessive amounts on a single occasion. This consumption pattern is especially associated with intentional and unintentional injuries. The young age of the population of many countries in the Americas also is associated with increased risk, because young people tend to drink more per occasion than older adults at an age when they are more likely to take other risks such as speeding in a car or engaging in unsafe sex.

Injuries contribute to more than 40% of alcohol-related mortality and life-years lost to disability in the Americas (Rehm and Monteiro, 2005). While fatal injuries are one of the most measurable health consequences of acute alcohol intoxication, much less is known about nonfatal injuries.

An important cause of injuries is violent behavior and aggression. Alcohol is known to increase aggression in both men and women, but the strength of this relationship differs from culture to culture. To date, it has been difficult to establish comparisons of domestic violence across countries, because different questions and indicators have been used in studies, and because of the general taboos and secrecy surrounding violence between couples. Moreover, the role of alcohol in partner violence has been largely ignored. There is a need to increase knowledge and understanding of the relationship between alcohol consumption and partner violence across different cultures, using comparable measures and methods, so that policies aimed at reducing partner violence and addressing the role played by alcohol consumption are appropriate for the societies in which they are applied.

The most important predictor of alcohol consumption and related harms is gender. Men and women differ in the prevalence and frequency of drinking, as well as in the quantity of alcohol consumed per occasion and the severity of some alcohol-related harms, again with variations among countries and within countries. In addition to biological differences between men and women in the way alcohol is metabolized and how it alters cognitive functions (Graham et al., 1998), there are also cultural differences reflected in different gender relations, roles, and expectations from country to country and in different contexts. In Latin America, studies have found that between 4% and 15% of women are affected by sexual violence from a partner. However, international research on such gender and cultural variations has had major limitations, including differences in how alcohol consumption is measured; how lifetime abstainers are distinguished from former drinkers; how heavy episodic drinking is defined for men and women; and how problems are defined, categorized, or reported, all of which makes it difficult to interpret differences between sexes and across countries.

In response to the need to generate Regional data on alcohol consumption in the general population that is comparable and that has a gender perspective, in 2004 the Pan

American Health Organization supported a multicentric study on gender, alcohol, culture, and harm (Taylor et al., 2007), which built on the international study called GENACIS (Gender, Alcohol and Culture: an International Study). Six countries from the Americas (Argentina, Canada, Costa Rica, Mexico, Uruguay, and the United States) participated in the GENACIS project, collecting information on alcohol consumption and alcohol-related problems from general population samples, using comparable variables and indicators. With PAHO's support, three other countries (Belize, Nicaragua, and Peru) collected new data using the same variables and indicators. In addition, Brazil funded a new survey using the same survey instrument. These countries represent a wide variation of social and economic development (including high-, middle-, and low-income countries), access to services, per capita income, gap between the poorest and the richest in each country, and societal gender roles (reflected in different human development indexes and gender development indexes).

This book expands on findings from the multicentric study by focusing specifically on alcohol consumption and partner violence. Each country chapter analyzes data using the same variables related to alcohol consumption and partner aggression, but interprets results considering each country's cultural framework. This book presents, for the first time, a comparative and international analysis of alcohol consumption and partner aggression with a gender perspective. It demonstrates that despite the large differences between countries and cultures, there are some commonalities and trends across countries regarding the relationship between alcohol and partner violence.

In particular, the findings described here indicate that partner violence is associated with younger ages in all countries, and that partners in common-law relationships were especially at risk in most countries. Women reported being victims of more severe aggression than men reported, and female victims reported greater fear, anger and upset. With regard to alcohol, men in all countries were more likely than women to have been drinking at the time of the partner aggression incident. Both men and women who were victims or perpetrators of partner aggression were more likely to be drinkers than abstainers and, among drinkers, were more likely to report drinking larger amounts per occasion.

At the same time, given the variations found across countries in the prevalence of violent behavior by men against women, the role of cultures' and societies' expectations about gender and about alcohol's effects also play a role in this relationship. These findings have implications for policies, awareness campaigns, and services for men and women involved in partner aggression.

Spain undertook the same survey in 2002 in Cantabria, Galicia, and Valencia (Sanchez et al., 2004). Although the data from Spain were not included in this book, it is interesting to note that findings in that country echoed some elements of a "Latin culture," reflecting

Spain's historical and cultural relationship with Latin America, despite the fact that Spanish society is much more similar to the United States and Canada in terms of social and economic development. This means that despite higher levels of education, Spanish women are much less likely than Spanish men to contribute financially to the family's income, and for most women, staying home (as housewives) is still the most common job. And yet, alcohol consumption is more prevalent in Spain's general population than in any country of Latin America (thus following the European pattern of regularly drinking with meals), being slightly higher in men than in women, and with excessive consumption being more prevalent among male drinkers (following the same pattern seen in Latin America of young people drinking excessively during weekends). However, the gender gap is narrowing, and among younger age groups there is a higher prevalence of excessive episodic drinking among women than among men. With regard to aggressive behaviors, while the levels of aggression in Spain were lower than in some Latin American countries, the association with alcohol was the same as that presented in the chapters of this book. In addition, a significant percentage of male aggressors (39%) did not feel their actions were a problem, did not recognize their severity and did not feel guilty about them. There was a clear association between levels of alcohol consumption and frequency of physical aggression against an intimate partner. These findings highlight the importance of cultural perceptions about aggression and alcohol consumption in societies in which gender relations are changing.

We hope this book will contribute to a greater awareness of the extent of alcohol consumption and its attendant problems in the Region, specifically domestic violence, and that it will lead to the development of effective alcohol policies and the provision of services to men and women with alcohol-related problems, not only in the countries included here but in all the Region's countries. In light of the evidence of the relationship between partner violence and heavy alcohol consumption, effective policies to reduce heavy episodic consumption of alcohol need to be promoted as an integral part of policies and programs to reduce domestic violence. Regardless of the level of development or culture, it is clear that action is needed to address alcohol-related partner violence.

Maristela G. Monteiro
Senior Advisor on Alcohol and Substance Abuse
Pan American Health Organization

Marijke Velzeboer-Salcedo
Senior Advisor on Gender, Ethnicity, and Health
Pan American Health Organization

References

Sanchez L, et al.(2004). Estudio Internacional sobre Género, Alcohol y Cultura "Proyecto GENACIS. Sociedad Española de Toxicomanías, Valencia.

Graham K, Wilsnack R, Dawson D, Vogeltanz N. (1998). Should alcohol consumption measures be adjusted for gender differences? *Addiction*, 93(8), 1137–1147.

Rehm J, Monteiro M. (2005). Alcohol consumption and burden of disease in the Americas –implications for alcohol policy. *Pan American Journal of Public Health* 18 (4/5) 241–248.

Rehm J, Room R, Monteiro M, Gmel G, Graham K, Rehn N, Christopher T. Sempos, Frick U, Jernigan D Alcohol as a risk factor for global burden of disease. In: Ezzati M, Lopez AD, Rodgers A, Murray CJL (eds) Quantification of Health Risks: Global and Regional Burden of Disease due to Selected Major Risk Factors. Vol 1, 959–1108, 2004, WHO, Geneva.

Taylor B, Rehm J, Caldera JT, Bejarano J, Cayetano C, Kerr-Correa F, Piazza M, Gmel G, Graham K, Greenfield T, Laranjeira R, Lima MC, Magri R, Monteiro M, Mora MEM, Munné M, Romero MP, Tucci AM, Wilsnack S. (2007). Alcohol, gender, culture and harms in the Americas: PAHO multi-centric study final report. Pan American Health Organization, Washington DC.

Gender, Alcohol, and Culture: An International Study (GENACIS)[1]

A brief history, present work, and future initiatives—Benjamin Taylor, MSc; Sharon C. Wilsnack, PhD; and Jürgen Rehm, PhD

The Motivation

Gender is a strong predictor of alcohol use and alcohol-related problems. In studies worldwide, men are more likely than women to consume alcohol and to experience more problems related to their drinking, a gender gap that is one of the few universal gender differences in human social behavior. Although this gender gap has narrowed a bit in some societies, population subgroups, and historical periods, there is little evidence that it is disappearing (Holmila and Raitasalo, 2005; Wilsnack and Wilsnack, 1997).

Despite the universality of gender differences in drinking behavior, the *magnitude* of the difference varies greatly across societies and historical eras, suggesting that whatever biological differences underlie men's greater consumption of alcohol compared to women, cultural influences can substantially modify them (Graham et al., 1998; Wilsnack et al., 2000). Thus, the study of how women's and men's drinking behaviors differ across a variety of cultural settings can make several important contributions: first, it can help to answer broader questions about how societies influence women and men to behave differently; second it can identify false assumptions about women's and men's drinking behaviors that may impair societies' efforts to identify and control alcohol-related problems; and third, it can identify gender-related drinking patterns and risk factors that, in turn, can inform the development of more effective, gender-sensitive approaches to prevention, treatment, and policy formulation (Wilsnack et al., 2005). As will be seen below, the Gender, Alcohol, and Culture: An International Study (GENACIS) project provides an extraordinary opportunity for improving our understanding of how gender and culture combine to affect alcohol consumption and related problems.

The Team

At the 1993 symposium of the Kettil Bruun Society for Social and Epidemiological Research on Alcohol (KBS)[2] in Krakow, Poland, 13 researchers from nine countries who were interested in research on women, gender, and alcohol use organized the International Research Group on Gender and Alcohol (IRGGA). Now boasting more than 140 members from more than 40 countries, IRGGA meets annually in conjunction with the yearly KBS symposium. Group members have published papers on methodo-

---

[1] Additional information about GENACIS can be found at the project's two websites: http://www.med.und.nodak.edu/depts/irgga (the general project website at the University of North Dakota) and http://www.genacis.org (in Lausanne, Switzerland, where the GENACIS codebook and other information related to data analysis are posted).
[2] For more information on the Kettil Bruun Society, please visit their website at www.arg.org/kbs/ .

logical aspects of gender and alcohol research (Graham et al., 1998) and secondary analyses of general population surveys (Haavio-Mannila et al., 1996; Vogeltanz-Holm et al., 2004; Wilsnack et al., 2000), including a three-year comparative study of alcohol use and related problems among women in nine European countries (Allamani et al., 2000; Gmel, Bloomfield, et al., 2000; Knibbe and Bloomfield, 2001). These studies notwithstanding, the limited set of comparable questions and measures available in existing data sets was recognized as a major impediment to conducting international comparative analyses of men's and women's drinking behavior. In response, GENACIS, a truly international initiative, was born.

The Project

In 1998, IRGGA members began designing the Gender, Alcohol, and Culture: An International Study (GENACIS), a multinational study intended to collect and analyze data from new surveys in many countries, using similar questions, measures, and survey methods (Wilsnack and Wilsnack, 2002). As of February 2008, 47 countries were participating in the study, including nations in Africa, South and Central America, North America, Europe, and Asia. An undertaking of this scope clearly requires many types of support, and the work to date has been made possible through grants and other support from the United States National Institute on Alcohol Abuse and Alcoholism (part of the National Institutes of Health), the European Union, the World Health Organization, the Pan American Health Organization (specifically for the GENACIS Multicentric Project, described below), and government agencies and other organizations that have funded GENACIS surveys in their home countries. The GENACIS database currently holds information from more than 160,000 respondents worldwide, making it one of the largest and most culturally diverse studies of alcohol use to date.

Survey Measures

For each content area of the common GENACIS questionnaire (drinking variables plus seven domains of potential antecedents and consequences), members created a minimum set of "core" questions and a larger set of "expanded core" questions that would provide more extensive and detailed information. Most questions and measures in the GENACIS questionnaire were taken from well-validated survey instruments and, wherever possible, from internationally field-tested instruments. Under the supervision of each country's survey director and other senior survey staff, and prior to being used in the survey, all GENACIS questions were translated into the target country's language and then back-translated to check for translation accuracy and cultural appropriateness of the items. If surveys needed to use more than one language, the questionnaire was translated into the most commonly understood language, and then interviewers were selected and trained so that they could translate the questionnaire for other language groups.[3]

---

[3] The countries participating in the GENACIS multicentric study as of February 2008 were: Argentina, Australia, Austria, Belize, Brazil, Canada, Costa Rica, Czech Republic, Denmark, Finland, France, Germany, Hungary, Iceland, India, Ireland, Isle of Man, Israel, Italy, Japan, Kazakhstan, Mexico, the Kingdom of the Netherlands, New Zealand, Nicaragua, Nigeria, Norway, Peru, Russia, Spain, Sri Lanka, Sweden, Switzerland, Uganda, United Kingdom, United States of America, and Uruguay.

The expanded questionnaire included detailed questions about *alcohol consumption and alcohol-related problems*, which were designed to measure drinking patterns and total volume of alcohol consumed, as well as self-perceived and more objective indicators of alcohol-related problems. Questions about drinking-related problems drew on studies evaluating models of alcohol-related harm (Gmel, Rehm, et al., 2000; Greenfield, 1998; Rehm et al., 1999) and combined three types of indices: self-perceived problems, disapproval as perceived by others, and more objective indicators such as drunk driving offenses. These questions and the questions about alcohol consumption included all the items from the Alcohol Use Disorders Identification Test (AUDIT) (Saunders et al., 1993), which allowed respondents to be scored on that internationally validated measure.

Other questionnaire sections included measures of *drinking contexts and companions, social pressures about drinking, intimate relationships, health and lifestyle*, and some *demographic* variables. Specifically important for this book, and because reducing violence toward women is a high priority internationally (European Commission, 2000; World Health Organization, 1999), the GENACIS surveys included detailed questions about *violence and victimization*.

Survey Implementation
Survey characteristics
The GENACIS surveys varied somewhat in their sampling frame (some were regional in scope; others, national), age range of samples, and mode of administration. That said, survey directors were strongly encouraged to meet minimum requirements: (1) a sample size of at least 1,000 that includes women and men; (2) multi-stage random sampling; (3) either a national sample or, in large countries such as India, sample an entire province or region that includes both urban and rural areas, corresponds to a governmental unit for which there are aggregate statistics, and includes a large population of drinkers; (4) strenuous effort to attain a 70% or higher completion rate; and (5) inclusion of all questions from the common GENACIS questionnaire, with the exception of any questions judged by the survey leader and staff to be culturally inappropriate for their country (such exclusions were rare). Most GENACIS surveys involved face-to-face interviews; some were conducted via telephone interviews or postal surveys.

Data Management
GENACIS data is centrally managed at the Swiss Institute for the Prevention of Alcohol and Drug Problems (SIPA) in Lausanne, Switzerland, under the direction of Dr. Gerhard Gmel. After the data is initially cleaned in each country and then further cleaned and edited at SIPA, each country's data set is merged with the central data base that contains the data from all other GENACIS surveys. SIPA staff members send

either a complete edited GENACIS data base or subsets of countries and variables (to be analyzed for specific publications) to GENACIS members, who conduct analyses at their home institutions. Three monographs, a special issue in a journal, and more than 100 articles and book chapters have been based on GENACIS data since the project's inception.

The PAHO Multicentric Study: A Focus on the Americas

The PAHO Multicentric Study is an arm of the GENACIS project that operates in North, South, and Central America. It is designed to include more of the Region's countries in the project and addresses key issues on alcohol and health in the Americas. The collaborating countries in the PAHO initiative are Argentina, Belize, Brazil (with both a national sample and a São Paulo sample), Canada, Costa Rica, Mexico, Nicaragua, Peru, Uruguay, and the United States of America. The PAHO project's main objective is to gain a detailed epidemiological picture of alcohol consumption and related outcomes in the Americas, with the first report recently published as an overview of this work (Taylor et al., 2007). Work already done has led to an increased awareness of alcohol consumption and alcohol-related problems, both in terms of public policy formulation and of survey methodology issues. Workshops and meetings have been held in participating countries to enable cultural and educational transfer among participants.

Work done as part of the PAHO project also contributed to the Brasilia Declaration, the result of a three-day meeting of the first annual Pan American Conference on Alcohol Public Policies, held in Brasilia, Brazil, in 2005. This meeting included a presentation and discussion among leaders of the multicentric project using GENACIS-related data and the formulation of priorities for policies on alcohol in the Americas. The Brasilia Declaration (Monteiro, 2007) recommended that:

- Preventing and reducing alcohol consumption-related harm be considered as public health priorities for action in all countries of the Americas.
- Regional and national strategies be developed, incorporating culturally-appropriate, evidence-based approaches to reduce alcohol consumption-related harm.
- These strategies be supported by improved information systems and additional scientific studies on the impact of alcohol and the effect of policies on alcohol on the national and cultural contexts of the countries in the Americas.
- A Regional network of national counterparts, nominated by Member States, be established with the Pan American Health Organization's technical cooperation and support to work towards reducing alcohol-related harm.
- Alcohol policies whose effectiveness has been established by scientific research be implemented and evaluated in all countries of the Americas.
- Priority areas of action include: heavy drinking occasions, overall alcohol consumption, alcohol and women (including pregnant women), alcohol and indigenous peoples, alcohol and youth, alcohol and other vulnerable populations, alcohol and violence, alcohol and intentional and unintentional injuries, underage drinking, and alcohol-use disorders.

These six recommendations are the scope within which the GENACIS Multicentric Project seeks to gain knowledge and understanding; they also provide part of the impetus for this publication.

Future Initiatives

GENACIS continues to hold yearly workshops before the annual meeting of the Kettil Bruun Society for Social and Epidemiological Research on Alcohol. Groups of members are exploring possible funding for new GENACIS surveys in countries not yet represented, with China and additional countries in Africa and Latin America being of particular interest.

In addition, co-investigators of a new National Institute on Alcohol Abuse and Alcoholism five-year grant meet twice each year to plan and present new analyses. These grant-supported analyses are using multilevel modeling and other advanced statistical techniques to investigate combined gender and cultural differences in drinking behavior and its adverse effects; how drinking and its effects are modified by socio-economic conditions, social status, social roles (including gender roles), and drinking contexts; and how drinking is linked to social pressures to control drinking, intimate relationships, and intimate partner violence. The individual-level measures of drinking patterns, drinking-related problems, and their possible antecedents and consequences are supplemented by societal-level measures (from archival sources and aggregated survey data), including measures of gender inequality and economic development. Findings will be disseminated in professional journals, research monographs, and at an international research conference to be hosted by GENACIS in the fourth year of the grant. It is anticipated that GENACIS activities will continue for many years to come. When all analyses and publications of interest to current and future members are completed, GENACIS data sets will be archived (probably at SIPA) for use by future researchers interested in global time trends in women's and men's drinking.

References

Allamani A, Voller F, Kubicka L, Bloomfield K. (2000). Drinking cultures and the position of women in nine European countries. *Substance Abuse*, 21, 231–247.

European Commission (May 2000). *Implementation by the European Community of the Platform for Action Adopted at the Fourth World Conference on Women in Beijing 1995*. Working document, European Commission.

Gmel G, Bloomfield K, Ahlström S, Choquet M, Lecomte T. (2000). Women's roles and women's drinking: A comparative study in four European countries. *Substance Abuse*, 21, 249–264.

Gmel G, Rehm J, Room R, Greenfield TK. (2000). Dimensions of alcohol-related social harm and health consequences in survey research. *Journal of Substance Abuse*, 12, 113–138.

Graham K, Wilsnack R, Dawson D, Vogeltanz N. (1998). Should alcohol measures be adjusted for gender differences? *Addiction*, 93, 1137–1147.

Greenfield TK. (1998). Evaluating competing models of alcohol-related harm. *Alcoholism: Clinical and Experimental Research*, 22, 52S–62S.

Haavio-Mannila E, Harris TR, Klassen AD, Wilsnack RW, Wilsnack SC. (1996). Alcohol and sexuality among American and Finnish women. *Nordisk Sexologi*, 13, 129–146.

Holmila M, Raitasalo K. (2005). Gender differences in drinking: Why do they still exist? *Addiction*, 100, 1763-1769.

Knibbe RA, Bloomfield K. (2001). Alcohol consumption estimates in surveys in Europe: Compa-rability and sensitivity for gender differences. *Substance Abuse*, 22, 23-38.

Monteiro MG. (2007). *Alcohol and Public Health in the Americas: A Case for Action.* Washington, D.C.: Pan American Health Organization.

Rehm J, Frick U, Bondy S. (1999). Reliability and validity analysis of an alcohol-related harm scale for surveys. *Journal of Studies on Alcohol*, 60, 203-208.

Saunders J, Aasland O, Babor T, De la Fuente J, Grant M. (1993). Development of the Alcohol Use Disorders Identification Test (AUDIT): WHO Collaborative Project on Early Detection of Persons with Harmful Alcohol Consumption-II. *Addiction*, 88, 791-804.

Taylor B, Rehm J, Aburto J, Bejarano J, Cayetano C, Kerr-Correa F, Ferrand M, Gmel G, Graham K, Greenfield T, Laranjeira R, Lima M, Magri R, Monteiro M, Medina Mora M, Munné M, Romero M, Tucci A, Wilsnack S. (2007). Alcohol, Gender, Culture and Harms in the Americas: PAHO Multicentric Study Final Report. Washington, D.C.: Pan American Health Organization.

Vogeltanz-Holm ND, Neve RJM, Greenfield TK, Wilsnack RW, Kubicka L, Wilsnack SC, Fleming, JM, Spak F. (2004). A cross-cultural analysis of women=s drinking and drinking related problems in five countries: Findings from the International Research Group on Gender and Alcohol. *Addiction Research and Theory*, 12, 31-40.

Wilsnack RW, Vogeltanz ND, Wilsnack SC, Harris TR, et al. (2000). Gender differences in alcohol consumption and adverse drinking consequences: Cross-cultural patterns. *Addiction*, 95, 251-265.

Wilsnack RW, Wilsnack SC. (1997). Introduction. In R. W. Wilsnack and S. C. Wilsnack (Eds.), *Gender and Alcohol: Individual and Social Perspectives* (pp. 1-16). New Brunswick, NJ: Rutgers Center of Alcohol Studies.

Wilsnack RW, Wilsnack SC, Obot IS. (2005). Why study gender, alcohol and culture? In I. S. Obot & R. Room (eds.), *Alcohol, Gender and Drinking Problems: Perspectives from Low and Middle Income Countries* (pp. 1-23). Geneva: World Health Organization.

Wilsnack SC, Wilsnack RW. (2002). International gender and alcohol research: Recent findings and future directions. *Alcohol Research & Health*, 26, 245-250.

World Health Organization (1999). *WHO Multi-Country Study of Women's Health and Domestic Violence: Core protocol.* WHO/EIP/GPE/99.3. Geneva: World Health Organization

General Issues in Research on Intimate Partner Violence: An Overview[1] —*Sharon C. Wilsnack and Richard W. Wilsnack*

with Kathryn Graham (Canada), Myriam Munné (Argentina), Claudina E. Cayetano (Belize), Florence Kerr–Corrêa (Brazil), Maria Cristina Pereira Lima (Brazil), Sharon Bernards (Canada), Julio Bejarano (Costa Rica), Martha Romero Mendoza (Mexico), José Trinidad Caldera Aburto (Nicaragua), Marina Julia Piazza Ferrand (Peru), and Raquel Magri (Uruguay)

Extent of Intimate Partner Violence

It is difficult to arrive at a consensual estimate of the extent of intimate partner violence (IPV) within communities, societies, or cultures. Reasons for the difficulty include differing criteria for what constitutes a violent act (e.g., whether or not to include verbal acts such as name-calling and threats), differences in sample design (e.g., sampling only married partners, partners residing together, or also partners who are romantically or sexually involved but not cohabiting), greater attention given to violence perpetrated by male partners than by female partners, inconsistent reporting of violence by victims and perpetrators, and underreporting of IPV (which typically occurs to a greater extent in the criminal justice system but also to an unknown extent in surveys) (Boyle et al., 2004; Kilpatrick, 2004; Schafer et al., 2002).

Several efforts in recent years have attempted to identify cross-cultural patterns in rates and predictors of physical violence against intimate partners through multinational surveys (Andersson et al., 2007; Flake and Forste, 2006; Garcia-Moreno et al., 2006; Sadowski et al., 2004)[2] or by combining findings from single-site studies around the world (Archer, 2006; Krahé et al., 2005). The prevalence of physical violence toward female partners in these studies differs greatly from site to site. In the studies reviewed for this chapter, the lifetime prevalence of partner physical violence toward women ranged from a low of 2.7% in a German sample (Luedtke and Lamnek, 2002) to a high of 61% in a province of Peru (Garcia-Moreno et al., 2006)[3]. These wide prevalence rate differences may have resulted, to an unknown extent, from variations in sampling (e.g., national vs. regional vs. community samples; all women vs. women currently married or living with partners vs. women ever married or partnered), constraints on interviewing (such as interviewing only persons at home during daytime hours, interviewers' fear of entering potentially dangerous neighborhoods after dark), and variations

---

[1] The preparation of this chapter was supported in part by Grant R01 AA015775 from the National Institute on Alcohol Abuse and Alcoholism, National Institutes of Health, Department of Health and Human Services, United States Government.
[2] Because the research reported in this book focused on physical aggression and alcohol consumption in adult women and men who were married, cohabiting, or involved in non-cohabiting romantic relationships, we did not review studies that focused exclusively on pre-marital adolescents or on students. Thus, for example, the context for findings here would not include the International Dating Violence Study (Hines and Straus, 2007), which included only classroom samples of college students.
[3] The WHO Multi-country Study on Women's Health and Domestic Violence (Garcia-Moreno et al., 2006), cited frequently in this chapter, included the capital or other large city (and in seven countries a provincial site) in each of ten countries: Bangladesh, Brazil, Ethiopia, Japan, Namibia, Peru, Samoa, Serbia and Montenegro, Thailand, and the United Republic of Tanzania.

in definitions and measures of violence (e.g., emotional vs. physical vs. sexual violence; different time frames such as lifetime vs. recent occurrence). In general, "fragmented and unsystematic" cross-cultural data on partner physical violence (Krahé et al., 2005) have impeded progress in developing more effective interventions against such violence. From a more positive perspective, the wide variation in prevalence rates suggests that IPV is not inevitable, and encourages the search for increased knowledge about predictors of IPV that may be amenable to prevention efforts (Garcia-Moreno et al., 2006).

In order to maximize comparability across countries that may have different norms regarding verbal expressions of hostility and regarding cohabitation among unmarried persons, in this book we focus on (a) acts of physical aggression between (b) romantic or sexual partners who may or may not be residing together. IPV occurs between same-sex partners as well as between heterosexual partners (e.g., Balsam et al., 2005; Cameron, 2003; Madera and Toro-Alfonso, 2005; Miller et al., 2000). However, because of the small number of respondents who reported same-sex partners in the surveys presented in this book and because much of our focus is on gender differences in aggressive behavior, which could vary by gender of target, we limit our analyses to respondents with opposite-sex partners.

IPV by Men and Women

In most countries outside North America and Europe, partner violence is seen as a behavior predominantly perpetrated by male partners against female partners (e.g., Ellsberg, 2000; Flake and Forste, 2006; Heise et al., 1999; cf. Moraes and Reichenheim, 2002; Reichenheim et al., 2006). Accordingly, with the exception of early research conducted by Straus and colleagues in the United States (see Kaufman, Kantor and Asdigian, 1997; Straus, 1993, 1995), research in most countries has focused predominantly on men assaulting women. However, several recent general population surveys in western societies have found that women reported similar or slightly higher rates of aggression and violence toward their partners as men did (Anderson, 2002; Archer, 2000; AuCoin, 2005; Caetano, McGrath et al., 2005; Richardson, 2005; Williams and Frieze, 2005; cf. Tjaden and Thoennes, 2000). This apparent gender equity has been variously questioned. For one thing, a major problem with most measures of partner violence is that they do not allow proactive and unprovoked acts of aggression to be distinguished from aggressive behaviors that are reactive or done in self-defense (e.g., Johnson and Ferraro, 2000; Krahé et al., 2005). Moreover, a consistent pattern in research in several countries is that IPV severe enough to cause injury is more likely to be carried out by men against women (Archer, 2000; Cascardi et al., 1992; Mihorean, 2005; Mirrlees-Black, 1999; Straus, 1995; Swart et al., 2002; Tjaden and Thoennes, 2000). It is estimated that IPV accounts for 40% to 60% of female homicides in many countries (Garcia-Moreno, Heise et al., 2005; Krug et al., 2002). In Buenos Aires province in Argentina, 68% of the 1,284 women murdered between 1997 and 2003 were killed by their husband, partner, or ex-partner (Chejter, 2005). In the United States in 2002, in homicides resulting from IPV, 76% of the victims were women (Fox and Zawitz, 2004). In Canada, between 1975 and 2004, 77% of victims of spousal homicide were women (Johnson, 2006). Finally, gender differences in violence may be smaller in general population samples than in institutional samples (e.g., in clinics or shelters), and men may be more likely than women to engage in IPV that involves sexual abuse or stalking, or that leads to involvement of the criminal justice system (Saunders, 2002).

In Latin American countries, violence carried out by men against women has been a source of concern among governmental organizations and social sectors. In recent surveys, residents of several cities have stated that male-to-female violence is a major source of concern. In fact, male violence toward women is seen as one of the greatest threats to public health, causing pain and many premature deaths (Castro and Riquer, 2003; Orpinas, 1999).

Analyses or summaries of *multinational* data to date have typically obtained (or reported) findings only about male assaults on female partners (Flake and Forste, 2006; Garcia-Moreno et al., 2006; Krug et al., 2002; Sadowski et al., 2004). Fewer multinational studies have reported evidence of partner physical violence against both sexes (e.g., Andersson et al., 2007; Archer, 2006; Krahé et al., 2005), and some studies have found that the perpetration of violence is not more prevalent among men than among women. However, studies that have not found much higher rates among men have typically had special characteristics, including relying on data mainly from wealthier nations in Europe, North America, and Australasia (Archer, 2000; Caetano, Field et al., 2005; Magdol et al., 1997) or obtaining male data only from men who are home during working hours and not likely to be representative of a country's general male population (Andersson et al., 2007).

Health, Social, and Economic Costs and Consequences

It is well understood in countries around the world that intimate partner violence against women imposes enormous social costs, not only in harm to health and families, but also in harm to employment and in high costs for related health care, law enforcement, and lost economic productivity. It is difficult to estimate these costs in monetary terms, and such estimates have generally been made only for a few of the largest and wealthiest economies. In the United States, for example, an estimated US$ 4 billion was spent on health care costs related to intimate partner violence in 1995 (National Center for Injury Prevention and Control, 2003). For Latin American countries, there are very few such estimates, but available estimates illustrate the magnitude of social costs. In Colombia, for instance, Sanchez and colleagues (2004) estimated that in 2003 the country's economy as a whole lost 0.85% of its gross domestic product (GDP), or roughly US$ 675 million, from wage losses due to family violence, and that the Government of Colombia spent US$ 73.7 million that year (about 0.6% of its budget) to prevent and detect family violence and provide services to survivors (see also Morrison et al., 2007). Morrison and Orlando (1999) estimated that women's reduced earnings related to domestic violence in 1996 cost Chile's economy US$ 1.56 billion (more than 2% of the country's GDP) and cost Nicaragua's economy US$ 29.5 million (about 1.6% of its GDP).

The non-monetary health and social costs of intimate partner violence in the Americas may be even greater. In addition to the well-documented adverse effects of IPV on pregnancy and pregnancy outcome (discussed below), studies in many countries have found associations between IPV and numerous physical and mental health problems in women. Based on data from 15 sites worldwide, including sites in Brazil and Peru, García-Moreno, Jansen, and colleagues (2005) found that women with lifetime experiences of physical and/or sexual violence were more likely to report poor or very poor health. In Mexico City in 1995, 50% of women who sought treatment in the hospital emergency departments sampled presented with injuries resulting from "marital disputes" (probably under-representing IPV among non-married partners) (Ascencio,

1999). A study in Managua, Nicaragua, found that women who experienced severe partner physical violence were twice as likely as women who had not been abused to be hospitalized and to undergo surgery (Morrison and Orlando, 1999); and data from Argentina suggest high health care costs associated with adverse health consequences of IPV (Teubal, 2006). The WHO Multi-Country Study (Garcia-Moreno, Jansen, et al., 2005) found that in all 15 sites women who had ever experienced physical or sexual violence from a partner scored higher on a measure of emotional distress and showed greater likelihood of having thought about or attempted suicide, after controlling for effects of age, education, and marital status. Women in Nicaragua who reported abuse were six times as likely as those who did not report abuse to experience emotional distress (Ellsberg, Caldera et al., 1999). And among women who had partners and lived in poor neighborhoods of Santiago, Chile, past-year experience of IPV was associated with significant elevations of depression and symptoms of post-traumatic stress disorder (Ceballo et al., 2004).

Research from the United States and Canada also indicates that women who have been victims of IPV have worse physical and mental health (Dutton et al., 2006; Plichta, 2004; Ratner, 1993; Trainor, 2002), including higher risks of depression, suicidal ideation and behavior, and substance abuse (Golding, 1999) compared with women who have not experienced IPV, and these consequences are greater for female than for male victims (Johnson, 2006; Trainor, 2002). In addition, IPV adversely affects women's employment through absenteeism, tardiness, and being forced to leave jobs (Swanberg et al., 2005). Health and employment effects of IPV on men have not been adequately evaluated; however, research from Canada suggests that women are more likely than men to take time off from work and to have been hospitalized due to partner violence (Mihorean, 2005).

Children of violent parents also experience adverse consequences. For example, a study of male adolescents in Medellin, Colombia, (Majia et al., 2006) found that witnessing family violence in the two years preceding the study was associated with increased violent behavior, reduced prosocial behavior, and increased substance abuse by the adolescent. From 1995 United States data, McDonald and colleagues (2006) estimated that more than 15 million children were living in households where IPV had occurred in the preceding year. Estimates from Canada (Dauvergne and Johnson, 2001) suggest that 37% of spousal violence cases were witnessed by children. Research has shown that exposure to IPV harms children's mental and behavioral health, including increased risks of anxiety, depression, post-traumatic stress, and aggression toward others (Dauvergne and Johnson, 2001; Kitzmann et al., 2003; Wolfe et al., 2003). Children in homes where violence occurs also have increased risks of being victims of physical abuse themselves (Ernst et al., 2006; Stover, 2005).

IPV and Marital Status

It is sometimes tacitly assumed that IPV is mainly a problem of married couples, who may have longer exposure to risks of violence. Recent research suggests that this is generally not true. Research in the United States and Canada, for example, consistently finds that rates of male violence toward female partners are higher in cohabiting couples who are not married than in married couples (Brownridge and Halli, 2000; Caetano, McGrath, et al., 2005; Jasinski, 2001; Johnson, 2006; Kenney and McLanahan, 2006; Lipsky et al., 2005). The risk that male partners will kill their female partners is also greater in cohabiting couples than in married couples (Shackleford, 2001). Most surveys in Latin America also find higher rates of IPV among cohabiting couples than among married couples. Flake and Forste's (2006) study of five Latin American countries (Colombia, the Dominican Republic, Haiti, Nicaragua, and Peru) found that married women were considerably less likely than cohabiting women to be physically abused. This effect was strongest in the Dominican Republic, where cohabiting women were twice as likely as married women to be abused. Higher rates of IPV among cohabiting women than among married women have also been reported in single-country studies in Chile (Urzua et al., 2001; cf. Cebello et al., 2004), Mexico (Ascencio, 1999), and Peru (Flake, 2005). A survey conducted nationwide in Costa Rica in 2003 (Sagot and Guzman, 2004) found that women's lifetime risk of suffering sexual and physical violence was highest among women who were married or living with a partner.

Many surveys have found that risks of experiencing IPV are also elevated among women who are separated or divorced (e.g., Bachman and Saltzman, 1995; Johnson, 2006; Vest et al., 2002), but cross-sectional surveys cannot show whether the violence preceded or followed the breakup. Causal relationships probably exist in both temporal sequences: IPV is known to increase the likelihood of subsequent divorce or separation (DeMaris, 2000; Ramisetty-Mikler and Caetano, 2005; Zlotnick et al., 2006); and longitudinal studies in the United States have shown that women separated but not divorced from partners subsequently experience increased risks of IPV (Koziol-McLain et al., 2001) and increased risks of being killed by their partners (Campbell et al., 2003). In Canada, half of the women reporting spousal assault by a past partner said that the assault occurred after the separation, and a substantial proportion reported increased severity of aggression after separation (Johnson, 2006). In general, it is likely that the associations between divorce (and other marital statuses) and IPV differ across countries with different laws and societal norms regarding marriage and divorce.

IPV and Pregnancy

Studies in several countries in the Americas have examined how pregnancy modifies risks of IPV. In a Costa Rican study (Núñez-Rivas et al., 2003), one-third of a sample of 118 pregnant women reported experiencing violence from their partners. Mothers who had suffered acts of partner violence were three times as likely as other mothers to have a low birthweight newborn. Similarly, a study in Mexico City found that 31% of a sample of pregnant women reported having experienced partner violence (Doubova et al., 2007). A study of pregnant women in public maternity wards in Rio de Janeiro (Moraes and Reichenheim, 2002) found that 18% of the women reported having experienced physical abuse by their male partner during the pregnancy; and 20% of pregnant public health care users in São Paulo reported having experienced IPV during their pregnancy (Durand and Schraiber, 2007). Somewhat lower rates of IPV were reported by pregnant women in Mexico City (7.6%) (Díaz-Olavarrieta et al., 2007), Morelos, Mexico, (10.6%) (Castro et al., 2003) and León, Nicaragua (13.4%) (Valladares et al., 2005). The WHO Multi-Country Study (Garcia-Moreno, Jansen, et al., 2005) found that the proportion of ever-pregnant women who reported having been physically abused during at least one pregnancy ranged from 4% to 12% in the majority of the 15 sites. Across all sites, more than 90% of the abusers were the biological fathers of the children being carried. Data from a hospital-based domestic violence treatment unit in Buenos Aires suggest that 75% of alleged "spontaneous abortions" of women in the treatment unit were in fact the result of physical partner aggression during pregnancy (Centro de Informática, 2006).

Evidence from United States studies does not consistently show that pregnancy either prevents or provokes assaults by male partners (Jasinski, 2001; Saltzman et al., 2003), although women's risk of being killed by partners may rise during pregnancy (Krulewitch et al., 2001; Shadigian and Bauer, 2005). Most surveys find that between 5% and 10% of United States women have experienced IPV during pregnancy (Espinosa and Osborne, 2002; Gazmararian et al., 1996; Koenig et al., 2006). Pregnant women are more likely to experience violence if they are relatively young (Gazmararian et al., 1995; Jasinski, 2001; Parker et al., 1994) and if the pregnancy was unwanted or poorly timed, at least from the male partner's point of view (Cokkinides and Coker, 1998; Gazmararian et al., 1996; Goodwin et al., 2000; Jasinski, 2001; Saltzman et al., 2003). One recent study of pregnant, low-income women in Alabama (Li et al., 2008) found that the woman's use of alcohol was associated with increased risk of IPV, after controlling for a number of other individual and neighborhood characteristics.

There is little uncertainty about the effects of IPV during pregnancy: studies in many countries consistently find that pregnant women who experience IPV are more likely to have adverse pregnancy outcomes, including preterm delivery, low birthweight infants, and higher rates of infant and maternal morbidity and mortality (Arcos et al., 2001; Ascencio, 1999; Åsling-Monemi et al., 2003; Boy and Salihu, 2004; Hasselmann and Reichenheim, 2006; Heise et al., 1999; Morrison and Orlando, 1999; Murphy et al., 2001; Nasir and Hyder, 2003; Núñez-Rivas et al., 2003; Valladares Cardoza, 2005).

Social Contexts of IPV
Culture of Violence and Gender-Role Inequality in Latin America

Despite considerable diversity and variability across different Latin American countries and population subgroups, studies of domestic violence in Latin America have identified two cultural characteristics of most Latin American countries that may contribute to this region's high rates of intimate partner violence: (a) a history of war and social violence, and (b) rigid and patriarchal gender roles (see Flake and Forste, 2006). Many Latin American countries have a long history of wars and civil or other conflicts, which may desensitize citizens to acts of violence, create a culture permissive of violence, and legitimize violence in relationships and families as a form of social control (e.g., Buvini et al., 1999: McWhirter, 1999; Silber, 2004). The gender-role concepts of *machismo* and *marianismo* are also powerful influences on the socialization of men and women in many Latin American countries. "Machismo as an ideology exaggerates the differences between men and women, emphasizing male moral, economic, and social superiority over women...(and defining) masculine identity in terms of dominance and aggression" (Ellsberg et al., 2000, p. 1606). "Marianismo refers to the expectation that women embrace the veneration of the Virgin Mary in that they are capable of enduring any suffering inflicted upon them by males...(and) be submissive, dependent, sexually faithful to their husbands, and...take care of household needs and dedicate themselves entirely to their husbands and children" (Flake and Forste, 2006, p. 20). These rigidly differentiated gender roles reinforce and perpetuate male dominance and female submission, reflected in extreme forms in male aggression and violence toward female partners.

The contributions of historical violence and patriarchal gender roles to patterns of physical partner aggression in individual countries are discussed in greater detail in specific country chapters in this book.

Lower Socioeconomic Status and Poverty

Low education, unemployment, and low income have been associated with increased risks of IPV in many countries of the Americas, including Brazil (Deslandes et al., 2000; Moraes and Reichenheim, 2002; Reichenheim et al., 2006), Chile (Ceballo et al., 2004; Larrain, 1993), Haiti (Gage, 2005), Mexico (Castro et al., 2003; Figueroa et al., 2004; Rivera-Rivera et al., 2004), Nicaragua (Ellsberg, Peña et al., 1999, 2000), and Peru (Flake, 2005; Gonzales de Olarte and Gavilano Llosa, 1999). In many Latin American countries, women who are more empowered educationally, economically, and socially tend to be the most protected from risks of partner violence (see, e.g., Archer, 2006; Gage, 2005; cf. Morrison and Orlando, 1999). If male violence toward female partners is viewed in part as an attempt to resolve a crisis of male identity, unemployment and poverty can be seen as conditions which create or contribute to such crises. Thus, associations between lower socioeconomic status and higher rates of IPV may be partly explained by men's maladaptive use of partner violence to cope with economic threats to their sense of male identity and power (see Bejarano, in this volume).

North American research is generally consistent with that in Latin America. Canadian and American women living in poverty or on low incomes are more likely to be abused by their male partners (Cunradi et al., 2002; Fox et al., 2002; Johnson, 2006; Rennison and Welchans, 2000; Schumacher et al., 2001; Vest et al., 2002). Among low-income women, those who have had to seek and depend on public welfare payments are at greater risk of IPV (Fairchild et al., 1998; Honeycutt et al., 2001; Lown & Schmidt, 2006; Tolman and Raphael, 2000).

Explaining the consistent association of IPV with poverty in North American studies, however, is more complicated. On the one hand, IPV may tend to impoverish women by destabilizing their ability to get and keep jobs (for example, because of injuries and other related health problems from IPV) (Lown and Schmidt, 2006; Riger and Staggs, 2004; Yoshihama et al., 2006). Male partners often interfere with women's efforts to work (or go to school), perhaps in part because these efforts would threaten to reduce women's dependence on their partners (Lloyd and Talluc, 1999; Pearson et al., 1999; Tolman and Raphael, 2000). On the other hand, reduced income may lead to increased risks of IPV. There is a growing body of research in the United States and Canada that shows that male unemployment is associated with subsequently increased risks of male violence against female partners (Brzozowski, 2004; Caetano, McGrath et al., 2005; Fox et al., 2002; Johnson, 1996; Kyriacou et al., 1999), and it may also increase risks of subsequent female violence against male partners (Caetano, McGrath et al., 2005; Newby et al., 2003). At least one study has found that increases in women's income and employment may reduce their subsequent risks of being victims of IPV (Gibson-Davis et al., 2005).

Intergenerational Continuity of Violence

Another context of IPV that has received considerable attention is the intergenerational continuity of violence. It is widely believed and claimed that children from violent families are more likely to grow up to become perpetrators or victims of IPV, although the reasons for such effects of childhood experiences have been more debated than demonstrated. Furthermore, tests of the claimed connections have often failed to distinguish differences in how children experienced violence (e.g., as victims of abuse by parents vs. as witnesses of parental IPV), differences in how childhood experiences affect being a perpetrator versus a victim of intimate adult violence, and gender differences in the effect of violent childhood experiences. In addition, studies of intergenerational continuity often have not had representative general population samples, have had to rely on recall of childhood experiences, and have paid little attention to historical changes (e.g., in marital and gender roles and tolerance of IPV) (see, e.g., Lackey, 2003; Stith et al., 2000).

Despite these methodological limitations, one relatively consistent research finding on intergenerational effects is that men who experienced abuse and/or witnessed parental violence as children are more likely to be violent to their partners. This finding has been reported in studies in Mexico (Castro et al., 2003), Nicaragua (Ellsberg et al., 1999), and for clinical and court samples (Schumacher et al., 2001) and general population samples in the United States (Herrenkohl et al., 2004; Margolin et al., 2003; Whitfield et al., 2003). Several studies in Latin America also report intergenerational effects on victimization by violent spouses. Studies in Argentina (Corsi, 2006), Chile (Morrison and Orlando, 1999), Haiti (Gage, 2005), Mexico (Castro et al., 2003; Rivera-Rivera et al., 2004, 2006; Villarreal, 2007), and Peru (Flake, 2005) have found that experiencing abuse and/or witnessing parental violence in childhood increased women's risks of victimization by a partner in adulthood. Some studies in the United States have also found that either being physically abused by parents or witnessing violence between parents increases the risk of becoming a victim of IPV, particularly for women (Lipsky et al., 2005; Renner and Slack, 2006; Stith et al., 2000; Whitfield et al., 2003). Other studies, however, failed to find intergenerational effects on IPV victimization (Schumacher et al., 2001; Sullivan et al., 2005) or found that experiences of parental violence make women more likely to become violent toward their partners (Herrenkohl et al., 2004; Heyman and Smith Slep, 2002; Sullivan et al., 2005).

Attempts to explain intergenerational transmission of violence have offered more ideas than evidence. It has been suggested that children who are witnesses or victims of parental violence learn to imitate, approve, and/or tolerate such behavior in intimate partnerships, or that such children are later more likely to develop hostility, antisocial behavior disorders, and problem drinking, which may then contribute to IPV (see, e.g., Renner and Slack, 2006; Stith et al., 2000; White and Widom, 2003). However, in the United States evidence that children have learned from parents to become violent toward partners has been relatively weak (Sellers et al., 2005; Simons et al., 1995), and evidence for other mediating factors has typically been gender-specific: parental violence may reduce men's commitment to their partners (Lackey, 2003) and may lead women to have poorer-quality relationships with their partners (Herrenkohl et al., 2004), resulting in greater risks of violence against partners. White and Widom (2003) found that intergenerational transmission of violence may be mediated by several factors among women (hostility, alcohol problems, and antisocial personality disorder), but only by antisocial personality disorder among men.

Alcohol Use and IPV

Relatively few studies outside North America and Europe have examined the association between alcohol use and IPV. The studies of multiple societies outside North America and Europe that have included measures of alcohol use have focused entirely on associations between men's drinking and men's violence toward their female partners (Flake and Forste, 2006; Jeyaseelan et al., 2004; Levinson, 1989). In general, these studies report that men's heavier drinking or intoxication is associated with increased risks that men will assault their female partners. Associations between alcohol use, alcohol abuse, or drunkenness by male partners and increased risks of violence toward female partners have also been reported in single-country studies in Chile (Urzua et al., 2001), Haiti (Gage, 2005), Mexico (Gómez-Dantés et al., 2006; Rivera-Rivera et al., 2004), Nicaragua (Morrison and Orlando, 1999), and Peru (Flake, 2005). A study of pregnant women in Rio de Janeiro (Moraes and Reichenheim, 2002) found that IPV was twice as common in households where there was alcohol abuse; however, it was unclear whether the alcohol abuse was that of the male partner, the female partner, or both.

Only a few non-Western, single-site studies have reported on how women's experiences of partner aggression are related to women's alcohol consumption; these include studies in South Africa (Jewkes et al., 2002) and Uganda (Koenig et al., 2003). To our knowledge, no multinational research or studies in Latin American countries have investigated how women's typical drinking patterns, or women's alcohol use at the time of partner aggression, affect women's likelihood of being victims or perpetrators of physical partner aggression.

Additional studies of IPV and alcohol use in countries represented in this book are reviewed in individual country chapters, and cross-country patterns in associations between alcohol use and physical partner aggression are discussed in the chapter "Comparison of Partner Physical Aggression across Ten Countries."

Summary: Unique Contributions of this Book

It is clear from this brief research overview that intimate partner violence is a major social and health problem in the Americas and that many important questions remain unanswered. Increased understanding of the predictors and consequences of partner violence is critical for designing effective approaches to prevention, intervention, and policy.

Although research in North America and Europe has identified associations between alcohol use (particularly by the male partner) and risks of intimate partner violence, relatively few studies outside North America and Europe have examined these associations. This book moves beyond previous research in several important respects:
    (a) the data are from general population samples, rather than from clinical samples, greatly increasing the extent to which findings can be generalized to entire populations;
    (b) experiences of physical partner aggression were reported by both men and women;

(c) women and men reported their experiences as both perpetrators and victims of physical partner aggression;
(d) drinking behavior of both men and women is analyzed in relation to acts of partner physical aggression perpetration and victimization;
(e) associations between drinking and partner aggression are analyzed with regard both to drinking during the partner aggression event, and to typical drinking patterns of both partners; and
(f) the use of comparable measures of alcohol use and partner aggression allow comparisons of findings across ten countries of the Americas.

Taken together, these analyses provide a more complete picture than has previously been available of how alcohol use by men and women in the Americas is linked to their experiences of partner physical aggression. This knowledge, in turn, may suggest more effective approaches to prevention of and intervention in the widespread and challenging problem of intimate partner violence in the Americas.

References

Anderson KL. (2002). Perpetrator or victim? Relationships between intimate partner violence and well-being. *Journal of Marriage and the Family*, 64, 851-863.

Andersson N, Ho-Foster A, Mitchell S, Scheepers E, Goldstein S. (2007). Risk factors for domestic physical violence: National cross-sectional household surveys in eight southern African countries. *BMC Women's Health*, 7 (11), 1-13.

Archer J. (2000). Sex differences in aggression between heterosexual partners: A meta-analytic review. *Psychological Bulletin*, 126, 651-680.

Archer J. (2006). Cross-cultural differences in physical aggression between partners: A social-role analysis. *Personality and Social Psychology Review*, 10, 133-153.

Arcos GE, Uarac UM, Molina VI, Repossi FA, Ulloa VM. (2001). Impacto de la violencia doméstica sobre la salud reproductiva y neonatal. *Revista Médica de Chile*, 129, 1413-1424.

Ascencio RL. (1999). The health impact of domestic violence: Mexico City. In Morrisson AR, Biehl ML. (eds.), *Too Close to Home: Domestic Violence in the Americas* (pp. 81-101). Washington, DC: Inter-American Development Bank (distributed by The Johns Hopkins University Press).

Åsling-Monemi K, Peña R, Ellsberg MC, Persson LA. (2003). Violence against women increases the risk of infant and child mortality: A case-referent study in Nicaragua. *Bulletin of the World Health Organization*, 81, 10-18.

AuCoin K. (Ed.) (2005). *Family Violence in Canada: A Statistical Profile*. Ottawa, Canada: Canadian Centre for Justice Statistics, Statistics Canada. www.statcan.ca. Catalogue no. 85-224-XIE.

Bachman R, Saltzman LE. (1995). *Violence Against Women: Estimates from the Redesigned National Crime Victimization Survey*. Washington, DC: U. S. Department of Justice, Office of Justice Programs. Online at *www.ojp.usdoj.gov/bjs/pub/pdf/femvied.pdf*

Balsam KF, Rothblum ED, Beauchaine TP. (2005). Victimization over the life span: A comparison of lesbian, gay, bisexual, and heterosexual siblings. *Journal of Consulting and Clinical Psychology*, 73, 477-487.

Boy A, Salihu HM. (2004). Intimate partner violence and birth outcomes. *International Journal of Fertility and Women's Medicine*, 49, 159-164.

Boyle A, Robinson S, Atkinson P. (2004). Domestic violence in emergency medicine patients. *Emergency Medicine Journal*, 21, 9–13.

Brownridge DA, Halli SS. (2000). "Living in sin" and sinful living: Toward filling a gap in the explanation of violence against women. *Aggression and Violent Behavior*, 5, 565–583.

Brzozowski J-A. *(2004). Spousal violence.* In J-A. Brzozowski (Ed.), *Family Violence in Canada: A Statistical Profile 2004* (pp. 5–10). Ottawa, Canada: Canadian Centre for Justice Statistics, Statistics Canada. www.statcan.ca. Catalogue no. 85-224-XIE.

Buvinić M, Morrison AR, Shifter M. (1999). Violence in the Americas: A framework for action. In Morrisson AR, M. L. Biehl (eds.), *Too Close to Home: Domestic Violence in the Americas* (pp. 3–34). Washington, DC: Inter-American Development Bank (distributed by The Johns Hopkins University Press).

Caetano R, Field CA, Ramisetty-Mikler S, McGrath C. (2005). The five-year course of intimate partner violence among White, Black, and Hispanic couples in the United States. *Journal of Interpersonal Violence*, 20, 1039–1057.

Caetano R, McGrath C, Ramisetty-Mikler S, Field CA. (2005). Drinking, alcohol problems and the five-year recurrence and incidence of male to female and female to male partner violence. *Alcohol: Clinical and Experimental Research*, 29, 98–106.

Cameron P. (2003). Domestic violence among homosexual partners. *Psychological Reports*, 93, 410–416.

Campbell JC, Webster D, Koziol-McLain J, Block C, Campbell D, Curry MA, et al. (2003). Risk factors for femicide in abusive relationships: Results from a multisite case control study. *American Journal of Public Health*, 93, 1089–1097.

Cascardi M, Langhinrichsen J, Vivian D. (1992). Marital aggression: Impact, injury, and health correlates for husbands and wives. *Archives of Internal Medicine*, 152, 1178–1184.

Castro R, Peek-Asa C, Ruiz A. (2003). Violence against women in Mexico: A study of abuse before and during pregnancy. American Journal of Public Health, 93, 1110–1116.

Castro R, Riquer F. (2003). Research on violence against women in Latin America: From blind empiricism to theory without data. Cad. *Saúde Pública*, 19, 135–146.

Ceballo R, Ramirez C, Castilla M, Caballero GA, Lozoff B. (2004). Domestic violence and women's mental health in Chile. *Psychology of Women Quarterly*, 28, 298–308.

Centro de Informática (2006). Dirección General de la Mujer del Gobierno de la Ciudad de Buenos Aires.

Chejter S. (2005). Un estudio estadístico sobre femicidios en la provincia de Buenos Aires. Femicidios e Impunidad. Buenos Aires: CECYM.

Cokkinides V, Coker A. (1998). Experiencing physical violence during pregnancy: Prevalence and correlates. *Family and Community Health*, 20, 19–37.

Corsi J. (2006). *La violencia hacia la mujer en el contexto doméstico.* Fundación Mujeres.

Cunradi CB, Caetano R, Schafer J. (2002). Socioeconomic predictors of intimate partner violence among White, Black, and Hispanic couples in the United States. *Journal of Family Violence*, 17, 377–389.

Dauvergne M, Johnson H. (2001). Children witnessing family violence. In Trainor C, Mihorean K. (eds.), *Family Violence in Canada: A Statistical Profile 2001* (pp. 19–26). Ottawa, Canada: Canadian Centre for Justice Statistics, Statistics Canada. www.statcan.ca. Catalogue no. 85-224-XIE.

DeMaris A. (2000). Till discord do us part: The role of physical and verbal conflict in union disruption. *Journal of Marriage and the Family*, 62, 683-692.

Deslandes SF, Gomes R, Silva CMFP. (2000). Caracterização dos casos de violência doméstica contra a mulher atendidos em dois hospitais públicos do Rio de Janeiro. (Characterization of the cases of domestic violence against women assisted in two public hospitals of Rio de Janeiro.) Cad. *Saúde Pública*, 16, 129-137.

Díaz-Olavarrieta C, Paz F, Abuabara K, Martínez Ayala HB, Kolstad K, Palermo T. (2007). Abuse during pregnancy in Mexico City. *International Journal of Gynecology and Obstetrics*, 97, 57-64.

Doubova SV, Gamanes-Gonzalez V, Billings DL, et al. (2007). Partner violence against pregnant women in Mexico City. Rev. *Saúde Pública* [online], 41 (4), 582-590.

Durand JG, Schraiber LB. (2007). Violencia na gestação entre usuárias de serviços públicos de saúde da Grande São Paulo: Prevalencia e fatores associados. *Revista Brasileira de Epidemiologia*, 10, 310-322.

Dutton MA, Green BL, Kaltman SI, Roesch DM, Zeffiro TA, Krause ED. (2006). Intimate partner violence, PTSD, and adverse health outcomes. *Journal of Interpersonal Violence*, 21, 955-968.

Ellsberg MC, Caldera T, Herrera A, Winkvist A, Kullgren G. (1999). Domestic violence and emotional distress among Nicaraguan women. *American Psychologist*, 54, 30-36.

Ellsberg MC, Peña R, Herrera A, Liljestrand J, Winkvist A. (1999). Wife abuse among women of childbearing age in Nicaragua. *American Journal of Public Health*, 89, 241-244.

Ellsberg M, Peña R, Herrara A, Liljestrand J, Winkvist A. (2000). Candies in hell: Women's experiences of violence in Nicaragua. *Social Science and Medicine*, 51, 1595-1610.

Ernst AA, Weiss SJ, Enright-Smith S. (2006). Child witnesses and victims in homes with adult intimate partner violence. *Academic Emergency Medicine*, 13, 696-699.

Espinosa L, Osborne K. (2002). Domestic violence during pregnancy: Implications for practice. *Journal of Midwifery and Women's Health*, 47, 305-317.

Fairchild DG, Fairchild MW, Stoner S. (1998). Prevalence of adult domestic violence among women seeking routine care in an American Indian and/or Alaska Native health care facility. *American Journal of Public Health*, 88, 1515-1517.

Figueroa MD, Millán-Guerrero RO, Estrada-López M, Isais-Millán R, Bayardo-Quezada C, Trujillo-Hernández B, Tene CE. (2004). Maltrato físico en mujeres. *Gaceta Médica de México*, 140, 481-484.

Flake DF. (2005). Individual, family, and community risk markers for domestic violence in Peru. *Violence Against Women*, 11, 353-373.

Flake DF, Forste R. (2006). Fighting families: Family characteristics associated with domestic violence in five Latin American countries. *Journal of Family Violence*, 21, 19-29.

Fox GL, Benson ML, DeMaris AA, Van Wyk J. (2002). Economic distress and intimate violence: Testing family stress and resource theories. *Journal of Marriage and the Family*, 64, 793-807.

Fox JA, Zawitz MW. (2004). Homicide trends in the United States. Washington, D. C.: U.S. Department of Justice, Bureau of Justice Statistics. At *www.ojp.usdoj.gov/bjs/homicide/homtrnd.htm*

Gage AJ. (2005). Women's experience of intimate partner violence in Haiti. *Social Science and Medicine*, 61, 343-364.

Garcia-Moreno C, Heise L, Jansen HAFM, Ellsberg M, Watts C. (2005). Public health: Violence against women. *Science*, 310, 1282-1283.

Garcia-Moreno C, Jansen HAFM, Ellsberg M, Heise L, Watts C. (2005). WHO Multi-Country Study on Women's Health and Domestic Violence. Geneva: World Health Organization.

Garcia-Moreno C, Jansen HAFM, Ellsberg M, Heise L, Watts CH, on behalf of the WHO Multi-Country Study on Women's Health and Domestic Violence Against Women Study Team (2006). Prevalence of intimate partner violence: Findings from the WHO multi-country study on women's health and domestic violence. *Lancet*, 368, 1260-1269.

Gazmararian JA, Adams MM, Saltzman LE, Johnson CH, Bruce FC, Marks JS, et al. (1995). The relationship between pregnancy intendedness and physical violence in mothers of newborns. *Obstetrics and Gynecology*, 85, 1031-1038.

Gazmararian JA, Lazorick S, Spitz AM, Ballard TJ, Salzman LE, Marks JS. (1996). Prevalence of violence against pregnant women. *JAMA*, 275, 1915-1920.

Gibson-Davis GM, Magnuson K, Gennetian LA, Duncan GJ. (2005). Employment and the risk of domestic abuse among low-income women. *Journal of Marriage and the Family*, 67, 1149-1168.

Golding JM. (1999). Intimate partner violence as a risk factor for mental disorders: A meta analysis. *Journal of Family Violence*, 14, 99-132.

Gómez-Dantés H, Vázquez-Martínez JL, Fernández-Cantón SB. (2006). La violencia en las mujeres usuarias de los servicios de salud en el IMSS y la SSA. *Salud Publica de Mexico*, 48 (Supplement 2), S279-S287.

Gonzales de Olarte E, Gavilano Llosa P. (1999). Does poverty cause domestic violence? Some answers from Lima. In Morrison AR, Biehl M L. (eds.), *Too Close to Home: Domestic Violence in the Americas* (pp. 35-49). Washington, DC: Inter-American Development Bank (distributed by The Johns Hopkins University Press).

Goodwin MM, Gazmararian JA, Johnson CH, Gilbert BC, Saltzman LE, the PRAMS Working Group. (2000). Pregnancy intendedness and physical abuse around the time of pregnancy: Findings from the Pregnancy Risk Assessment Monitoring System, 1996-1997. *Maternal and Child Health Journal*, 4, 85-92.

Hasselmann MH, Reichenheim ME. (2006). Parental violence and the occurrence of severe and acute malnutrition in childhood. *Pediatric and Perinatal Epidemiology*, 20, 299-311.

Heise L, Ellsberg M, Gottemöller, M. (1999). Ending violence against women. *Population Reports*, 27 (4), Series L, No. 11. Baltimore, MD: Population Information Program, Johns Hopkins University School of Public Health.

Herrenkohl TI, Mason WA, Kosterman R, Lengua LJ, Hawkins JD, Abbott RD. (2004). Pathways from physical childhood abuse to partner violence in young adulthood. *Violence and Victims*, 19, 123-136.

Heyman RE, Smith Slep AM. (2002). Do child abuse and interparental violence lead to adulthood family violence? *Journal of Marriage and the Family*, 64, 864-870.

Hines DA, Straus MA. (2007). Binge drinking and violence against dating partners: The mediating effect of antisocial traits and behaviors in a multinational perspective. *Aggressive Behavior*, 33, 441-457.

Honeycutt TC, Marshall LL, Weston R. (2001). Toward ethnically specific models of employment, public assistance, and victimization. *Violence Against Women*, 7, 126-140.

Jasinski JL. (2001). Pregnancy and violence against women: An analysis of longitudinal data. *Journal of Interpersonal Violence*, 16, 712-733.

Jewkes R, Levin J, Penn-Kekana L. (2002). Risk factors for domestic violence: Findings from a South African cross-sectional study. *Social Science and Medicine*, 55, 1603-1617.

Jeyaseelan L, Sadowski LS, Kumar S, Hassan F, Ramiro L, Vizcarra B. (2004). World studies of abuse in the family environment -- Risk factors for physical intimate partner violence. *Injury Control and Safety Promotion*, 11, 117-124.

Johnson H. (1996). *Dangerous Domains: Violence against Women in Canada*. Toronto, Canada: Nelson.

Johnson H. (2006). Measuring Violence against Women: Statistical Trends 2006. Ottawa, Canada: Canadian Centre for Justice Statistics, Statistics, Canada.

Johnson MP, Ferraro KJ. (2000). Research on domestic violence in the 1990s: Making distinctions. *Journal of Marriage and the Family*, 62, 948-963.

Kaufman Kantor G, Asdigian NL. (1997). Gender differences in alcohol-related spousal aggression. In Wilsnack RW, Wilsnack SC. (eds.), *Gender and Alcohol: Individual and Social Perspectives* (pp. 312-334). New Brunswick, NJ: Rutgers Center of Alcohol Studies.

Kenney CT, McLanahan SS. (2006). Why are cohabiting relationships more violent than marriages? *Demography*, 43, 127-140.

Kilpatrick DG. (2004). What is violence against women? Defining and measuring the problem. *Journal of Interpersonal Violence*, 19, 1209-1234.

Kitzmann KM, Gaylord NK, Holt AR, Kennedy ED. (2003). Child witnesses to domestic violence: A meta-analytic review. *Journal of Consulting and Clinical Psychology*, 71, 339-352.

Koenig LJ, Whitaker DJ, Royce RA, Wilson TE, Ethier K, Fernandez MI. (2006). Physical and sexual violence during pregnancy and after delivery: A prospective multistate survey of women with or at risk for HIV infection. *American Journal of Public Health*, 96, 1052-1059.

Koenig MA, Lutalo T, Zhao F, Nalugoda F, Wabwire-Mangen F, Kiwanuka N, Wagman J, Serwadda D, Wawer M, Gray R. (2003). Domestic violence in rural Uganda: Evidence from a community-based study. *Bulletin of the World Health Organization*, 81, 53-60.

Koziol-McLain J, Coates CJ, Lowenstein CR. (2001). Predictive validity of a screen for partner violence against women. *American Journal of Preventive Medicine*, 21, 93-100.

Krahé B, Bieneck S, Möller I. (2005). Understanding gender and intimate partner violence from an international perspective. *Sex Roles*, 52, 807-827.

Krug EG, Dahlberg LL, Mercy JA, Zwi AB, Lozano R. (eds.) (2002). *World Report on Violence and Health*. Geneva: World Health Organization.

Krulewitch CJ, Pierre-Louis ML, de Leno-Gomez R, Guy R, Green R. (2001). Hidden from view: Violence deaths among pregnant women in the District of Columbia, 1988-1996. *Journal of Midwifery and Women's Health*, 46, 4-10.

Kyriacou DN, Anglin D, Taliaferro E, Stone S, Tubb T, Linden JA, et al. (1999). Risk factors for injury to women from domestic violence. *New England Journal of Medicine*, 341, 1892-1898.

Lackey C. (2003). Violent family heritage, the transition to adulthood, and later partner violence. *Journal of Family Issues*, 24, 74-98.

Larrain S. (1993). *Estudio de Frezuencia de la Violencia Intrafamiliar y la Condición de la Mujer in Chile.* Santiago, Chile: Pan American Health Organization.

Levinson D. (1989). *Family Violence in Cross-Cultural Perspective.* Newbury Park, CA: Sage.

Li Q, Kirby RS, Sigler RT, Hwang SS, LaGory ME, Goldenberg RL, Wilsnack SC, Wilsnack RW. (2008). Maternal alcohol use and other individual/household and neighborhood determinants of intimate partner violence among low-income pregnant women in Alabama. Presented at the 31st Annual Meeting, Research Society on Alcoholism, Washington, DC, June, 2008.

Lipsky S, Caetano R, Field CA, Larkin GL. (2005). Psychosocial and substance-use risk factors for intimate partner violence. *Drug and Alcohol Dependence,* 78, 39-47.

Lloyd S, Talluc N. (1999). The effects of male violence on female employment. *Violence Against Women,* 5, 370-392.

Lown EA, Schmidt LA. (2006). Interpersonal violence among women seeking welfare: Unraveling lives. *American Journal of Public Health,* 96, 1409-1415.

Luedtke J, Lamnek S. (2002). Schläge in jeder dritten Familie. Agora, 1, 8-9. Cited in Krahé et al., 2005.

Madera SR, Toro-Alfonso J. (2005). Description of a domestic violence measure for Puerto Rican gay males. *Journal of Homosexuality,* 50, 155-173.

Magdol L, Moffitt TE, Caspi A, Newman DL, Fagan J, Silva PA. (1997). Gender differences in partner violence in a birth cohort of 21-year-olds: Bridging the gap between clinical and epidemiological approaches. *Journal of Consulting and Clinical Psychology,* 65, 68-78.

Majia R, Kliewer W, Williams L. (2006). Domestic violence exposure in Colombian adolescents: Pathways to violent and prosocial behavior. *Journal of Traumatic Stress,* 19, 257-267.

Margolin G, Gordis EB, Medina AM, Oliver P. (2003). The co-occurrence of husband-to-wife aggression, family-of-origin aggression, and child abuse potential in a community sample: Implications for parenting. *Journal of Interpersonal Violence,* 18, 413-440.

McDonald R, Jouriles EN, Ramisetty-Mikler S, Caetano R, Green E. (2006). Estimating the number of American children living in partner-violent families. *Journal of Family Psychology,* 20, 137-142.

McWhirter PT. (1999). La Violencia privada: Domestic violence in Chile. *American Psychologist,* 54, 37-40.

Mihorean K. (2005). Trends in self-reported spousal violence. In K. AuCoin (Ed.), *Family Violence in Canada: A Statistical Profile* (pp. 13-33). Ottawa, Canada: Canadian Centre for Justice Statistics, Statistics Canada. *www.statcan.ca.* Catalogue no. 85-224-XIE.

Miller AJ, Bobner RF, Zarski JJ. (2000). Sexual identity development: A base for work with same-sex partner abuse. *Contemporary Family Therapy,* 22, 189-200.

Mirrlees-Black C. (1999). *Domestic Violence: Findings from a New British Crime Survey Self-Completion Questionnaire.* Home Office Research Study 191. London: Home Office. Online at *www.homeoffice.gov.uk/rds/pdfs/hors191.pdf.*

Moraes C L, Reichenheim ME. (2002). Domestic violence during pregnancy in Rio de Janeiro, Brazil. *International Journal of Gynecology and Obstetrics,* 79, 269-277.

Morrison A, Ellsberg M, Bott S. (2007). Addressing gender-based violence: A critical review of interventions. *The World Bank Research Observer,* 22, 25-51.

Morrison AR, Orlando MB. (1999). S*ocial and economic costs of domestic violence: Chile and Nicaragua*. In Morrison AR, Biehl ML. (eds.). Too Close to Home: Domestic Violence in the Americas (pp. 51-80). Washington, DC: Inter-American Development Bank (distributed by the Johns Hopkins University Press).

Murphy CC, Schei B, Myhr TL, Du Mont J. (2001). Abuse: A risk factor for low birth weight? A systematic review and meta-analysis. *CMAJ*, 164, 1567-1572.

Nasir K, Hyder AA. (2003). Violence against pregnant women in developing countries: Review of evidence. *European Journal of Public Health*, 13, 105-107.

National Center for Injury Prevention and Control. (2003). *Costs of Intimate Partner Violence Against Women in the United States*. Atlanta, GA: Centers for Disease Control and Prevention.

Newby JH, Urbano RJ, McCarroll JE, Martin LT. (2003). Spousal aggression by US Army female soldiers toward employed and unemployed civilian husbands. *American Journal of Orthopsychiatry*, 73, 290-295.

Núñez-Rivas H, et al. (2003). Physical, psychological, emotional, and sexual violence during pregnancy as a reproductive-risk predictor of low birthweight in Costa Rica. *Pan American Journal of Public Health*, 14 (2), 75-83.

Orpinas P. (1999). Who is violent?: Factors associated with aggressive behaviors in Latin America and Spain. *Rev Panam Salud Pública*, 5 (4-5), 391-411.

Parker B, McFarlane J, Soeken K. (1994). Abuse during pregnancy: effects on maternal complications and birthweight in adult and teenage women. Obstetrics and Gynecology, 84, 323-328.

Pearson J, Thoennes N, Griswold EA. (1999). Child support and domestic violence: The victims speak out. *Violence Against Women*, 5, 427-448.

Plichta SB. (2004). Intimate partner violence and physical health consequences. *Journal of Interpersonal Violence*, 19, 1296-1323.

Ramisetty-Mikler S, Caetano R. (2005). Alcohol use and intimate partner violence as predictors of separation among US couples: A longitudinal model. *Journal of Studies on Alcohol*, 66, 205-212.

Ratner PA. (1993). The incidence of wife abuse and mental health in abused women in Edmonton, Alberta. *Canadian Journal of Public Health*, 84, 246-249.

Reichenheim ME, Moraes CL, Szklo A, Hasselmann MH, Ramos De Souza E, Lozana JDA, Figueiredo, V. (2006). The magnitude of intimate partner violence in Brazil: Portraits from15 capital cities and the Federal District. *Cadernos de Saúde Pública*, 22, 425-437.

Renner LM, Slack KS. (2006). Intimate partner violence and child maltreatment: Understanding intra- and inter-generational connections. *Child Abuse and Neglect*, 30, 599-617.

Rennison CM, Welchans S. (2000). *Intimate Partner Violence*. Washington: U. S. Department of Justice, Bureau of Justice Statistics Special Report, NCJ 178247. Online at *www.ojp.usdoj.gov/bjs/pub/pdf/ipv.pdf*

Richardson DS. (2005). The myth of female passivity: Thirty years of revelations about female aggression. *Psychology of Women Quarterly*, 29, 238-247.

Riger S, Staggs SL. (2004). Welfare reform, domestic violence and employment: What do we know, what do we need to know? *Violence Against Women*, 6, 1039-1065.

Rivera-Rivera L, Allen B, Chávez-Ayala R, Ávila-Burgos L. (2006). Abuso físico y sexual durante la niñez y revicitimización de las mujeres Mexicanas durante la edad adulta. *Salud Publica de Mexico*, 48 (Supplement 2), S268-S278.

Rivera-Rivera L, Lazcano-Ponce E, Salmerón-Castro J, Salazar-Martínez E, Castro R, Hernández-Avila M. (2004). Prevalence and determinants of male partner violence against Mexican women: A population-based study. *Salud Publica de Mexico*, 46, 113-122.

Sadowski LS, Hunter WM, Bangdiwala SI, Muñoz SR. (2004). The world studies of abuse in the family environment (WorldSAFE): A model of a multi-national study of family violence. *Injury Control and Safety Promotion*, 11, 81-90.

Sagot M, Guzman L. (2004). Research Final Report. Program Nº 824-A1-908: *Prevention of Violence against Women in Costa Rica. Project Nº 824-A1-545: National Survey on Violence against Women.* San José: University of Costa Rica, Research Center on Women Studies.

Saltzman L, Johnson C, Gilbert B, Goodwin M. (2003). Physical abuse around the time of pregnancy: An examination of prevalence and risk factors in 16 states. *Maternal and Child Health Journal*, 7, 31-43.

Sanchez F, Llorente MV, Chaux E, Garcia L, Ojeda D, Ribero R, Salas LM. (2004). *Los Costos de la Violencia Intrafamiliar en Colombia.* Bogota, Colombia: Universidad de los Andes, Centro de Estudios sobre Desarrollo Económico.

Saunders DG. (2002). Are physical assaults by wives and girlfriends a major social problem? A review of the literature. *Violence Against Women*, 8, 1424-1448.

Schafer J, Caetano R Clark CL. (2002). Agreement about violence in U. S. couples. *Journal of Interpersonal Violence*, 17, 457-470.

Schumacher JA, Feldbau-Kohn S, Smith Slep AM, Heyman RE. (2001). Risk factors for male-to-female partner physical abuse. *Aggression and Violent Behavior*, 6, 281-352.

Sellers CS, Cochran JK, Branch KA. (2005). Social learning theory and partner violence: A research note. *Deviant Behavior*, 26, 379-395.

Shackleford TK. (2001). Cohabitation, marriage, and murder: Woman-killing by male romantic partners. *Aggressive Behavior*, 27, 284-291.

Shadigian EM, Bauer ST. (2005). Pregnancy-associated death: A qualitative systematic review of homicide and suicide. *Obstetrical and Gynecological Survey*, 60, 183-190.

Silber IC. (2004). Mothers/fighters/citizens: Violence and disillusionment in post-war El Salvador. *Gender and History*, 16, 561-587.

Simons RL, Wu C, Johnson C, Conger RD. (1995). A test of various perspectives on the intergenerational transmission of domestic violence. *Criminology*, 33, 141-172.

Stith SM, Rosen KH, Middleton KA, Busch AL, Lundeberg K, Carlton RP. (2000). The intergenerational transmission of spouse abuse: A meta-analysis. *Journal of Marriage and the Family*, 62, 640-654.

Stover CS. (2005). Domestic violence research: What have we learned and where do we go from here? *Journal of Interpersonal Violence*, 20, 448-454.

Straus MA. (1993). Physical assaults by wives: A major social problem. In Gelles RJ, Loseke D. (eds.), *Current Controversies on Family Violence* (pp. 67-87). Newbury Park, CA: Sage.

Straus MA. (1995). Trends in cultural norms and rates of partner violence: An update in 1992. In Stith SM, Straus MA. (eds.), *Understanding Partner Violence: Prevalence, Causes, Consequences, and Solutions* (pp. 30-33). Minneapolis, MN: National Council on Family Relations.

Sullivan TP, Meese KJ, Swan SC, Mazure CM, Snow DL. (2005). Precursors and correlates of women's violence: Child abuse traumatization, victimization of women, avoidance coping, and psychological symptoms. *Psychology of Women Quarterly*, 29, 290-301.

Swanberg JE, Logan TK, Macke C. (2005). Intimate partner violence, employment, and the workplace. *Trauma, Violence, and Abuse*, 6, 286-312.

Swart L, Stevens MSG, Ricardo I. (2002). Violence in adolescents' romantic relationships: Findings from a survey amongst school-going youth in a South African community. *Journal of Adolescence*, 25, 385-395.

Teubal, R. (2006). Abordaje de la violencia intrafamiliar en el ámbito intrahospitalario. In R. Teubal et al., *Violencia familiar, trabajo social e instituciones* (pp. 171-178). Buenos Aires: Paidós.

Tjaden P, Thoennes N. (2000). Prevalence and consequences of male-to-female and female-to-male intimate partner violence as measured by the National Violence Against Women Survey. *Violence Against Women*, 6, 142-161.

Tolman RM, Raphael J. (2000). A review of research on welfare and domestic violence. *Journal of Social Issues*, 56, 655-682.

Trainor C. (ed.) (2002). *Family Violence in Canada: A Statistical Profile.* Ottawa, Canada: Canadian Centre for Justice Statistics, Statistics Canada. www.statcan.ca. Catalogue no. 85-224-XIE.

Urzua R, Ferrer M, Gutierrez C, Larrain S. (2001). *Deteccion y analisis de la prevalencia de la violencia intrafamiliar.* Santiago, Chile: Centro de Analisis de Politicas Publicas, Universidad de Chile.

Valladares Cardoza E. (2005). Partner violence during pregnancy, psychosocial factors and child outcomes in Nicaragua. *http://urn.kb.se/resolve?urn=urn:nbn:se:umu:diva-578* (2007-12-31).

Valladares E, Peña R, Persson LÅ, Högberg U. (2005). Violence against pregnant women: Prevalence and characteristics. A population-based study in Nicaragua. *BJOG: An International Journal of Obstetrics and Gynaecology*, 112, 1243-1248.

Vest JR, Catlin TK, Chen JJ, Brownson RC. (2002). Multistate analysis of factors associated with intimate partner violence. *American Journal of Preventive Medicine*, 22, 156-164.

Villarreal A. (2007). Women's employment status, coercive control, and intimate partner violence in Mexico. *Journal of Marriage and the Family*, 69, 418-434.

White HR, Widom CS. (2003). Intimate partner violence among abused and neglected children in young adulthood: The mediating effects of early aggression, antisocial personality, hostility and alcohol problems. *Aggressive Behavior*, 29, 332-345.

Whitfield CL, Anda RF, Dube SR, Felitti VJ. (2003). Violent childhood experiences and the risk of intimate partner violence as adults. *Journal of Interpersonal Violence*, 18, 166-185.

Williams SL, Frieze IH. (2005). Patterns of violent relationships, psychological distress, and marital satisfaction in a national sample of men and women. *Sex Roles*, 52, 771-784.

Wolfe DA, Crooks CV, Lee V, McIntyre-Smith A, Jaffe PG. (2003). The effects of children's exposure to domestic violence: A meta-analysis and critique. *Clinical Child and Family Psychology Review*, 6, 171-187.

Yoshihama M, Hammock AC, Horrocks J. (2006). Intimate partner violence, welfare receipt, and health status of low-income African American women. *American Journal of Community Psychology*, 37, 95-109.

Zlotnick C, Johnson DM, Kohn R. (2006). Intimate partner violence and long-term psychosocial functioning in a national sample of American women. *Journal of Interpersonal Violence*, 21, 262-275.

Common Survey Methods and Analyses Conducted for Each Country Chapter—Sharon Bernards and Kathryn Graham

This chapter describes the common methodology used to collect survey data from men and women in each of the 10 countries included in this book: Argentina (survey conducted in 2002), Belize (2005), Brazil (2006-2007), Canada (2004-2005), Costa Rica (2003), Mexico (2005), Nicaragua (2005), Peru (2005), the United States (2001, women only), and Uruguay (2004). The chapter also describes variations from the common survey protocol used by certain countries and details country-specific methods provided in individual country chapters; it also describes the analyses conducted for each country chapter.

Surveys

In most countries, interviewers surveyed respondents in person at the selected households. Interviews in Canada were conducted by telephone, and the United States survey consisted of 28% telephone and 72% in-person interviews. As described in the country chapters, most samples were selected using random sampling methods and involved national or large regional samples. Table 1 shows the geographic areas surveyed, the age range of survey respondents, the unweighted sample size for each country, and the percent of current drinkers for men and women.

TABLE 1. Age range, geographic area of sample, unweighted sample size, and percent of current drinkers, by sex, GENACIS study, participating countries in the Americas.

Country and age range	Geographic area of sample	Males N	Males Current drinkers (%)	Females N	Females Current drinkers (%)
Argentina (18–65)	City and province of Buenos Aires	402	91.5	598	73.8
Uruguay (18–65)	Several cities	376	81.1	624	60.3
Brazil (18–97)	Metropolitan São Paulo	867	60.1	1216	30.0
Peru (18–64)	Lima, Ayacucho	516	82.4	1015	61.1
Costa Rica (18–92)	Greater metropolitan area of San José	416	68.5	857	42.8
Nicaragua (15–87)	Bluefields, Estelí, Juigalpa, León and Rivas	614	43.4	1416	10.5
Belize (18–98)	National	1,911	50.6	2074	18.9
Mexico (12–65)	Tijuana, Ciudad Juárez, Monterrey and Querétaro	529	70.6	429	40.9
United States (21–94)	National (48 states)	0	NA	1126	65.8
Canada (18–76)	National (10 provinces)	5,661	81.7	8072	74.6

Measures

All participating countries used the GENACIS core questionnaire, with some countries modifying some of the measures. Respondents were asked about their alcohol consumption and a variety of related issues, including consequences of drinking, drinking contexts, health, relationships, and partner violence. Table 2 shows the measures included in this book's analyses.

TABLE 2. Standard format for measuring variables and variations adopted by specific countries.

VARIABLE	Standard format	Variations from the standard format
Demographics		
Gender	Respondent was asked "What is your gender?"	**Belize:** Determined by interviewer for respondents interviewed in person; interviewer asked respondent the gender of other people in household. **Canada:** Gender was determined by interviewer and verified with two questions later in survey **Mexico:** Determined by interviewer
Age	Calculated from respondent's year or date of birth.	**Belize:** "Last week Sunday, what was your age?" **Mexico:** "How old are you?"
Marital status	Respondents were asked for their current *marital status* (married, cohabiting/common law, divorced, separated, single or never married and widowed).	**Canada:** Common law included people who initially gave their marital status as single but indicated in response to a subsequent question that they lived with a romantic partner
Employment status	Response options varied by country to reflect the employment situation in each country. Responses were categorized where possible into the following categories: • In labour force (working for pay, self–employed, employed but temporarily not working — e.g. maternity/paternity leave) • Unemployed involuntarily or not working due to long term illness/disability • Not in labor force (homemaker or caring for the family, unemployed voluntarily for other reasons) • Student • Retired (retired, receiving a pension)	**Mexico:** Based on last 30 days **Belize:** Did not include retired as an employment category *Country–specific definition of "in labor force":* **Belize:** income recipient **Brazil:** In addition to working for pay included additional categories of retired and working for pay, informal work **Canada:** Working full time or working part time (even if also retired, student or caring for family), maternity/paternity leave **Peru:** In addition to working for pay included additional categories of on strike, living from or renting properties

TABLE 2. (continued)

VARIABLE	Standard format	Variations from the standard format
Alcohol Consumption Measures		
Drank any alcohol past 12 months	Based on questions of number of drinking days and number of drinks per occasion in past year (see below). Zero drinking days or zero drinks per occasion recorded as non–drinker	**Brazil:** Based on responses to: Which is the alcoholic beverage of your preference? and How long has it been since you drank any alcoholic beverage? **Canada, Mexico:** "Did you have any drink containing alcohol in the past 12 months?"
Frequency of drinking — average number of drinking days (drinkers only)	Respondents were asked how often they drank any type of alcoholic beverage using the following scale: never (excluded), less than once a month (coded as 6 days per year), 1–3 days a month (coded as 24 days), 1–2 days a week (78 days), 3–4 days a week (182 days) and 5–7 days a week (312 days). Respondents were also asked how often they drank specific types of alcoholic beverages (beer, wine, spirits and other local drinks). The highest frequency given for overall or beverage–specific responses was used	**United States:** Did not use beverage specific responses to calculate measure **Mexico:** Response options included 3 or more a day, twice a day, once a day, 5–6 times a week **Belize, Brazil, Canada, Peru:** Response options included 5 or 6 days a week and every day **Argentina, Costa Rica, Mexico, Nicaragua, United States, Uruguay:** Response options included once in last 12 months; twice in last 12 months; 3 to 6 times in last 12 months; 7 to 11 times in last 12 months (all of which responses were coded as 6 days per year)
Average number of drinks per occasion (drinkers only)	On those days when you had any kind of beverage containing alcohol how many drinks did you usually have per day? Responses were open ended. 30 or more drinks coded as 30 for analyses.	**Brazil:** Response options were 1-2 drinks, 3-4, 5-6, 7-9, 10 or more drinks which were coded as 1.5, 3.5, 5.5, 8 and 11.5 for analyses **Belize, Canada, Peru:** Responses of 30 or more drinks were coded as 30 by interviewer **Argentina, Canada:** less than 1 coded as 1
Average annual volume\total number of drinks per year (drinkers only)	Calculated by multiplying beverage specific frequency and quantity responses (number of days consumed beer X number of beers consumed each day + number of days consumed wine X number of glasses of wine consumed + etc. for each beverage type).	**United States:** Reported two measures in country chapter: 1) number of drinking days multiplied by generic usual quantity in past 12 months; and 2) using beverage specific questions based on past 30 days multiplied by 12

TABLE 2. (continued)

VARIABLE	Standard format	Variations from the standard format
Drank 5 or more drinks on at least one occasion in past year (drinkers only)	Respondents were asked how often they drank *five or more alcoholic drinks* on any occasion in the past year. This item was dichotomized into drank five or more/did not drink five or more.	**United States:** Asked about six or more drinks per occasion **Argentina, Costa Rica, Mexico, Nicaragua and Uruguay:** Used a graduated frequency measure (i.e. how often the respondent drank 12 drinks to less than 20 drinks; 8 drinks to less than 12; 5 drinks to less than 7; etc. to 1 drink to less than 3 drinks) to calculate the dichotomous measure of whether the respondent drank five or more drinks.
Intimate Partner Agression		
Aggression by an intimate partner	Respondents were asked "What is the most physically aggressive thing done to you during the last 2 years by someone who is or was in a close romantic relationship with you (such as a wife, husband, boyfriend, girlfriend)?" For coding of responses see next item, "Type of aggression."	**Canada:** A close romantic relationship was defined as "someone such as a spouse/partner, lover, or someone you are or were dating or going out with." **Mexico:** Respondents were asked "Has someone with whom you have or have had a sentimental relationship, such as your spouse, partner, boyfriend/girlfriend ever done any of the following things to you?" Then the respondent was asked about the most violent act experienced over the last two years.
Type of aggression by a partner	Based on responses to the question described above, the following acts were examined within each country: push/shove; slap; grab/squeeze/restrain; punch; throw something/throw something at; beat up; all other physical acts. Examples of acts coded into the "other" category were poke, scratch, choke, bite, broke a bone, kicked, hit and used a weapon. The GENACIS core question included an explicit instruction not to include sexual aggression and rape (covered later in the questionnaire).	**Brazil, Canada, Mexico, Nicaragua:** No instruction was given by the interviewer to the respondent regarding sexual aggression (i.e. either to include or exclude it). **Mexico:** The word "pistol" was used instead of "weapon" **USA:** Included an extra category "severe forms of aggression" which included broken bones, threatened with a weapon and shot at with a gun **Canada, Nicaragua, Peru, United States:** Open–ended responses were coded using preset categories. Some open–ended responses included more than one act, in which case the most severe of the acts was used. Beat up included the term beat/beat up, beat with an object, as well as text indicating the notion of repeated acts that hurt or several acts that hurt which were done at the same time.

TABLE 2. (continued)

VARIABLE	Standard format	Variations from the standard format
Severity of partner's aggression	"On a scale of 1 to 10 where 1 is minor aggression and 10 is life threatening aggression, how would you rate the level of this aggressive act?"	**Mexico:** Not asked. **Canada:** "...how would you rate their aggression towards you?" **United States:** Used the term "endangerment" rather than "severity" when reporting results.
Level of fear	"How scared were you just after the incident happened?" (1 – not at all to 10 – very).	**Mexico:** Not asked.
Level of upset	"How upset were you just after the incident happened?" (1 – not at all to 10 – very).	**Belize:** Not asked. **Mexico:** Not asked.
Level of anger	"How angry were you just after the incident happened?" (1 – not at all to 10 – very).	**Belize:** Not asked. **Mexico:** Not asked.
Medical attention	"Did you seek medical attention from a doctor, nurse, paramedic or other health professional either at the time the person did this to you or in the next day or so?"	**Belize:** Not asked. **United States:** Not asked
Alcohol consumption at the time of the incident	"Had you or the other person been drinking before this incident?" Response options were: Both, respondent only, other person only and neither	**Canada:** "Had you, the other person, both of you or neither of you been drinking when the incident occurred?"
Aggression toward an intimate partner		**Not measured in surveys in Belize, Mexico, and the United States.**
Aggression toward an intimate partner by respondent	"What is the most physically aggressive thing you have done during the last 2 years **to someone** who is or was in a close romantic relationship with you (such as a wife, husband, boyfriend, girlfriend)?"	**Canada:** A close romantic relationship was defined as "someone such as a spouse/partner, lover, or someone you are or were dating or going out with."
Type of aggression by respondent	[see details above for Type of aggression by a partner]	[see details above for Type of aggression by a partner]
Severity of respondent's aggression	On a scale of 1 to 10 where 1 is minor aggression and 10 is life threatening aggression, how would you rate the level of this aggressive act?	**Canada:** "...how would you rate your aggression toward the other person?"
Level of fear	How scared were you just after the incident happened? (1 - not at all to 10 - very).	

TABLE 2. (continued)

VARIABLE	Standard format	Variations from the standard format
Level of upset	How upset were you just after the incident happened? (1 - not at all to 10 - very).	
Level of anger	How angry were you just after the incident happened? (1 - not at all to 10 - very).	
Alcohol consumption at the time of the incident	Had you or the other person been drinking before this incident? Response options were: Both, respondent only, other person only and neither	**Canada:** "Had you, the other person, both of you or neither of you been drinking when the incident occurred?"

Analyses

Analyses were limited to adults aged 18 years and older (with the exception of the United States sample, where the age was 21 years and older); as shown in Table 1, upper age limits varied from country to country. Wherever possible analyses were limited to heterosexual partner aggression, because aggression by a male toward a female partner is likely to be different from aggression by a female partner to another female or by a male partner to another male partner. To that end, respondents who indicated they were gay or homosexual, that they had had sex mostly or only with same-sex partners in the past 12 months, and/or that the partner involved in the aggression was the same sex were excluded from the analyses. No sexual orientation information was available for Uruguay.

Data from Brazil, Canada, Mexico and the United States were weighted to adjust for sampling designs. The weight for Brazil was adjusted for oversampling of persons aged 60 years and older. The weight for Canada was adjusted for undersampling of persons in households with multiple adults and slight oversampling in the smaller provinces. The weight for Mexico was similarly adjusted for lower probability of selection for respondents from multi-adult households. The weight applied to the United States data was adjusted for oversampling of women who consumed four or more drinks per week, as well as for variations in non-response rates by sampling unit and major demographic characteristics. No weights were used in the analyses for other countries.

The same set of analyses was conducted for each country, with exceptions made for questions omitted in specific countries (as noted in Table 2). In addition, results from specific countries were not reported when the number of available cases was fewer than 20. In most countries, the number of divorced and separated respondents were insufficient to analyse as separate categories; therefore, these two categories were combined. Widowed respondents were excluded from analyses of marital status due to the small number of widowed respondents in most countries.

Comparable analyses are presented in each country chapter. Table 3 summarizes the results presented in each country chapter, the test of significance used, and the criterion for significance. It also indicates where the results are located within each chapter (e.g., figure number, text). For example, the percent of male and female respondents who reported being the victim or perpetrator of partner violence is shown in Figure 1 in all chapters except the United States chapter, where this information is provided in the text, because the U.S. included only female respondents and asked only about victimization. Every attempt was made to make the results in each chapter easily interpretable by readers who have varying backgrounds in research and statistics.

Similarly, basic tests for statistical significance were used in order to allow for a variety of fairly straightforward comparisons of interest. For some measures, pairwise comparisons were made between male and female victims, male and female aggressors, male victims and female aggressors, and female victims and male aggressors. Statistically, significant differences were determined using chi–square tests, analysis of variance (ANOVA) controlling for age, or logistic regression controlling for age. In general, a probability (p) value < .05 was considered evidence of statistical significance. However, as indicated in Table 3, where large numbers of post hoc tests were conducted, a lower p-value of < .01 was set as the criterion for significance to adjust for the increased possibility of findings being significiant due to chance.

TABLE 3. Results presented in each country chapter, type of significance test used, and criterion for statistical significance.

Results presented	Test of significance	Significance criterion	Location of results in chapters (Figure No. or text)
Percent of: •Female respondents who were victims •Female respondents who were aggressors •Male respondents who were victims •Male respondents who were aggressors Note: "Pairwise" differences referred to in the following analyses involve comparisons between these four gender by victim/aggressor groupings.	Chi–square test of significance of pairwise differences between: % male vs. female victims; % male vs. female aggressors; % female victims vs. male aggressors; % male victims vs. female aggressors.	p < .05	1 US: in text
Percent of respondents in each age–gender group who were victims or aggressors; mean age for the four gender by victim/aggressor groups.	Descriptive information included in each chapter. Testing for significant differences between specific age categories done only in the comparative chapter.		2 US: 1
Percent of men and women in each marital status group who were victims or aggressors.	Chi–square tests of significance of pairwise differences between marital status groups.	p < .01	3 US: 2

TABLE 3, (continued)

Results presented	Test of significance	Significance criterion	Location of results in chapters (Figure No. or text)
Percent reporting each type of aggressive act (e.g., pushing, slapping, etc.) for the four gender by victim/aggressor groups.	Chi square tests of pairwise differences for each type of aggression	$p < .01$	4 US: 3
Mean ratings of severity, fear, anger and upset for each of the four gender by victim/aggressor groups.	ANOVA (controlling for age) of mean rating for pairwise differences	$p < .05$	5 US: 4 in text Mexico: excluded
Percent of male and female victims who sought medical attention	Chi square test comparing percent of male vs. female victims who sought medical attention.	$p < .05$	In text
Percent who reported respondent only, partner only, both or no one drinking at time of incident for each of the four gender by victim/aggressor groups.	Chi-square test of pairwise differences for one or both drinking vs. no one drinking.	$p < .05$	6 US: 4 Mexico: 5
Mean severity ratings by whether one or both drinking versus no one drinking for each of the four gender by victim/aggressor groups.	ANOVA (controlling for age) of mean rating of severity by one or both drinking versus no one drinking.	$p < .05$	In text US: 5
Percent experiencing victimization/aggression (for each of the four groups) by whether respondent drank alcohol in past 12 months.	Logistic regression (controlling for age) predicting victimization/aggression done separately for men and women by whether drank alcohol in past 12 months.	$p < .05$	In text
Percent experiencing victimization/perpetration (for each of the four groups) among current drinkers who drank five or more drinks compared to drinkers who did not drink five drinks.	Logistic regression[1] (controlling for age) predicting victimization/aggression done separately for men and women by whether or not drank five drinks.	$p < .05$	7 US, Mexico: 6 Nicaragua: Excluded
Mean number of days, usual number of drinks and annual total number of drinks for current drinkers in each of the four gender by victim/aggressor groupings compared to no aggression.	Logistic regression[2] (controlling for age) predicting victimization/aggression done separately for men and women by each alcohol consumption measure.	$p < .05$	8, 9 and 10 US, Mexico, Nicaragua: 7, 8, 9

[1] Canada, the United States: Multinomial logistic regression predicting victimization/aggression in which one or both had been drinking and victimization/aggression with no one drinking (compared to no victimization/aggression).
[2] Canada, Mexico, the United States: Multinomial logistic regression predicting whether experienced victimization/aggression in which one or both had been drinking and victimization/aggression with no one drinking (compared to no victimization/aggression).

In order to be concise, respondents who reported physical aggression by a partner are referred to as "victims," and respondents who reported physical aggression toward a partner are referred to as "aggressors." It should be noted, however, that it is impossible to determine what initiated an incident of aggression by or toward a partner. For example, a respondent (designated as an "aggressor") who reported physical aggression toward a partner may, in fact, have been acting in self-defense in response to aggression by a partner and could, therefore, be the victim in that particular incident. The percent of respondents reporting only aggression by a partner, only aggression toward a partner, and aggression both by and toward a partner are described within each country chapter, but all other analyses were conducted separately for aggression by a partner and aggression toward a partner. It is important to note that some respondents who reported physical aggression by and toward a partner were describing a single incident, while others were describing two separate incidents that may or may not have involved the same partner.

Limitations

The limitations applicable to the analyses for most or all countries are discussed here; limitations relating to a specific country are discussed within that country's chapter. First, questions focused only on physical aggression, excluding emotional or psychological abuse or threats; moreover, most surveys explicitly excluded sexual aggression. Second, some respondents were both victims and aggressors (i.e., they reported that they had been a victim of an aggressive act by a partner as well as been aggressive toward a partner). The time frame for different questions varied: specifically, respondents were asked for their current age and marital status and past year drinking patterns, whereas the partner aggression questions relate to the two years preceding the survey. Finally, despite the precaution of excluding specific analyses if fewer than 20 cases were available, results which are based on low numbers of cases should be interpreted with caution, as noted in individual chapters.

UNHAPPY HOURS:

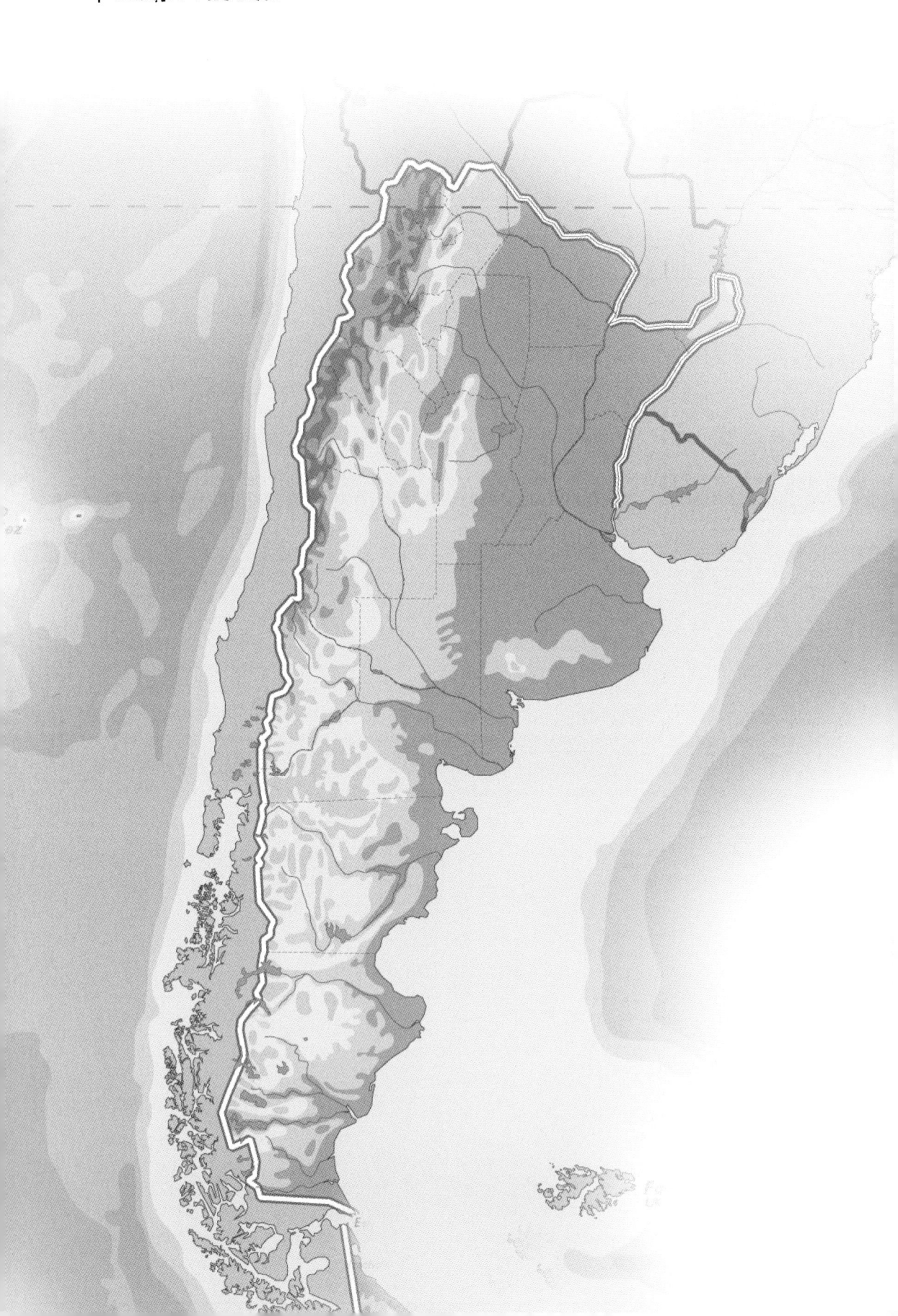

Argentina: Alcohol and Partner Physical Aggression in Buenos Aires Province and City —*Myriam I. Munné*

Introduction
Awareness of intimate partner violence has increased in Argentina in recent years. While partner aggression has been the subject of research for more than 40 years in Canada and the United States (Centro de Encuentros Cultura y Mujer, 1995), it has only been in the past 20 years or so that a group of professionals in Argentina has been working in this field. As this effort began, a small number of individuals were resposible for breaking down the barriers imposed by prejudices and myths surrounding this issue (Giberti, 1992). Once awareness of partner violence as a serious social issue grew, the Government of Argentina created institutions to build a knowledge base regarding this problem.

Addressing violence against women involves confronting pervasive stereotypes and myths related to partner aggression. One example of a widespread myth in Argentina is that the aggressors are alcoholics, uneducated, and from the lower social strata (Ferreira, 1994). In addition, there has been a widely held belief that women who are victims of physical aggression by a spouse somehow provoked the aggression. For example, when faced with a case of a battered woman, some officials of the judicial system will ask the woman: "What have you done to him for him to batter you?" (Munné, 1999). In this way, the myth that a woman provokes the abuse is established and reinforced, further deepening the process of victimization. The victim then accepts these myths and begins to judge herself within this framework.

Legislation
After years of debate, in 1995, the National Congress enacted Law 24.417, known as the Protection from Family Violence Law. This law makes it possible for any victim of domestic violence to report the situation to the family courts assigned for this purpose, without the assistance of a lawyer or intervention by the police. The fact that no lawyer is required allows the population segments of lowest income to gain access to the judiciary system and enables the judges to take precautionary measures in those cases in which domestic violence is confirmed. The aggressor can be denied access to the home, and the custody and corresponding alimonies in cases of couples with children can be arranged. The law also requires all public entities (e.g., schools and hospitals) to report cases of domestic violence to the courts. The National Council of Youth and Family and the Ministry of Justice, Security, and Human Rights are responsible for keeping data related to domestic violence incidents. Additionally, the law includes provisions for the creation of a multidisciplinary team of professionals to evaluate risks and to issue reports on family interactions to the civil court where

these are judged to be needed. Although Law 24.417 is a significant step in Argentina's legislation in the protection from family violence, it has not been sufficiently publicized, and its existence is therefore not known to many who might benefit from the direct access to the family courts system that it provides.

Community-level Programs

In 1989, the city government of Buenos Aires created the Women's Office, which has a 24-hour help line and specialized units for the assistance and treatment of domestic violence. In 1992, the National Women's Council was created as an entity reporting directly to the office of Argentina's President. It has incorporated domestic violence as a priority focus and develops activities and programs targeted to preventing violence and providing assistance to victims of violence. In 1999, the Council created the National Program for the Care, Evaluation, and Monitoring of Violence against Women. The Council also developed a manual to serve as a guide for intervention in situations of domestic violence and has organized seminars—including one on public policies, health, and family violence—in various parts of the country in an effort to raise public awareness about this issue. It is also responsible for monitoring adherence to related international conventions to which the country is a signatory.

In December 1998, Argentina's Attorney General created the Office for Assistance to Victims of Crime. This entity provides legal, psychological, and social counseling; conducts follow-up on victims of all types of crimes; and carries out research in this area. In 2006, the Ministry of the Interior created an office where victims of violence who report their situation to the police can receive professional assistance. In addition, the federal police created a center to provide assistance to victims of domestic violence, and, in Buenos Aires province, several police stations staffed by female police officers have been created. There are also several nongovernmental organizations that provide counselling and treatment, as well as conduct research related to various domestic violence issues.

Statistics on Spousal Violence

Unfortunately, the dearth of reliable statistics regarding domestic violence in Argentina does not allow an accurate measurement of the problem's magnitude (Equipo Latinoamericano de Justicia y Género, 2005). In their absence, available information, while fragmented, nonetheless sheds some light on the general situation.

A study carried out by the University of La Plata and the Center for Studies of Culture and Women found that 1,284 females were murdered between 1997 and 2003 in Buenos Aires province, with most victims (70%) being killed by someone they knew. In 68% of cases, the aggressor was the woman's husband, partner, or ex-partner (Chejter, 2005).

Records from social services agencies also provide some indication of the scope of the problem. The women's office of the city government of Buenos Aires reported receiving 12,417 calls in 2006 asking for advice on how to cope with domestic violence situations. That same year, the women's office provided support to 3,700 women in its centers, and 253 were assisted in its shelters (Dirección General de la Mujer, 2006). Most of the victims assisted were in the 24-44-year-old age group, and 77.5% had children.

Reports on domestic violence from the women's office indicate that aggressors belong to all social classes, and 85.7% of aggressors were employed. A telephone help line for children who are victims of or witnesses to acts of domestic violence registered 2,182 calls in 2006 for the city of Buenos Aires alone.

According to the Civil Court, the number of domestic violence cases (including on men, women, and children) reported to this body has increased from 996 in 1995 to 3,992 in 2005. The victims were mainly women, increasing from 749 in 1995 to 2,000 in 2005, although the number of male victims has also increased (32 cases in 1995 to 166 in 2005) (Equipo Latinoamericano de Justicia y Género, 2005). A team of psychologists, social workers, and attorneys working under the Ministry of Justice, Security, and Human Rights handles around 300 new cases of domestic violence each month in the city of Buenos Aires. According to statistics from the Office for Assistance to Victims of Crime under the Attorney General of Argentina, 140 new civil cases related to domestic violence received assistance in 2006.

In Buenos Aires province, the General Department of Coordination of Gender Policies of the provincial-level Ministry of Security reported that between March and November 2006, it saw 20,000 cases of victims of family violence and that 90% of them were women; 7,200 were formal complaints and 12,400 were civil reports (Ministerio de Relaciones Exteriores, Comercio Internacional y Culto 2007).

Women who have themselves been convicted of crimes may be particularly likely to be victims of partner aggression. For example, a survey carried out by the Federal Penitentiary Service found that 90% of female prisoners had been victims of domestic violence (Dirección Nacional de Política Criminal, 2006). In addition, partner aggression affects pregnant women. Data from a Buenos Aires city hospital which has a treatment unit for domestic violence cases suggested that 75% of alleged "spontaneous abortions" were, in fact, the result of a physical aggression during pregnancy (Dirección General de la Mujer, 2006).

The Drinking Context
Although alcohol consumption is widespread in Argentina, until recently very little research had been carried out on this topic. In the first national study on the use of psychoactive substances (Míguez, 1999), 66.2% of people aged 18–65 reported consuming alcohol within the last 30 days (78.8% among males and 54.4% among females). Abuse rates were seven times higher among males than among females. The average number of drinks consumed by those who reported drinking at least once a week within the past year was 4.2 (5.1 for males and 2.5 for females). Alcohol abuse was defined as intake higher than 70g of absolute alcohol daily. The rate of alcohol abuse among those who reported drinking at least once a week within the last year was 13.2% (18.1% for males and 4.7% for females). Socially vulnerable young people (i.e., those with low educational and socioeconomic level) had higher rates of abuse. Data from the second national study (Secretaria de Programación para la Prevención de la Drogadicción y Lucha contra el Narcotráfico, 2004a) showed that alcohol abuse had increased since 1999 among young people and among adolescents aged 12–15 years, although the legal drinking age in Argentina is 18. In this study, the lifetime prevalence of use of alcohol was 40% among females and 38% among males.

Alcohol Involvement in Partner Aggression

Alcohol consumption is considered a risk factor that enhances the probability of violence against women (Fiorito, 2006). Research suggests that alcohol is associated with intimate partner violence because alcohol problems and abusive drinking patterns lead to and exacerbate intimate partner conflicts, alcohol intoxication disrupts attention and judgment, and therefore it intensifies existing conflict and aggression (Leonard, 2001).

Information on alcohol involvement in partner aggression in Argentina is scarce. The first national study of use of psychoactive substances among individuals seeking emergency hospital services was carried out in 2003 (Secretaría de Programación para la Prevención de la Drogadicción y Lucha contra el Narcotráfico, 2004b). In this sample of 14,885 patients, 8.2% of the consultations were related to alcohol and other drugs. Alcohol was the main substance related to the consultation (83.7%), followed by marijuana and tranquilizers (around 10%). Of the consultations involving alcohol, 56.8% were related to violence, including domestic violence.

Although there are no official data regarding the prevalence of alcohol use among perpetrators of partner aggression, this figure is estimated to be about 30% in Latin American countries (Ferreira, 1994). Frequently, an association between domestic violence and alcohol has been uncovered at treatment centers responding to the needs of women who have been the victims of domestic violence. According to case data from one center administered by the Women's Office in the city of Buenos Aires, of a total of 239 women, 68% of their partners abused alcohol (Dirección General de la Mujer, 2006). Professionals working in other similar centers throughout Buenos Aires city and province also reported that alcohol abuse was very common among male perpetrators. In addition, in some domestic violence treatment centers for males, if the individual is alcohol-dependent, he is not included in the group but rather sent to alcohol addiction treatment (Fiorito, 2006). Research indicates that excessive alcohol consumption and partner physical aggression may reflect a man's underlying need for power and control, with alcohol serving as a weapon to reinforce dominance in an intimate male-female relationship (Gondolf, 1995).

It is also very frequent during treatment of male aggressors to observe the justification of violent acts as a result of alcohol consumption (Fiorito, 2006). In some cases, the men report not remembering their violent acts due to their drinking. Based on experience with cases at the Office for Assistance to Victims of Crime, it appears that victims and aggressors often cite alcohol as the causal factor for violent acts (Munné, 1999, 2005). This pattern became evident during an interview with one 45-year-old housewife who had been married for 10 years who reported that her husband had threatened to kill her. During the interview, she stated: "the thing is that he drinks and becomes very violent." She added that he had always been violent and frequently beat and insulted her. On several occasions, these incidents led to hospital visits. She recalled that several times she requested that he receive treatment for his problems with alcohol, believing that in this way she could solve the situation at home. She expressed a sense of "pity because he drinks." She described how once he lost control and threw several pieces of cutlery at her. Her fear led her to call the police, who ignored her plight, saying that her husband was only drunk and they did not want to arrest him. In this particular case, the police's consideration of the incident as being "a question of drunkards" rather than afamily violence problem served only to further exacerbate the woman's vulnerability.

It is important to note that Argentina's legislation does not establish the use of alcohol as either aggravating or attenuating responsibility for crimes. The current standard is that of intent, which is determined through psychiatric examination of the accused. The current trend resulting from psychiatric examinations indicates that the influence of alcohol prior to committing a crime holds no implications for the subject's guilt or punishment (Baigún and Zaffaroni, 1997).

Methods

In 2002, Argentina participated in the collaborative Gender, Alcohol, and Culture: An International Study (GENACIS) project as one of the developing countries receiving funding for this purpose by the World Health Organization.

Sample and Survey

The sample was selected from Buenos Aires city and province, a region which together represents approximately 50% of the population in Argentina. The sampling frame in the Federal Capital and Greater Buenos Aires was based on tract areas (urban blocks or quarters) stratified by school district in the city of Buenos Aires and by partidos (subdivisions) in Greater Buenos Aires. In the remainder of Buenos Aires province, the 167 towns with populations of 2,000 or more population were classified by size and region before being sampled. Sampling involved three stages: sampling of areas and buildings, sampling of households when there was more than one household in the same building, and sampling of an individual in the household. Respondents included urban males and females between the ages of 18 and 65 years old. There were 1,000 completed interviews.

Fieldwork staff consisted of a director, three area supervisors, and 30 interviewers who were psychologists, anthropologists, sociologists, and social workers. Almost all interviewers were women, and a few were students. Data were collected using face-to-face interviews. Interviewers received training in both general and study-specific interviewing techniques and on issues related to privacy and confidentiality. Role-playing techniques were used for parts of the questionnaire that might be sensitive or otherwise problematic. Interviewers were provided with lists of available community resources that deal with alcohol and drug problems and agencies working in the area of domestic violence. This information was shared with respondents who inquired about how they might obtain help for themselves or other persons with problems in these areas. The interviewers were trained in special techniques enabling them to explain that the survey was aimed at the general population. This was an important step, in view of the fact that even if alcohol consumption is engrained in Argentine culture, many individuals, upon hearing the word "alcohol," might have reacted by asserting that they are not "alcoholics" and thus would not be eligible to participate in the survey. This reflects the social image of alcohol in Argentina, even among well-educated people, in which the concept of alcohol dependency carries a cultural stigma.

It is also important to note the country's underlying socio-political context during the time the study was conducted. Argentina had been facing an acute economic crisis, and the feeling of social vulnerability was very high. The financial situation at the household level was unstable, the rate of violent crimes was on the rise, and the population was very concerned about security issues.

Measures

All GENACIS partner aggression questions were used. Responses to the questions about the most severe type of partner aggression were open-ended and then coded into categories by the interviewer. One male victim and one male aggressor were excluded from these analyses because their partners involved in the aggression were also male. All drinking variable questions from the GENACIS expanded core questions were used in the Argentina survey. Whether the respondent drank five or more drinks on one occasion in the past year was based on the graduated frequency question as described in the chapter "Common Survey Methods and Analyses Conducted for Each Country," which appears earlier in this book.

As reported in previous analyses of the GENACIS study (Munné, 2005b), males drank more frequently and more heavily than females. The youngest age group (18–29 years old) consumed the largest amounts of alcohol. Males reported more positive consequences of drinking as well as more negative consequences. Based on the Alcohol Use Disorders Identification Test (AUDIT) scores, 11.6% of the sample was considered to engage in harmful use of alcohol. Concerning social consequences of drinking, 9.9% of current drinkers reported three or more social consequences of drinking (27.3% for males aged 18–29 years old). Harmful effects of drinking on the respondent's relationships were considerable, especially with regard to marriage and intimate relationships and relationships with family members. An important finding regarding relationship problems was the response to the item "people annoyed you by criticizing your drinking." Rates of endorsing this item were the highest of all relationship problems (26.7% in the youngest age group of males). Other social harms investigated in this study were becoming involved in a fight while drinking, with 23.2% of young males reporting that this had happened to them. Table 1 shows the demographic characteristics and drinking pattern for the Argentine survey sample.

Results

As shown in Figure 1, more males (14.5%) than females (9.4%) reported being victims of physical aggression by a partner ($p < .05$). Approximately 8% of both females and males reported being physically aggressive toward a partner. The difference between the percent of males who reported being the victim of aggression by a partner was also significantly larger than the percent of females who reported being aggressive toward a partner ($p < .05$). As well, a larger proportion of females reported being the victim of aggression by a partner than males reported being aggressive toward a partner, but this difference did not meet the criterion for statistical significance. Of those who reported being involved in any partner aggression, 47.6% of males and 36.7% of females reported being a victim only; 7.9% of males and 29.1% of females reported being an aggressor only; and 44.4% of males and 34.2% of females reported aggression both by a partner and toward a partner.

TABLE 1. Age, marital status, employment status, and drinking pattern in the 12 months preceding the survey, for male and female respondents, GENACIS survey, Argentina, 2002.

	Males (N=402)		Females (N=598)	
	Number	Percent or mean	Number	Percent or mean
Age		38.2 years		41.0 years
18–24 years	79	19.7%	88	14.7%
25–34 years	98	24.4%	116	19.4%
35–44 years	95	23.6%	146	24.4%
45–54 years	69	17.2%	124	20.7%
55 years and older	61	15.1%	124	20.7%
Marital status				
Married	155	38.6%	274	45.8
Cohabiting/Living with partner	56	13.9%	102	17.1%
Divorced or separated	38	9.5%	75	12.7%
Never married	148	36.8%	117	19.6%
Widowed	5	1.2%	29	4.9%
Employment status				
Working for pay (includes temporarily not working due to illness or parental leave)	294	73.1%	264	44.0%
Voluntarily unemployed (homemaker or other reasons)	6	1.5%	227	38.0%
Involuntarily unemployed	54	13.4%	52	8.7%
Student	38	9.5%	33	5.5%
Retired	10	2.5%	23	3.8%
Drinking pattern (past 12 months)				
Drank any alcohol during past 12 months	368	91.5%	441	73.8%
Average number of drinking days (drinkers only)		120.7 days		61.8 days
Average number of drinks per occasion (drinkers only)		3.7 drinks		1.7 drinks
Average annual volume (drinkers only)		494.6 drinks		133.2 drinks
Drank five or more drinks on one or more occasions (drinkers only)	217	59.1%	65	14.7%

FIGURE 1. Percent of respondents who reported having been a victim or aggressor, by sex, GENACIS survey, Argentina, 2002.

Category	Percentage
Female victimization	9.4
Female aggression	8.4
Male victimization	14.5
Male aggression	8.2

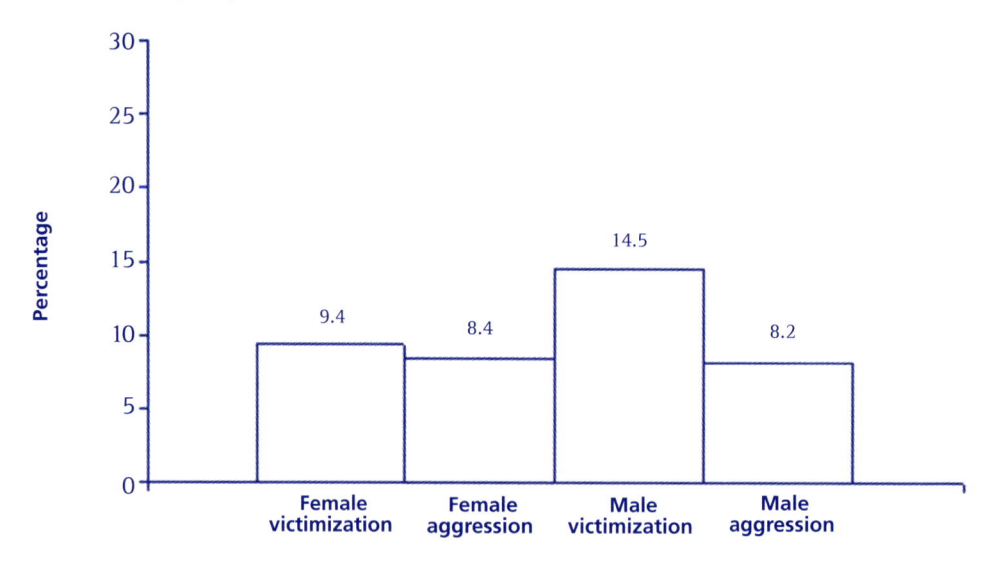

The average age of female victims was 34.0 years, and female aggressors 30.4 years. The average age of male victims and male aggressors were 29.8 years and 29.4 years, respectively. As shown in Figure 2, the percent of males and females reporting aggression by a partner and aggression toward a partner tended to decline with age.

FIGURE 2. Percent of respondents who reported having been a victim or aggressor, by age group and sex, GENACIS survey, Argentina, 2002.

Age group	Female victimization	Female aggression	Male victimization	Male aggression
18–24	19.3	25.0	25.3	12.7
25–34	11.2	9.5	23.7	17.5
35–44	8.9	8.2	11.6	4.2
45–54	7.3	1.6	4.4	2.9
55+	3.3	2.5	1.7	0.0

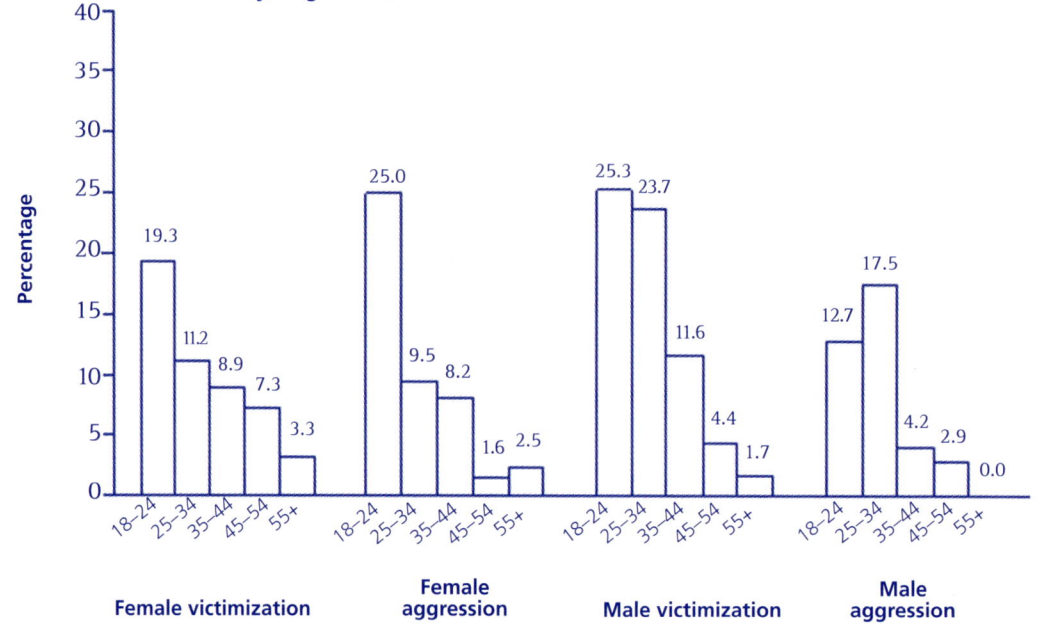

Partner aggression varied by marital status, but showed similarities between male and female victims and aggressors (see Figure 3). The percent reporting physical aggression involving a partner was higher among cohabiting men and women than among those who were married (p < .001 for all groups), and it was higher for those who were cohabiting than all other marital status groups for male aggressors (p < .01). Rates of partner aggression were lowest among married respondents, significantly lower than the rate for never-married male victims (p < .01), never-married female aggressors (p < .05), and divorced/separated female victims (p < .01). No other differences between marital status groups met the criterion for significance (set at p < .01 to adjust for the possibility of chance findings of significance due to the number of comparisons being made). These results should be treated with caution, however, due to the low number of cases within some marital status groups.

FIGURE 3. Percent of respondents who reported having been a victim or aggressor, by marital status and sex, GENACIS survey, Argentina, 2002.

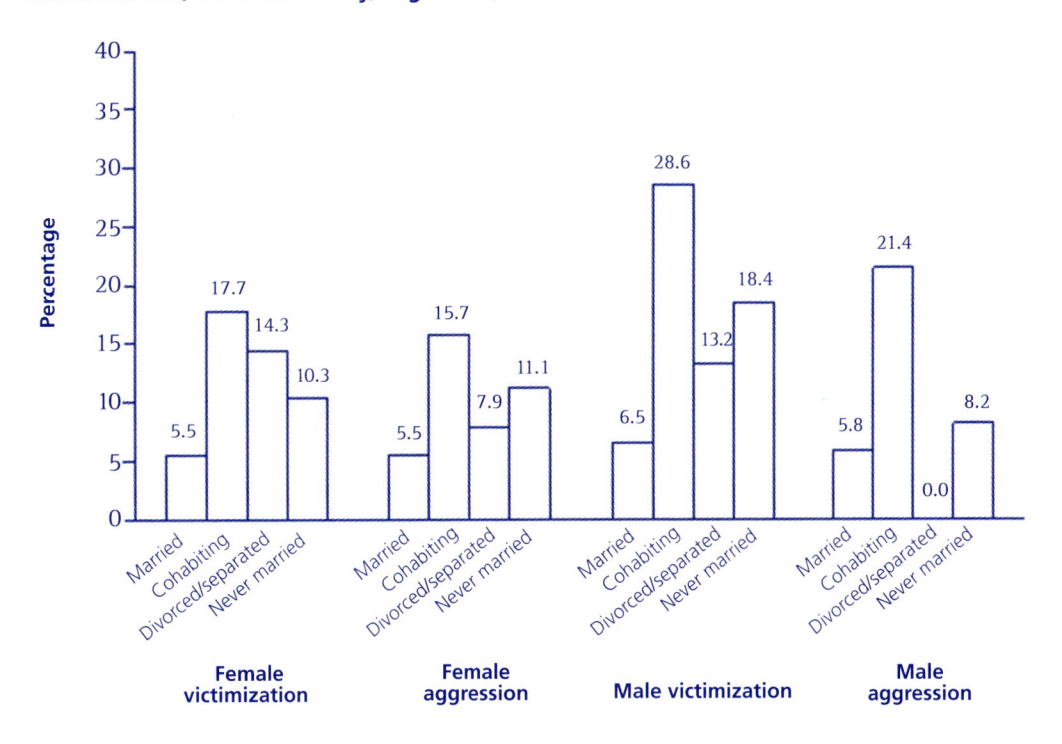

Group	Married	Cohabiting	Divorced/separated	Never married
Female victimization	5.5	17.7	14.3	10.3
Female aggression	5.5	15.7	7.9	11.1
Male victimization	6.5	28.6	13.2	18.4
Male aggression	5.8	21.4	0.0	8.2

As shown in Figure 4, the type of aggressive act most commonly reported was being pushed/shoved. Male victims were significantly more likely than female victims (p = .001) to report being slapped. In addition, female victims were more likely to report the more severe types of aggressions, such as being beaten up (10.7%), while no male victims reported being beaten up by a partner (p = .01) and no male aggressors reported beating up a female partner (although this difference compared with female victims did not meet the significance criterion). Other pair-wise differences in type of aggressive act between male and female victims and aggressors were not statistically significant (at a significance level of p < .01).

FIGURE 4. Type of aggressive act against females as reported by female victims and male aggressors, and against males as reported by male victims and female aggressors, GENACIS survey, Argentina, 2002.

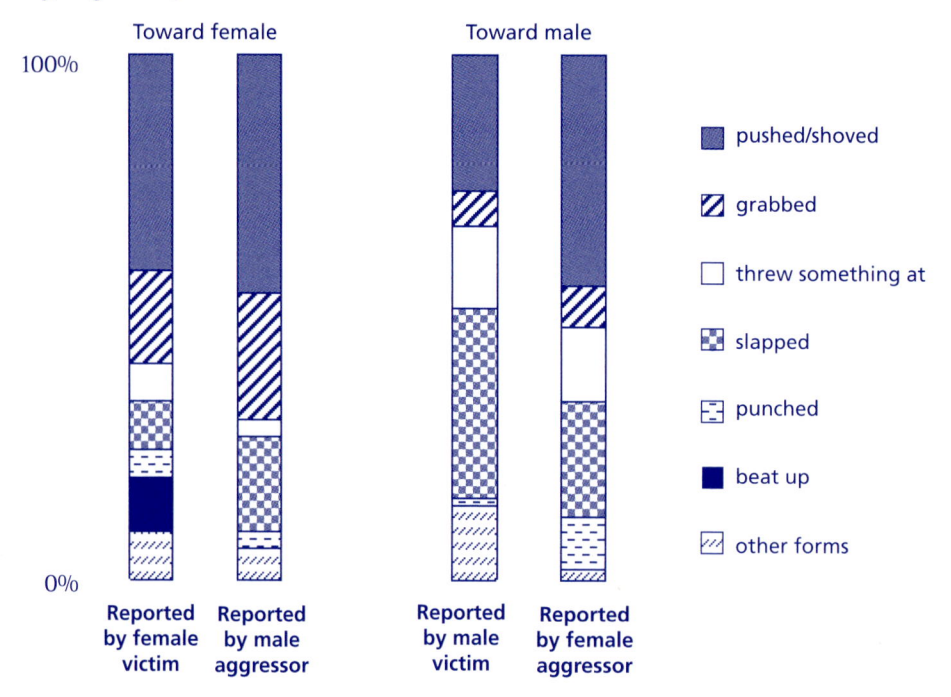

Figure 5 shows ratings of severity of aggression (on a scale from 1 to 10, with 10 being most severe) as well as ratings of how scared, upset, and angry the respondent felt at the time of the aggressive act. Male victims consistently gave the lowest ratings of the four groups on all measures (after controlling for age this difference was significant compared to female victims for all four ratings and compared to female aggressors for severity and anger). Anger ratings of female victims were significantly higher than those of male aggressors ($p < .01$). No other differences between male and female victims and aggressors met the criterion of $p < .01$ for statistical significance. Of those who reported any physical aggression by a partner, 4 women (out of 52) and no men (out of 56) reported seeking medical attention after the incident (a significant difference at $p < .05$).

FIGURE 5. Mean ratings of severity of aggression, fear, upset, and anger by male and female victims and aggressors, GENACIS survey, Argentina, 2002.

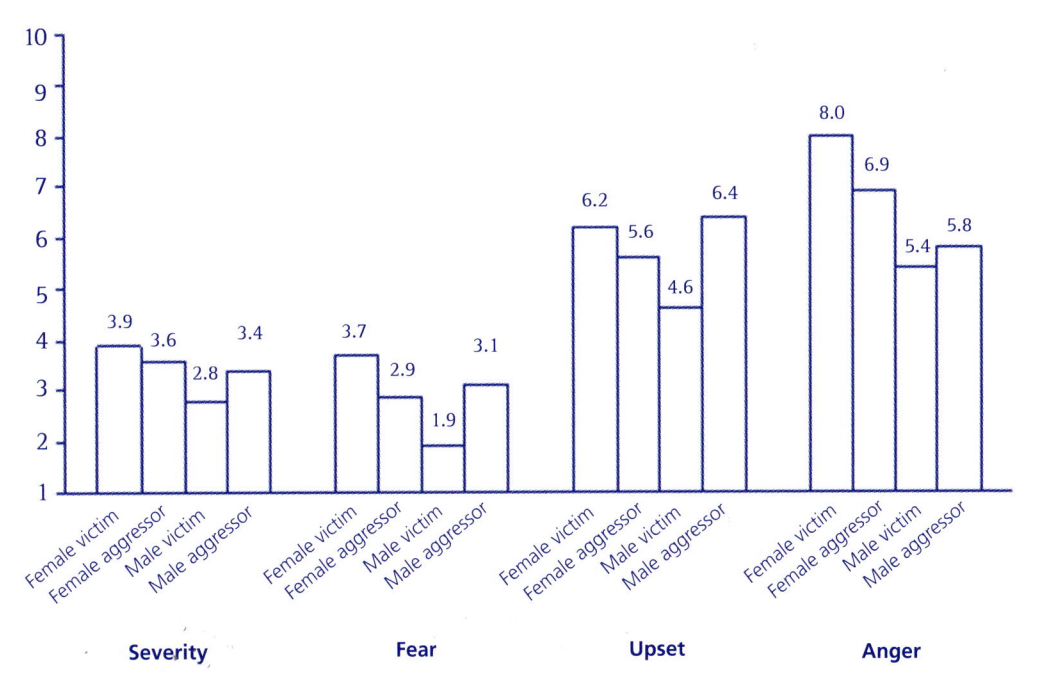

As shown in Figure 6, most respondents reported that no one was drinking at the time of partner aggression. When alcohol was involved, the aggressor was more likely to be male (as reported by both female victims and male aggressors); however, these results should be treated with caution due to the low numbers of cases. Male aggressors were more likely than female aggressors to have been the only partner drinking during the incident as reported by female and male victims ($p < .01$) and by male and female aggressors ($p < .01$). No other significant pairwise differences between male and female victims and aggressors were found.

FIGURE 6. Percent of incidents in which no partner had been drinking, both partners had been drinking, only the male partner had been drinking, or only the female partner had been drinking, as reported by male and female victims and aggressors, GENACIS survey, Argentina, 2002.

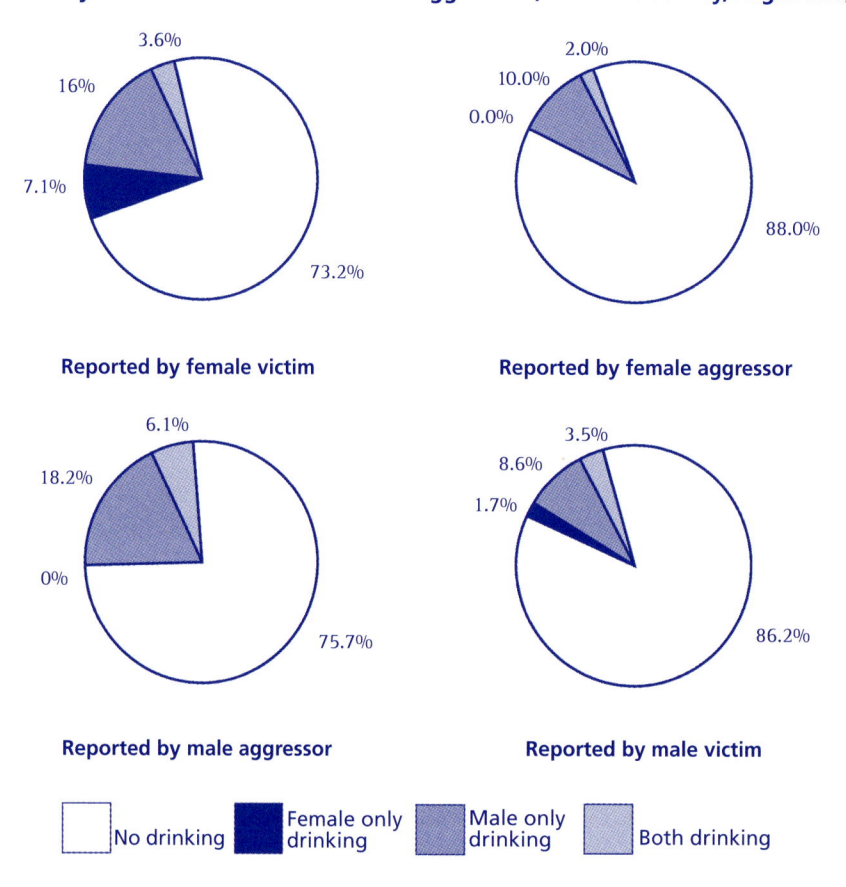

Reported by female victim: 73.2% No drinking, 7.1% Female only drinking, 16% Male only drinking, 3.6% Both drinking

Reported by female aggressor: 88.0% No drinking, 0.0% Female only drinking, 10.0% Male only drinking, 2.0% Both drinking

Reported by male aggressor: 75.7% No drinking, 0% Female only drinking, 18.2% Male only drinking, 6.1% Both drinking

Reported by male victim: 86.2% No drinking, 1.7% Female only drinking, 8.6% Male only drinking, 3.5% Both drinking

Legend: No drinking | Female only drinking | Male only drinking | Both drinking

The Relationship between Alcohol Consumption and Partner Aggression

The percent of victims and aggressors was higher among those who drank alcohol in the year before the survey than among those who abstained, with 10.7% of female drinkers reporting having been the victim of partner aggression and 8.8% reporting aggression toward a partner, versus 5.7 and 7.1%, respectively, for female abstainers; among male drinkers, 15.5% reported aggression by a partner and 9.0% reported aggression toward a partner versus 2.9% and 0.0%, respectively, for male abstainers. However, logistic regression of aggression (yes/no) on drinking status controlling for age produced no significant differences for the four groups of respondents.

Respondents' Drinking Pattern and Partner Aggression

The analyses in this section are limited only to respondents who consumed alcohol during the year preceding the survey.

Figure 7 shows the percentage of partner physical aggression reported by male and female victims and aggressors who drank five or more drinks at least once in the year before the survey compared to current drinkers who did not drink five or more drinks. In all cases the rate of partner aggression was higher for those who drank five or more drinks; however, logistic regression of whether partner aggression occurred on whether the respondent consumed five or more drinks controlling for age identified no significant differences.

FIGURE 7. Percent of respondents who reported victimization (aggression by a partner) or aggression (aggression toward a partner) by whether the respondent had consumed five or more drinks on an occasion or had never consumed five drinks on an occasion, by sex, GENACIS survey, Argentina, 2002.

	Never drank 5+	Drank 5+
Female victimization	10.1	13.9
Female aggression	8.0	13.9
Male victimization	9.4	19.8
Male aggression	4.7	12.0

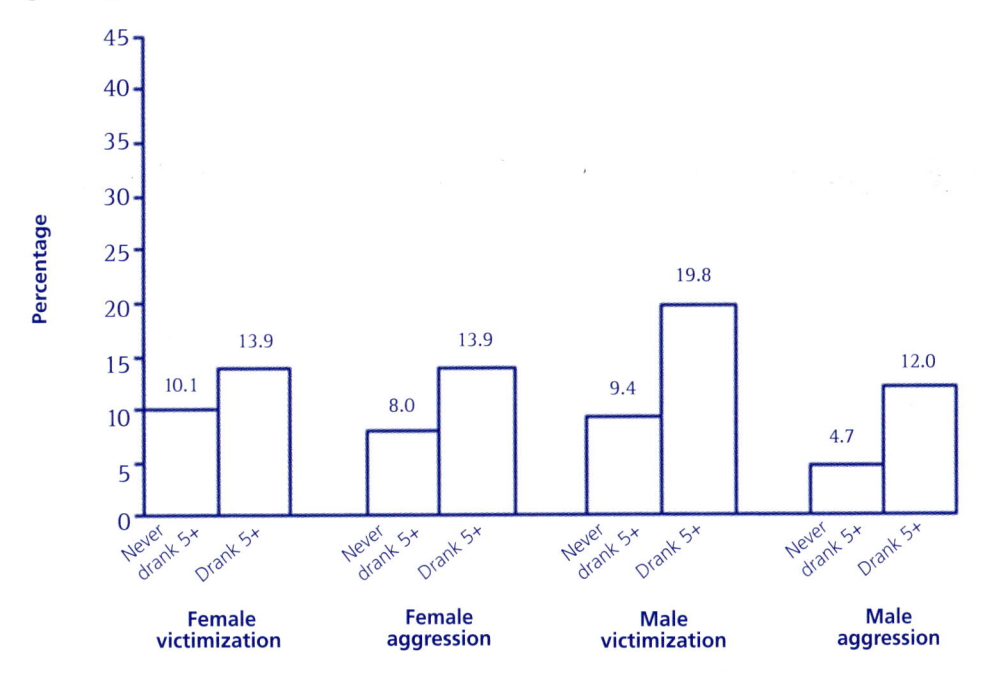

Figures 8, 9, and 10 show the average (mean) number of drinking days, the average usual number of drinks consumed on drinking days, and the average total number of drinks consumed in the year before the survey by whether the respondent was a victim of aggression by a partner and whether respondent was aggressive toward a partner. There was no evidence of aggression being associated with more frequent drinking; in fact, the frequency of drinking was actually lower for male and female victims and female aggressors. For all three measures of drinking pattern, the only significant finding was that the total number of drinks per year was higher for males who were aggressive toward a partner than for males who were not aggressive ($p < .05$ controlling for age).

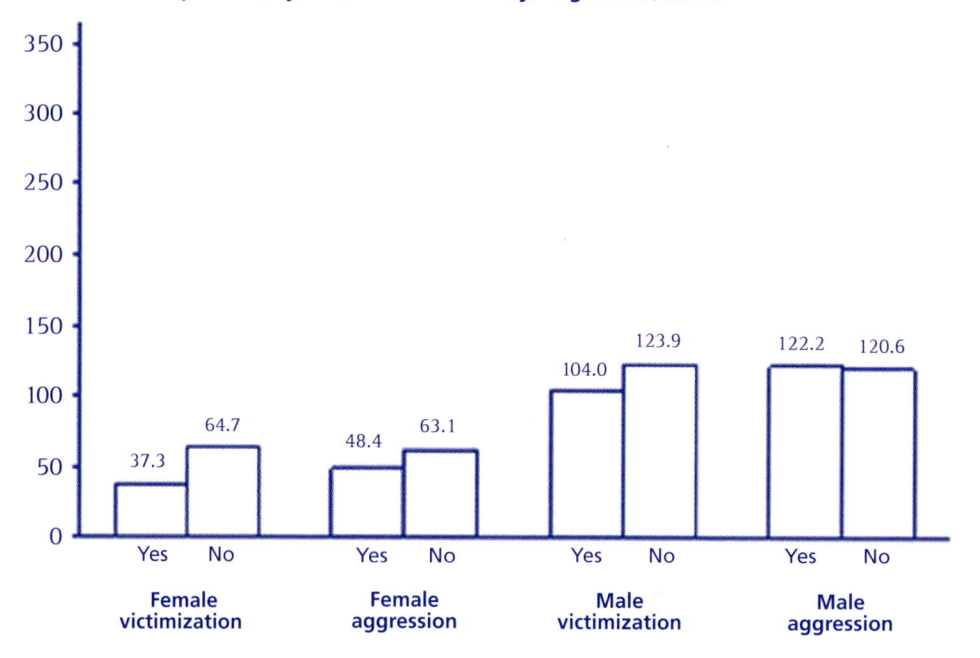

FIGURE 8. Mean number of drinking days in the year preceding the survey by whether the respondent had been a victim of partner aggression and whether the respondent had been aggressive toward a partner, by sex, GENACIS survey, Argentina, 2002.

	Yes	No
Female victimization	37.3	64.7
Female aggression	48.4	63.1
Male victimization	104.0	123.9
Male aggression	122.2	120.6

Argentina | 49

FIGURE 9. Mean number of drinks consumed on usual drinking occasions by whether the respondent had been a victim of partner aggression and whether the respondent was aggressive toward a partner, by sex, GENACIS survey, Argentina, 2002.

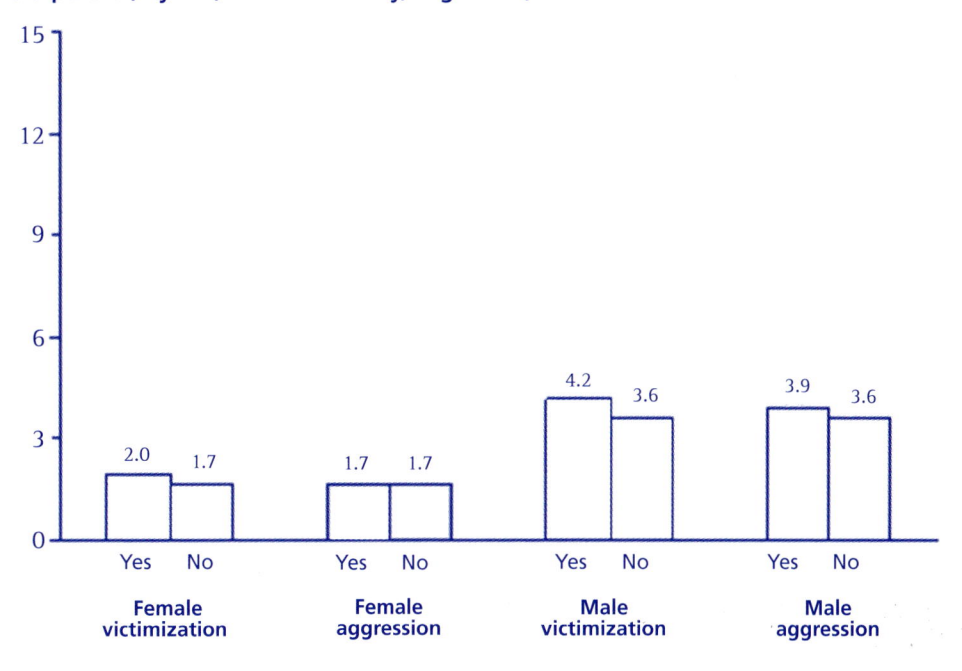

Female victimization	Female aggression	Male victimization	Male aggression
Yes: 2.0, No: 1.7	Yes: 1.7, No: 1.7	Yes: 4.2, No: 3.6	Yes: 3.9, No: 3.6

FIGURE 10. Overall mean number of drinks consumed annually by whether the respondent had been a victim of partner aggression and whether the respondent had been aggressive toward a partner, by sex, GENACIS survey, Argentina, 2002.

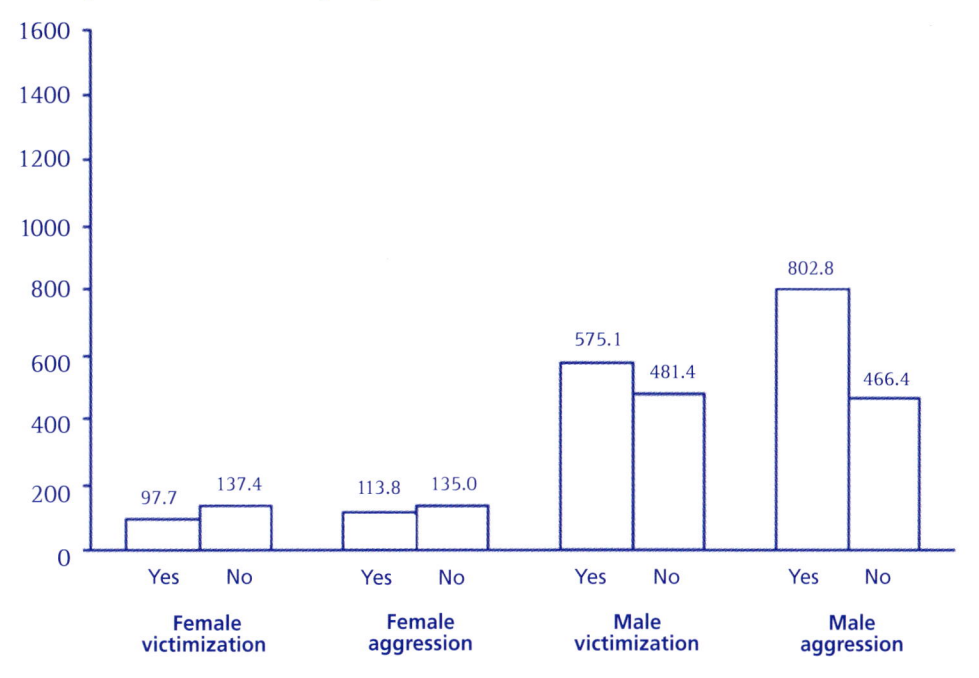

Female victimization	Female aggression	Male victimization	Male aggression
Yes: 97.7, No: 137.4	Yes: 113.8, No: 135.0	Yes: 575.1, No: 481.4	Yes: 802.8, No: 466.4

Discussion

Rates of partner aggression were lower than expected, especially those reported by female respondents. A possible explanation could be that women may be afraid to report physical aggression even though privacy and confidentiality were assured in the interviews. Although prevalence of partner aggression, especially aggression toward women, may be underestimated in the current study sample, the relationships between partner aggression and other variables nonetheless provide a greater understanding of partner aggression in Argentina.

The findings showed that aggression by a partner and aggression toward a partner tended to decline with age. This suggests that preventive measures should especially target young adults. In addition, findings from the present study reported previously (Munné, 2005b) as well as previous studies on alcohol consumption in Argentina, have found that young people were the group most at risk in terms of alcohol consumption and alcohol-related problems. Therefore, preventive measures focusing on the linkages between alcohol use and partner aggression should be particularly directed toward young people.

In relation to type of physical aggression, female victims reported experiencing more serious forms of aggression (e.g., being beaten up), rated the aggression as more severe than did male victims, and were more likely than male victims to require medical care. These results indicate that partner aggression is still a gender issue, in that women suffer from more severe forms of aggression. Even if numbers were very low, it is important to also note that of those who reported physical aggression by a partner only women reported seeking medical care following the incident.

As found in previous research in Canada (Graham and Wells, 2002), there were also gender differences in the emotional impact of aggression, with women tending to rate the impact of the aggressive act higher in terms of how scared, upset, or angry they felt after the episode, suggesting that women may be more likely than men to experience not only physical injury from partner aggression but psychological and emotional problems as well, and that these issues also need to be addressed as part of the services offered to female victims.

This study also provided insight into the role of alcohol consumption at the time of the aggressive incident. Although the majority of respondents reported that no one was drinking at the time of partner aggression, when drinking did occur, it was more likely to be the male who was drinking, especially in incidents in which the female was the victim (as reported by both female victims and male aggressors). This suggests that alcohol consumption is primarily a factor in male violence toward female partners, consistent with the impression from clinical studies noted earlier that males use alcohol consumption as an excuse to justify their violent acts, especially the most severe ones. It should be noted that these results should be treated with caution, however, due to the low number of cases.

The relationship between the respondent's drinking pattern and partner aggression was also explored in this study. Rates of partner aggression were higher for those who drank five or more drinks on one occasion at least once in the past year than for those who did not drink five drinks. This difference was consistent for male and female victims and aggressors, although individual comparisons did not meet the criterion for statistically significant differences after controlling for age. Frequency of drinking and usual number of drinks per occasion were not found to be significantly related to partner aggression; however, total number of drinks per year was significantly higher for males who reported being aggressive toward their partner than for males who reported no aggression toward a partner. These findings suggest that there is a need to further explore patterns of drinking in relation to partner aggression as well as the circumstances and contexts in which the drinking occurs. While these results provide some insight into the relationship between drinking patterns and partner aggression, more research is needed to explore the extent to which different alcohol patterns may facilitate violence in the Argentine context, especially among the heavier drinking segments of the population.

In terms of policy approaches, we are dealing with a complex phenomenon in that the relationship between alcohol and partner violence may operate through cultural beliefs about alcohol consumption and circumstances of drinking (Room, 2004). A better understanding of the role that alcohol plays in partner aggression will facilitate the development and implementation of appropriate preventive measures. One implication of the findings is that there is a need to train professionals in the alcohol abuse and domestic violence fields in order to equip them to be better able to cope with both issues simultaneously. For example, because police officers are often the first to respond to situations involving partner aggression, they would benefit from training that would enable them to address both issues related to partner aggression as well as issues related to exacerbation of this problem due to drinking, especially drinking by male aggressors. At the same time, there should be effective coordination between the designated agencies dealing with both issues. Given that these coexisting problems involve complexities requiring skilled management, all efforts should be made to foster a constructive and respectful dialogue among the involved social institutions in order to avoid harmful responses in dealing with the issues in conjunction.

Some limitations in the current study should be mentioned. The most important of these relates to sample size. In addition, the low rate of alcohol consumption at the time of the aggressive incident meant that some analysis, such as those comparing severity of incidents with and without alcohol, were not possible due to small numbers. Finally, it is unclear how questions on partner aggression and drinking at the time of aggression were interpreted. Argentina has traditionally been considered a "wet" culture in which alcohol is a part of daily life and drinking is the norm. However, drunkenness is socially condemned in certain segments in Argentine society (Munné, 2001). It may be that when interviewees were asked if they had been drinking before the incident of aggression, they were thinking of being drunk and might not have considered "drinking" as having cocktails with a meal, for example. For future research, use of qualitative data and the introduction of other improvements in measurement would be very useful in order to capture the most accurate picture possible of the role that alcohol plays in partner aggression.

References

Baigún D. and Zaffaron I. (1997) Código Penal y normas complementarias. Análisis doctrinario y jurisprudencia. Buenos Aires, José Luis Depalma Editor.

Centro de Encuentros Cultura y Mujer (CECYM) (1995) Centro de Encuentros Cultura y Mujer. Violencia Sexista. Control Social y resistencia de las mujeres.

Chejter S. (2005). Femicidios e impunidad. Centro de Encuentros de Cultura y Mujer.

Consejo Nacional de la Mujer Presidencia de la Nación (2006) Centro de Documentación.

Dirección Nacional de Política Criminal del Ministerio de Justicia de la Nación (2006) Informe estadístico.

Dirección General de la Mujer del Gobierno de la Ciudad de Buenos Aires (2006) Centro de Informática.

ELA Equipo Latinoamericano de Justicia y Género (2005). Informe sobre Género y Derechos Humanos. Vigencia y respeto de los derechos de las mujeres en Argentina

Fiorito O. (2006) Violencia masculina e ingesta alcohólica. Carrera Interdisciplinaria de Especialización en Violencia Familiar. Tesis.

Giberti Eva (1992) "La mujer y la violencia invisible". Buenos Aires, Editorial Sudamericana

Graham K, Wells S. (2002) The two World of aggression for men and women. *Sex Roles* 45 595–622.

Ferreira G. (1994). "La mujer maltratada. Un estudio de las mujeres víctimas de la violencia doméstica". Buenos Aires, Editorial Sudamericana.

Gondolf E. Alcohol abuse, wife assault and power needs. *Social Service Review* 69, 275–283

Leonard K. (2001) Domestic violence and alcohol. What is known and what to we need to know to encourage environmental interventions. Commissioned paper published in the proceedings of Alcohol Policy XII Conference, Alcohol and Crime, Research and Practice for Prevention, Washington, DC.

Míguez H. (1999) Estudio Nacional sobre sustancias adictivas de la República Argentina., Buenos Aires, Secretaría de Programación para la Prevención de la Drogadicción y Lucha contra el Narcotráfico.

Munné M. (1999) "Alcohol and domestic violence in Argentina: exploring the links and myths" paper presented at the 25th Annual Alcohol Epidemiology Symposium of the Kettil Bruun Society for Social and Epidemiological Research on Alcohol. Montreal, Canada May 31–June 4

Munné M. (2001) Drinking in tango lyrics: an approach to myths and meanings of drinking in Argentinian culture. *Contemporary Drug Problems*, 28, 415–439.

Munné M. (2005a) "Alcohol y violencia doméstica: Primeros resultados del Estudio Multicéntrico Alcohol, Género, Cultura y Daños" presented at 1st. Panamerican Conference on Alcohol Public Policies. Brasilia, Brasil. 28–30 November.

Munné M. (2005b) "Social Consequences of Alcohol Consumption in Argentina" in Alcohol, Gender and Drinking Problems, Perspectives from Low and Middle Income Countries. World Health Organisation. Department of Mental Health and Substance Abuse. Geneva
Oficina de Asistencia a la Víctima de la Procuración General de la Nación (2006) Informe Anual.

Room R. (2004) Intoxication and violence: a cultural perspective

Secretaría de Programación para la Prevención de la Drogadicción y Lucha contra el Narcotráfico (SEDRONAR) (2004a) Segundo estudio nacional sobre el consumo de sustancias psicoactivas. Secretaría de Prevención de la Drogadicción y Lucha contra el Narcotráfico. Buenos Aires.

Secretaría de Programación para la Prevención de la Drogadicción y Lucha contra el Narcotráfico (SEDRONAR) (2004b) El uso indebido de drogas y la consulta de emergencia. Primer Estudio Nacional. Secretaría de Prevención de la Drogadicción y Lucha contra el Narcotráfico. Buenos Aires.

UNHAPPY HOURS:

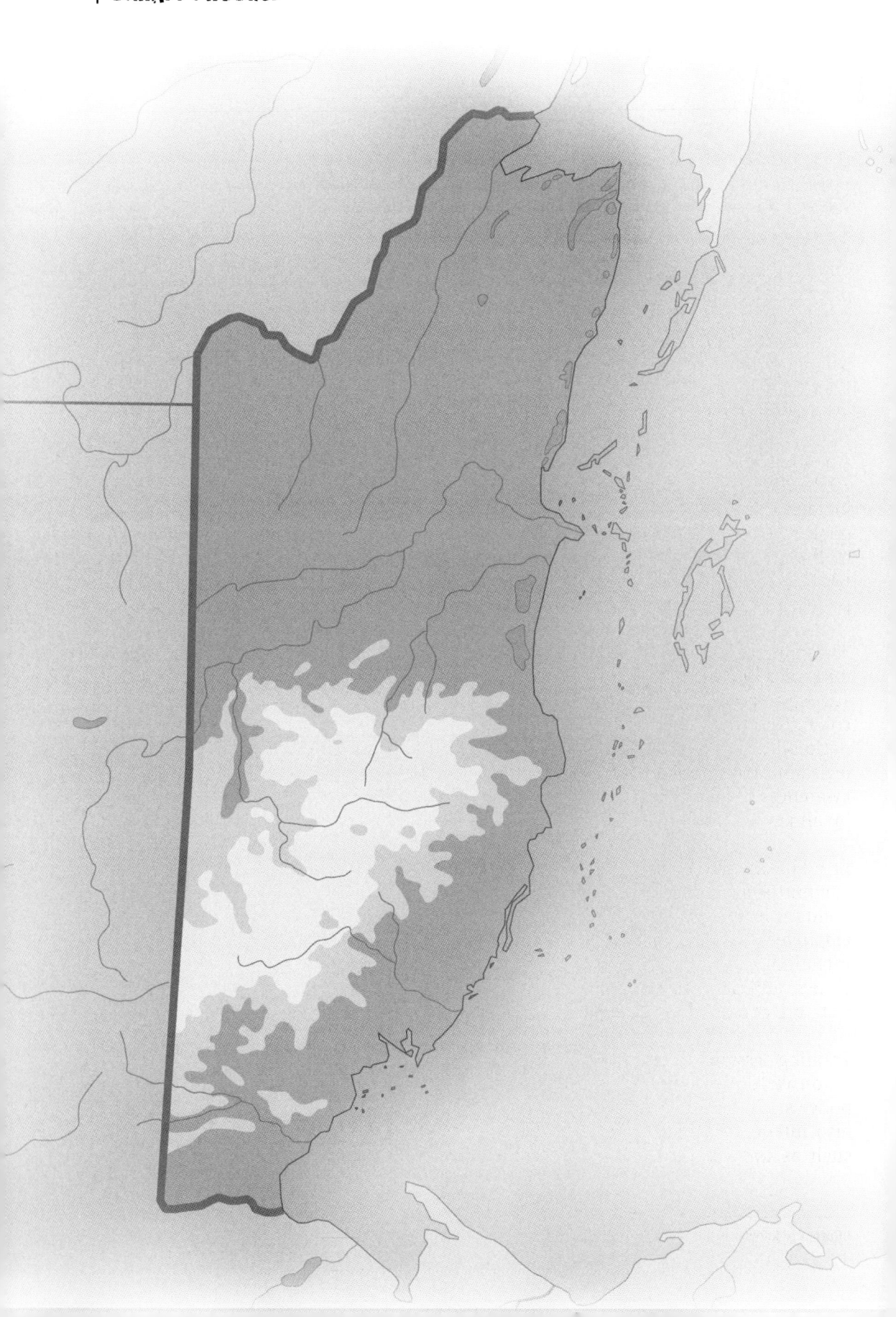

Belize: Alcohol and Partner Physical Aggression —*Claudina E. Cayetano and Kathryn Graham*

Introduction

Since the introduction in 1992 of the Domestic Violence Act—which defined domestic violence, including spousal rape in Belize—there has been considerable effort to place this issue on the public agenda. According to a report published by the Government of Belize in conjunction with the Pan American Health Organization (PAHO), "increased awareness and sensitivity to intra-family violence as public health and socioeconomic issues have emerged from a process of grassroots networking and advocacy" (Belize, Ministry of Health; PAHO, 2001).

An integrated model for addressing domestic violence was developed during the 1998-2002 period (Belize, Ministry of Health; PAHO, 2002) aimed at decreasing the incidence and prevalence of family violence. As a basis for developing this model, qualitative research was conducted in selected communities under the coordination of the Ministry of Health and the Women's Department of the Ministry of Human Development[1] with PAHO's technical assistance. The model includes detection, care, prevention, and promotion components.

A number of governmental and nongovernmental organizations have played important roles in addressing the impact of domestic violence on the Belizean population. Through the leadership of the Women's Department, a national family violence committee was created and tasked with the development and implementation of a national action plan with separate components focusing on family strengthening, legislation and policy development, resources development, and advocacy and public awareness. Various sectors contributed so that the family violence response was shared by all key sectors from the community to the national level.

In addition, the Ministry of Health and members of the national family violence committee developed a Domestic Violence Surveillance System in 1999. This system includes a National Gender-based Violence Registration Form to be completed by employees at institutions that come into contact with victims of domestic violence, including police departments, family courts and magistrates, health and hospital clinics, and the Human Services Department of the Ministry of Human Development. Data are compiled and analyzed by the Ministry of Health's Epidemiology Unit.

Training sessions to raise awareness about domestic violence issues among the population were also developed countrywide and as part of local networks. Currently, police stations in every district include a domestic violence unit. Family violence was also integrated into components of the educational curricula of training programs such as the nursing faculty and the police academy. In 2001, the Health Sector

---

[1] Currently known as the Ministry of Human Development and Social Transformation.

Domestic Violence Management Protocol was launched by the Ministry of Health. As described in this document (Belize, Ministry of Health; PAHO, 2001), the purpose of the protocol is to provide "health care providers with the necessary guidelines for the delivery of comprehensive attention to persons affected by family violence," and "a framework for the development of a family violence management protocol in other relevant sectors."

The 2006 Annual Report from the Women's Department of the Ministry of Human Development (Fonseca et al., 2007) highlighted the programs and services available for victims, as well as programs focused on prevention, education, personal development of women, and entrepreneurship. It also included advocacy for the new Domestic Violence Act of 2007, which embodies a policy of zero tolerance toward domestic violence and includes key modifications to the previous version, such as extending the definition of domestic violence to include physical, sexual, emotional, psychological, and/or financial abuse; more severe penalties for domestic violence offenses; and granting greater discretionary power to the police to intervene in domestic violence situations and to use evidence from police records if the victim is unwilling or unable to give evidence against the accused.[2]

Despite the growing number and intensity of campaigns promoting an environment that is free from violence, there persists in Belizean society a disturbing perception among some sectors that a husband is justified in physical aggression toward his wife for reasons such as her unfaithfulness, neglect of children, poor choices about spending money, refusal to have sex, and for not being attentive to her husband's needs (personal communication, psychiatric nurse practitioners, based on their assessments). Thus, women continue to experience problems from domestic abuse due to poverty and a lack of independent financial resources. Specifically, oftentimes women are forced to return to abusive home situations because they are unable to support themselves on their own.

Existing Knowledge of Rates of Partner Aggression in Belize

Since 1999, when the Ministry of Health initiated the Domestic Violence Surveillance System, it has undergone numerous revisions and modifications. It is currently considered a model system within the Caribbean subregion. The reporting form captures demographic information on the victim, information about the incident, the aggressor, the outcome of the incident, and information regarding referrals the victim and/or aggressor received. Of the agencies involved in the surveillance system, the Police Department consistently reports the largest proportion of cases. The Ministry of Health is also responsible for the entry of data provided by key partners in the network. The data are compiled and analyzed, and reports are produced on an annual basis.

In 2006, according to the Ministry of Health's Epidemiology Unit, 862 (89%) of the 968 cases reported to the authorities as part of the Domestic Violence Surveillance System involved partner aggression, with the remainder of incidents involving

---

[2] Government of Belize 8 March 2007 press release, available at http://www.belize.gov.bz/press_release_details.php?pr_id=4301.

violence toward children, parents, or other family members. Of the cases of partner aggression, 770 (89.3%) were related to a female victim and 92 (10.7%) to male victims. As shown in Table 1, the majority of reported cases occurred in Belize City and Orange Walk, especially among male victims. Approximately half of victims were Mestizo, about a third were Creole, and the remainder were of East Indian, Garifuna, Maya, other, or unknown ethnic groups.

TABLE 1. Characteristics of cases, by district, ethnic group, and sex, National Gender-based Violence Registration Form, Domestic Violence Surveillance System, Belize, 2006.

	All victims (N = 862)	Female (N = 770)	Male (N = 92)
	Percent	Percent	Percent
District			
Belize	46.2	44.4	60.9
Cayo	9.5	10.0	5.4
Corozal	18.6	20.0	6.5
Orange Walk	16.9	16.1	23.9
Stann Creek	3.9	4.2	2.2
Toledo	4.9	5.3	1.1
Ethnic group			
Creole	31.4	30.4	40.2
East Indian	6.3	6.2	6.5
Garifuna	3.1	2.9	5.4
Maya	5.9	6.5	1.1
Mestizo	50.2	50.6	46.7
Other	2.5	2.9	0.0
Unknown	0.4	0.5	0.0
Civil/marital status			
Married	31.3	31.0	33.7
Common law/living together	51.3	52.1	44.6
Separated/divorced	5.1	4.4	10.9
Single	10.2	11.9	10.9
Widowed	0.0	0.0	0.0
Relationship between victim and aggressor			
Husband/wife	32.5	32.3	33.7
Common law	50.6	51.0	46.7
Boyfriend/girlfriend	4.2	4.4	2.2
Ex-boyfriend/girlfriend	1.5	1.6	1.1
Ex-spouse	11.3	10.6	16.3
Type of violence (whether any of the following occurred)			
Emotional/verbal	71.0	70.9	71.7

TABLE 1. (continued)

	All victims (N = 862)	Female (N = 770)	Male (N = 92)
	Percent	Percent	Percent
Physical	61.5	64.7	34.8
Sexual	9.4	10.3	2.2
Economic	19.5	21.4	3.3
Neglect/abandonment	7.0	5.8	16.3
Other	2.8	2.5	5.4
Level of violence (mutually exclusive categories)			
Physical or sexual (may also include other forms)	64.2	67.5	35.9
Emotional or economic, but not physical or sexual (may also include other)	31.4	29.5	47.8
Other only	4.4	3.0	16.3
Chronicity of violence			
This was first incident in the victim's life	15.0	13.9	23.9
Previous incident occurred in past year	63.8	65.2	52.2

In terms of the civil or marital status of victims, about one-third of both male and female victims were married, and about one-half of female victims and slightly less than one-half of male victims were living in a common-law relationship. The same pattern was reflected in the relationship between the victim and aggressor. The average age of female victims was 30.1 years, while for male victims the average age was 36.9 years. Aggressors toward female victims were aged 33.4, on average, while aggressors toward male victims were 29.6 years of age, on average. According to these case files, 8.6% of female victims were pregnant at the time the aggression occurred.

As also shown in Table 1, over two-thirds of both males and females reported emotional or verbal abuse, and about two-thirds (65%) of females, but only 35% of males, reported being the victim of physical violence. Sexual and economic violence was more likely for female than for male victims, while male victims were more likely than female victims to report neglect or abandonment and other types of violence. As shown in the table, almost twice as many female as male victims reported physical or sexual violence (68% and 36%, respectively).

The results also indicated extensive chronicity of violence, with only 14% of females and 23.9% of males reporting that this was the first incident in their lives, and almost two-thirds of females and just over one-half of males reporting that a similar incident had happened in the past year. The system also includes information on referrals for victims and family members. In 2006, referrals were most commonly made to the family courts system (64.8%), followed by the police (15.5%), the Women's Department (13.9%), Human Services Department (6.3%), and psychiatric nurse practitioners (4.2%).

There is some evidence that the number of reported cases of domestic violence has dropped in recent years since reaching a high of 1,240 in 2003. In 2004, this number was 962, and in 2006 it was 968. However, it is difficult to ascertain whether the drop in cases is a result of national efforts to reduce domestic violence, changes in the recording system, or simply random variations. In terms of efforts to reduce violence, the change could be due to increased public awareness, since the Belize National Gender Policy was approved by Cabinet in 2002 and the surveillance system was strengthened in 2003. Both events followed extensive lobbying and advocacy. On the other hand, the reduction in cases may be at least partly related to the response that victims receive when requesting assistance. For example, there is only one shelter home in the country, located in Belize City, which means that women who reside in other districts do not have ready access to this facility and would need to be transported to this locale if the services of a shelter are required.

Although the surveillance system provides important information about domestic violence, it does not provide information about those cases that do not come to the attention of public authorities. The cases in the system appear to be those that are severe and possibly chronic. Thus, other approaches, such as general population surveys, can be useful in leading to a better understanding of the issue of partner aggression and in determining the potential for low-cost interventions to prevent chronic patterns of domestic violence from developing.

Alcohol Involvement in Partner Aggression

As described above, much progress has been made regarding the prevention, detection, and treatment of domestic violence. On the other hand, few efforts have been devoted to exploring the role of alcohol in domestic violence, especially partner aggression. Although a Belize National Gender Policy report (Johnson 2002) noted that "alcohol or other drug abuse features in the majority of cases" of domestic violence, alcohol and drug use have not been the specific focus of partner aggression interventions.

The importance of alcohol and drugs was confirmed by 2006 data from the surveillance system. Overall, the aggressor was noted as having consumed alcohol in 46.9% of incidents (50.3% of aggressors toward female victims, 18.5% of aggressors toward male victims), drugs in 9.5% of incidents (10.0% toward female victims, 5.4% toward male victims), and no alcohol or drugs in 25.2% of incidents (21.6% toward female victims, 55.4% toward male victims). No information about alcohol and drug use was available for 18.5% of incidents (18.2% toward female victims, 20.6% toward male victims).

The overall goal of the present research was to better understand physical aggression between married persons and others living in a common-law or romantic relationship in the general population of Belize, and the relationship between gender, partner physical aggression, and alcohol consumption.

Methods
Survey and Sample

The data were collected in 2005 using a random sampling approach in a national survey of 2,400 households. The survey was administered in a face-to-face interview, and all household[3] members, both male and female, 18 years and older, were eligible to participate. The individuals were interviewed privately away from other household members. Questionnaires were prepared in both English and Spanish, and a manual describing the survey's implementation was provided to interviewers.

A training-of-trainers exercise took place in Belize and included district supervisors who were permanent staff of the Central Statistical Office (CSO) with many years of experience in conducting surveys and in training field staff. The training, which was facilitated by an international consultant who was familiar with the implementation of the questionnaire in other countries, included conducting mock interviews. The trainers also participated in piloting the questionnaire and provided input into revisions to improve the final version for use in Belize. Households were selected randomly for the pilot testing and were not included as part of the final sample.

The sample comprised a two-stage design. In the first stage, each of the country's six administrative districts was subdivided into smaller Enumeration Districts (EDs) with an average size of 200 households each, from which a sample of urban and rural EDs was then selected. The second stage was the systematic random selection of households from within the selected EDs. A total of 120 EDs were sampled, and 20 households were randomly selected from each, thus yielding the sample size of 2,400 households (this represents 3.9% of the total households in Belize) (Belize, Central Statistics Office 2002). Interviewers were expected to make up to four attempts to call on households in order to obtain a response.

Of the total households in the sample, one or more persons from 1,990 households (82.9%) completed the interview, for a total of 2,074 females and 1,911 males. The remaining 17.1% of households were not included mainly due to vacant dwellings (5.3%) and non-contact (4.3%). The address was not found for 1.9% of the households, and in 1.8% of households (43 individuals) no one agreed to respond to the questionnaire.

The CSO district supervisors, and, occasionally, personnel from the Ministry of Health's Epidemiology Unit, were responsible for the overall supervision of the fieldwork in their respective districts with the assistance of field supervisors. Completed questionnaires were edited at the district level, while the data entry and processing were conducted at CSO headquarters using CSPro (Census and Survey Processing System software package).

The general characteristics of survey participants are shown in Table 2. Almost two-thirds (64%) of male respondents were aged 18-44, and about one-third (36%) were aged 45 and older. Female respondents were slightly younger, with approximately 68% belonging to the 18-44-year-old age group and 32% being aged 45 or older. The average age of male respondents was 40 years, and that of female respondents

---

[3] A household was defined as one or more persons (related or unrelated) living together; i.e. sleeping at least four nights a week in the dwelling and sharing at least one daily meal.

was 39 years. Approximately 40% of male and female respondents were married; approximately 20% were living with a partner; some 30% had never been married; and less than 10% were divorced, separated, or widowed. Approximately 50% of male respondents, but less than 20% of female respondents, reported drinking alcohol in the past 12 months, with male drinkers consuming alcohol on about five days a month on average and females about three days. Among drinkers, 68% of males and 43% of females reported consuming five or more drinks on at least one occasion in the past year. Among past-year drinkers, the average number of drinks on drinking occasions was 7.4 for males and 3.5 for females.

TABLE 2. Age, marital status, employment status, and drinking pattern in the 12 months preceding the survey, for male and female respondents, GENACIS survey, Belize, 2005.

	Males (N=1,911)		Females (N=2,074)	
	Number	Percent or mean	Number	Percent or mean
Age		40.2 years		39.0 years
18–24 years	381	20.0%	408	19.7%
25–34 years	432	22.6%	541	26.1%
35–44 years	417	21.8%	463	22.4%
45–54 years	310	16.2%	310	15.0%
55–64 years	172	9.0%	179	8.6%
65 years and older	197	10.3%	171	8.3%
Marital status				
Married	816	42.7%	839	40.5%
Cohabiting/Living with partner	405	21.2%	448	21.6%
Divorced or separated (includes married, but not in union)	51	2.7%	79	2.8%
Never married	593	31.1%	585	28.2%
Widowed	45	2.4%	123	5.9%
Employment status				
In labor force	1,443	76.0%	643	31.1%
Involuntarily unemployed	165	8.7%	84	4.1%
Not in labor force (homemaker, voluntarily unemployed, other)	221	11.6%	1,280	62.0%
Student	70	3.7%	59	2.9%
Drinking pattern (past 12 months)				
Drank any alcohol during past 12 months	964	50.6%	389	18.9%
Average number of drinking days (drinkers only)		62.7 days		35.2 days
Average number of drinks per occasion (drinkers only)		7.4 drinks		3.5 drinks
Average annual volume (drinkers only)		571.4 drinks		199.7 drinks
Drank five or more drinks on one or more occasions (drinkers only)	654	68.3%	169	43.4%

Measures that Differed from the Core Questions

As well as measures of alcohol consumption, the survey included only the following questions on partner aggression from the GENACIS questionnaire: whether the respondent had experienced physical aggression by a partner (but not whether respondent had been aggressive *toward* a partner), respondent's rating of severity of partner's aggression and rating of the respondent's fear at the time (both on scales of 1 to 10), type of aggression by partner, and whether the respondent or partner had been drinking at the time of the incident. Type of aggression was assessed using an open-ended format with responses coded into categories by the interviewers.

Results

As shown in Figure 1, a larger percentage of female than male respondents reported being the victim of physical aggression by a partner in the past two years ($p < .05$). The average age of female victims was 34.1 years, while the average age of male victims was 39.3 years. Figure 2 shows the rate of reporting of partner aggression by age group. As shown in this figure, the percent of male respondents who reported partner physical aggression tended to decline with increasing age (except for the lower rate among

FIGURE 1. Percent of respondents who reported having been a victim, by sex, GENACIS survey, Belize, 2005.

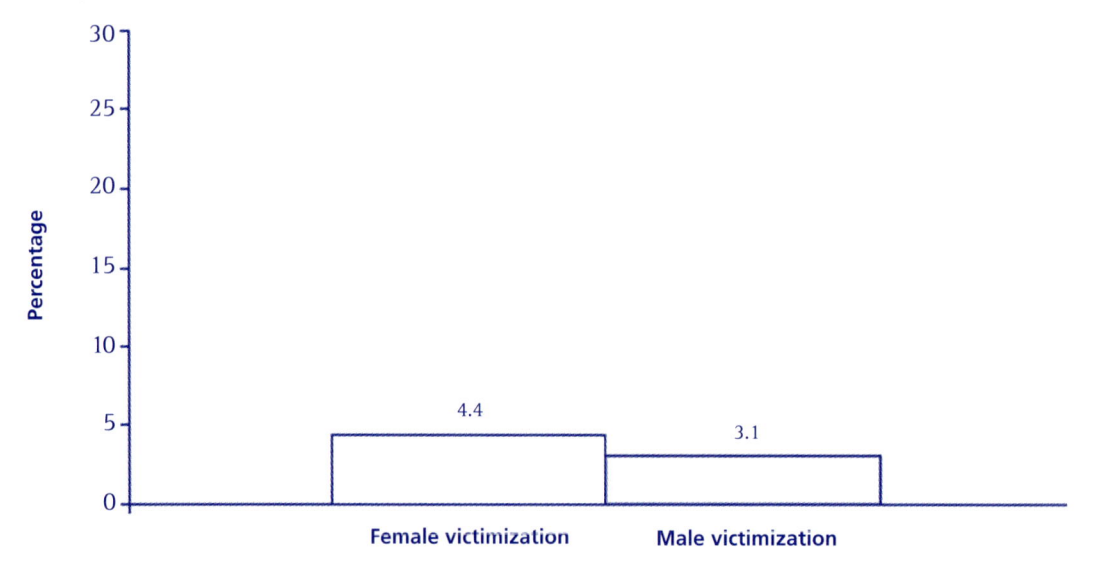

	Percentage
Female victimization	4.4
Male victimization	3.1

males aged 18–24), with the highest rate being reported among men in the 25–34-year-old age group; for female respondents, the rates increased until reaching a peak for the 35–44-year-old age group and then declined among females in the older age groups. On average, those who reported experiencing aggression by a partner were younger than those who reported no aggression (33.7 years for males experiencing aggression, versus 40.4 years for males who reported no aggression; 34.1 years for females with aggression, versus 39.3 years for females without aggression).

FIGURE 2. Percent of respondents who reported having been a victim, by age group and sex, GENACIS survey, Belize, 2005.

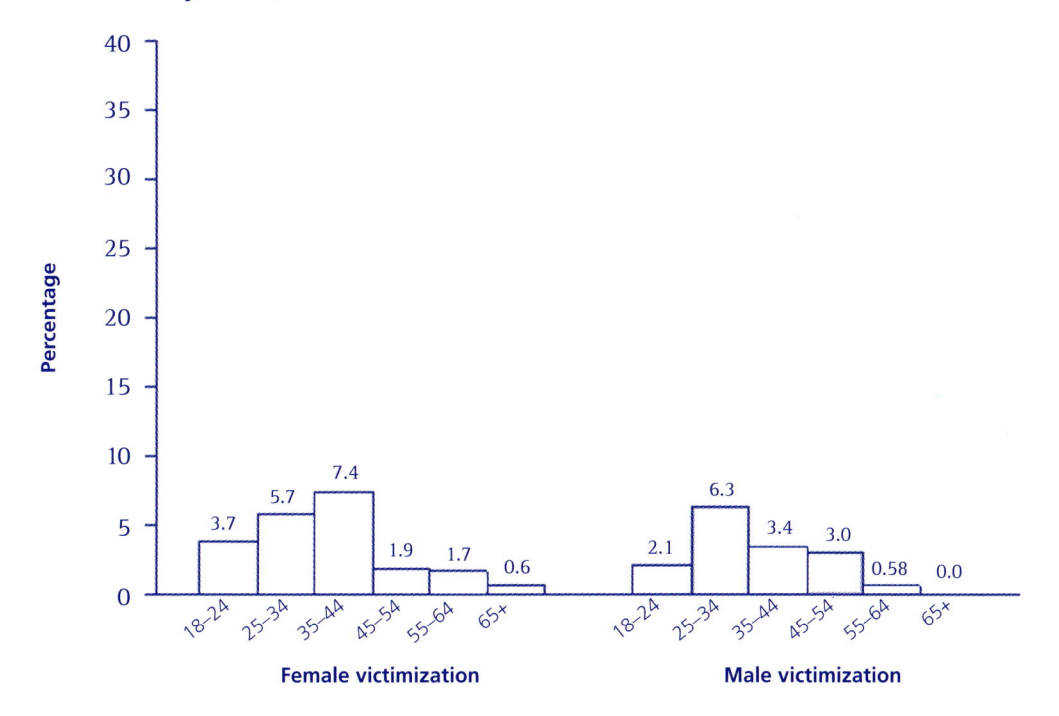

Female victimization:
- 18–24: 3.7
- 25–34: 5.7
- 35–44: 7.4
- 45–54: 1.9
- 55–64: 1.7
- 65+: 0.6

Male victimization:
- 18–24: 2.1
- 25–34: 6.3
- 35–44: 3.4
- 45–54: 3.0
- 55–64: 0.58
- 65+: 0.0

Figure 3 shows rates of partner physical aggression reported by males and females by their current marital status. The percentage of cohabiting males who reported aggression was higher than that for married males ($p < .001$), as was the percentage of cohabiting females versus married females ($p < .01$) and never–married females ($p < .01$). Results should be treated with caution, however, due to the low number of cases in some marital status groups, particularly for divorced or separated males and females.

As shown in Figure 4, males and females reported similar types of aggressive acts being done towards them by a partner, with pushing/shoving being the most common (39% of males, 37% of females). Exceptions are that a significantly larger percentage of females than males reported being beaten up (23.3% versus 5.1%), and a significantly larger percentage of males (15.3%) than females (2.2%) reported acts that were coded as other (including kicking, hitting, and using a weapon).

FIGURE 3. Percent of respondents who reported having been a victim, by marital status and sex, GENACIS survey, Belize, 2005.

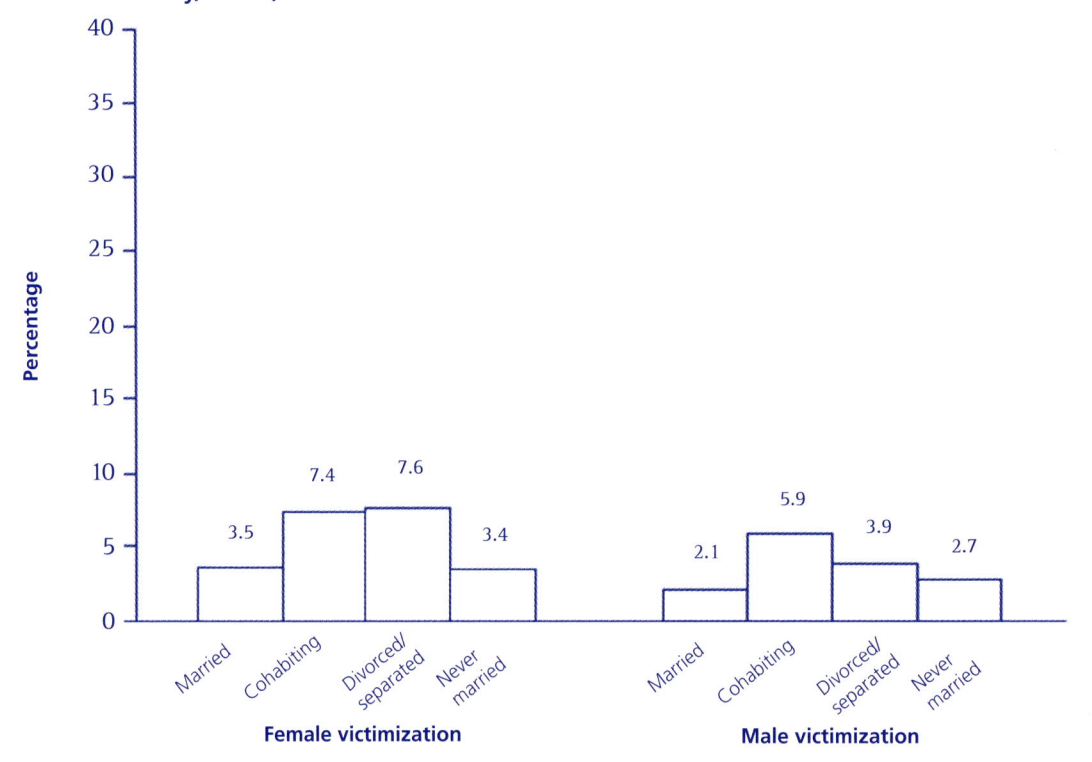

FIGURE 4. Type of aggressive act against females and males as reported by victims, by sex, GENACIS survey, Belize, 2005.

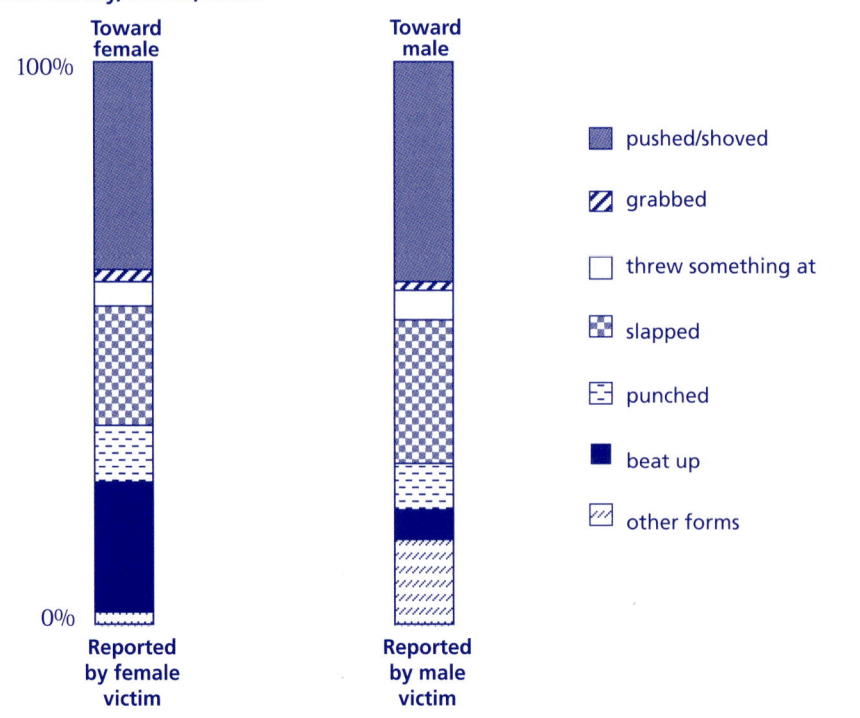

Ratings by males and females of the level of severity of the aggression and how scared the respondent felt at the time (both on a scale from 1 to 10) are shown in Figure 5. Mean ratings were significantly higher for females than for males for both measures ($p < .001$).

FIGURE 5. Mean ratings of severity of aggression and fear by male and female victims, GENACIS survey, Belize, 2005.

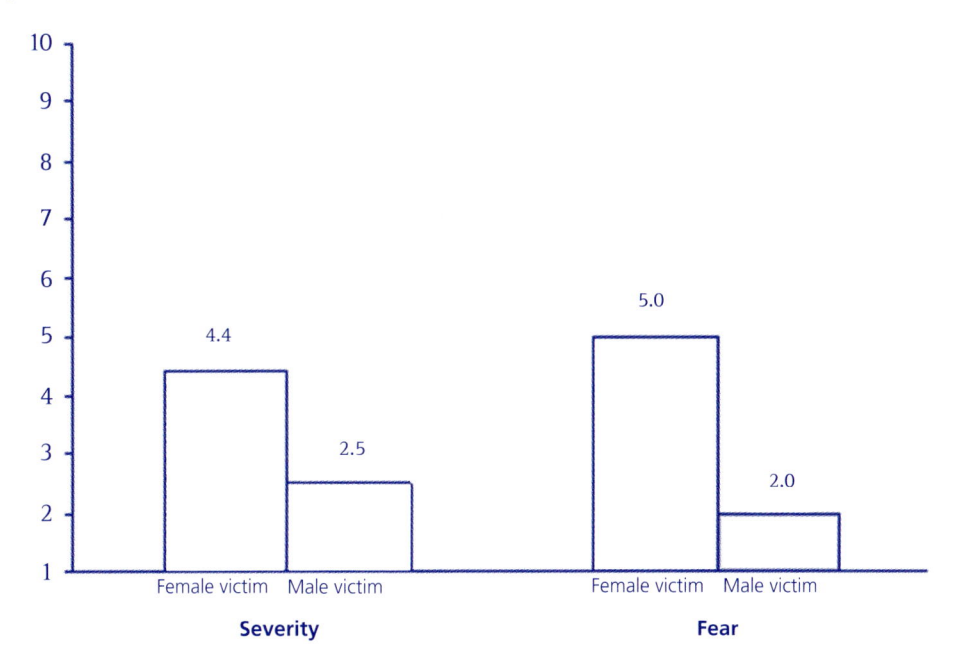

	Female victim	Male victim
Severity	4.4	2.5
Fear	5.0	2.0

As shown in Figure 6, 53% of female and 41% of male victims indicated that one or both partners had been drinking alcohol at the time of the incident of physical aggression. More females than males reported that only the aggressive partner was drinking ($p < .001$), and more males than females indicated that only the respondent (i.e., the victim) was drinking ($p = .001$). In other words, whether a male or a female was the victim, in the majority of incidents involving alcohol, the male was the only partner who was drinking.

The percent of incidents in which the aggressive partner was the only drinker (40% male only and 10.7% female only, as reported by the victim) was higher than the percent of incidents in which the victim reported being the only drinker (23.2% male only and 4.5% female only)—that is, both men and women were more likely to be the only drinker when they were the aggressor than when they were the victim; however, these differences did not reach the criterion for statistical significance. There were no other significant differences between males and females in reports of who was drinking.

For both male and female respondents, there was a trend that was not statistically significant for severity ratings to be higher for incidents in which one or both partners was drinking (5.0 for females, 2.8 for males) than for incidents in which no one was drinking (3.8 for females, 2.1 for males.

FIGURE 6. Percent of incidents in which no partner had been drinking, both partners had been drinking, only the male had been drinking, or only the female had been drinking, as reported by male and female victims, GENACIS survey, Belize, 2005.

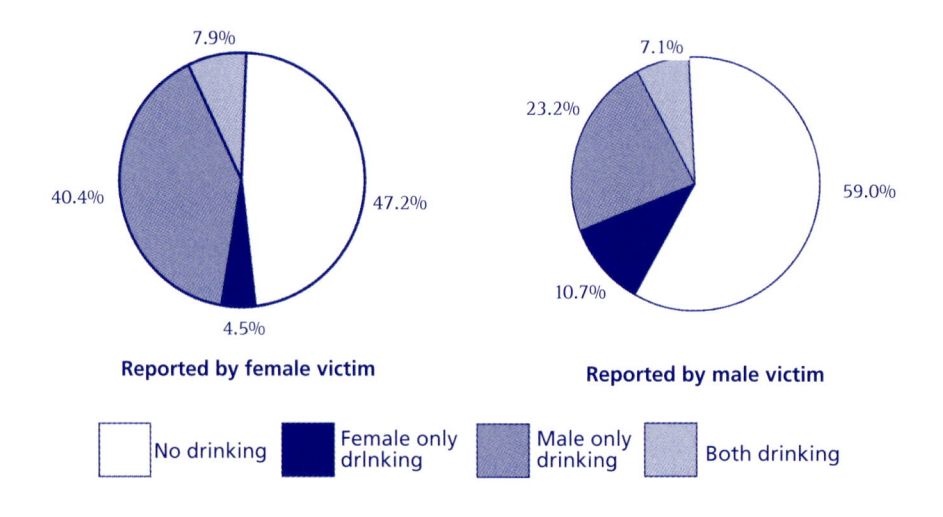

Reported by female victim: 47.2%, 7.9%, 40.4%, 4.5%
Reported by male victim: 59.0%, 7.1%, 23.2%, 10.7%

No drinking | Female only drinking | Male only drinking | Both drinking

The Relationship between Alcohol Consumption and Partner Aggression

The percent of female respondents who reported aggression by a partner was 8.5% among drinkers versus 3.4% for abstainers, while the percent of male respondents reporting aggression by a partner was 5.6% among drinkers versus 0.5% for abstainers. This difference was significant (p < .001) for both male and female respondents in logistic regression of partner aggression on drinker status controlling for age.

Respondents' Drinking Pattern and Partner Aggression

As shown in Figure 7, among female and male respondents who drank alcohol in the 12 months prior to the survey, rates of being the victim of physical aggression by an intimate partner were higher for those who drank five or more drinks on at least one occasion than for those who had not consumed five drinks at one time. However, these differences did not meet the criterion for statistical significance in logistic regression analyses of partner physical aggression on whether or not five or more drinks were consumed controlling for age.

Figure 8 shows the mean number of drinking days, Figure 9 shows the average number of drinks consumed per occasion, and Figure 10 shows the total number of drinks consumed in the past year for female and male victims of partner aggression, compared to females and males who had not been the victim of partner aggression. None of these comparisons was significant (controlling for age).

FIGURE 7. Percent of respondents who reported victimization (aggression by a partner) by whether respondents had consumed five or more drinks on an occasion or had never consumed five drinks on an occasion, by sex, GENACIS survey, Belize, 2005.

	Never drank 5+	Drank 5+
Female victimization	6.8	10.7
Male victimization	4.6	6.1

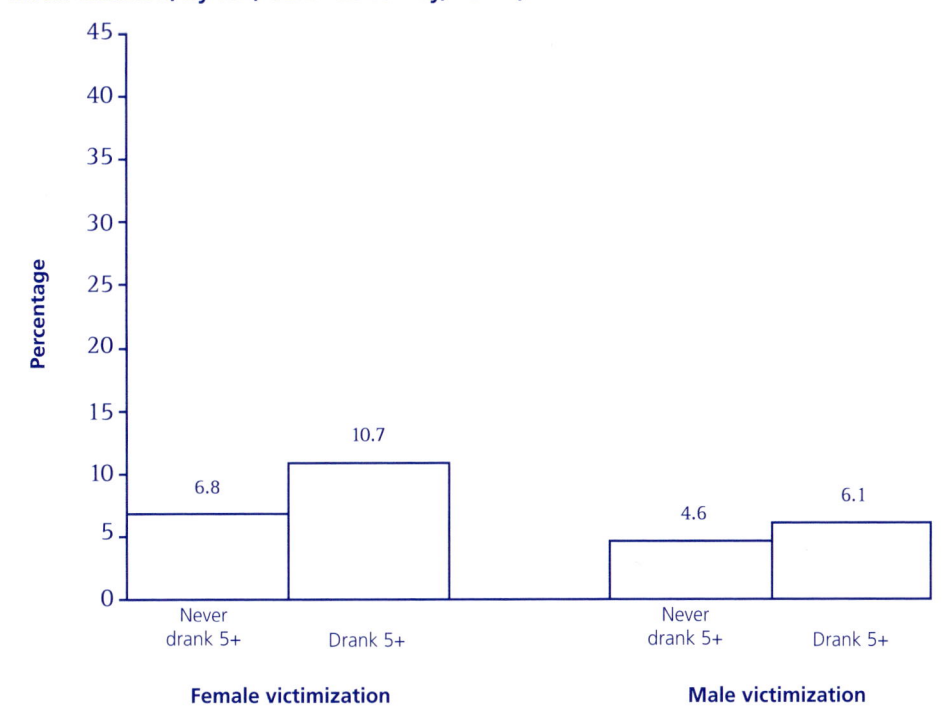

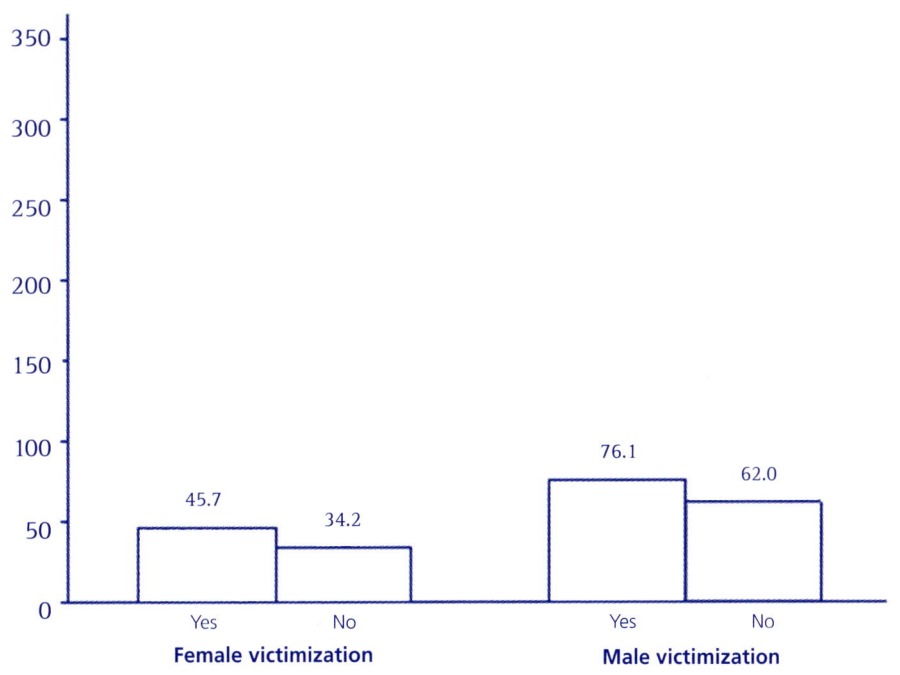

FIGURE 8. Mean number of drinking days in the year preceding the survey by whether the respondent had been a victim of partner aggression, by sex, GENACIS survey, Belize, 2005.

	Yes	No
Female victimization	45.7	34.2
Male victimization	76.1	62.0

FIGURE 9. Mean number of drinks consumed on usual drinking occasions by whether the respondent had been a victim of partner aggression, by sex, GENACIS survey, Belize, 2005.

Female victimization: Yes 3.7, No 3.5
Male victimization: Yes 6.7, No 7.5

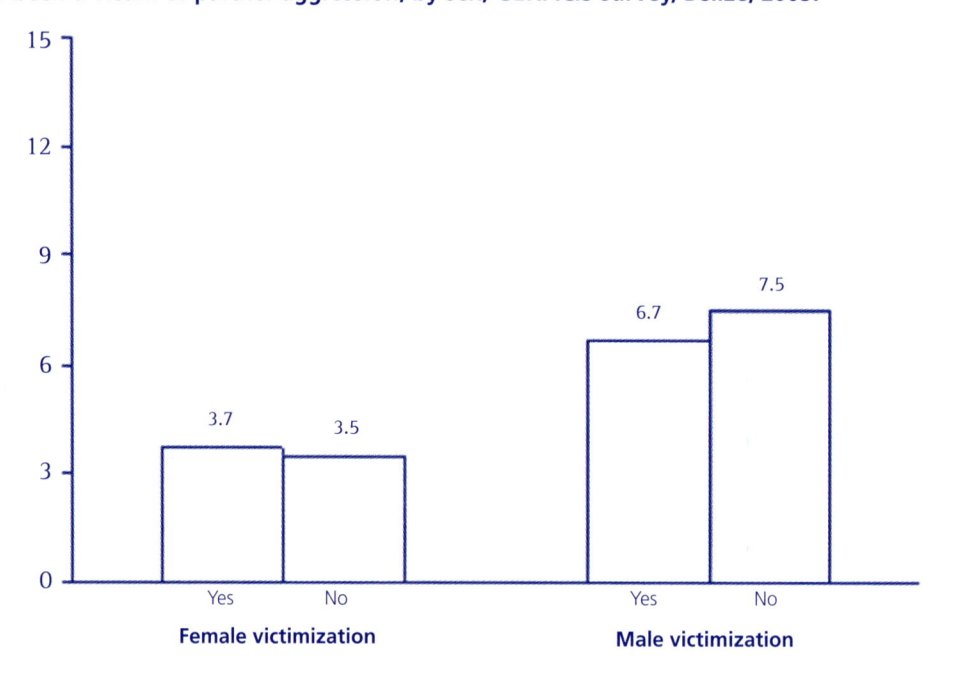

Figure 10. Overall mean number of drinks consumed annually by whether the respondent had been a victim of partner aggression, by sex, GENACIS survey, Belize, 2005.

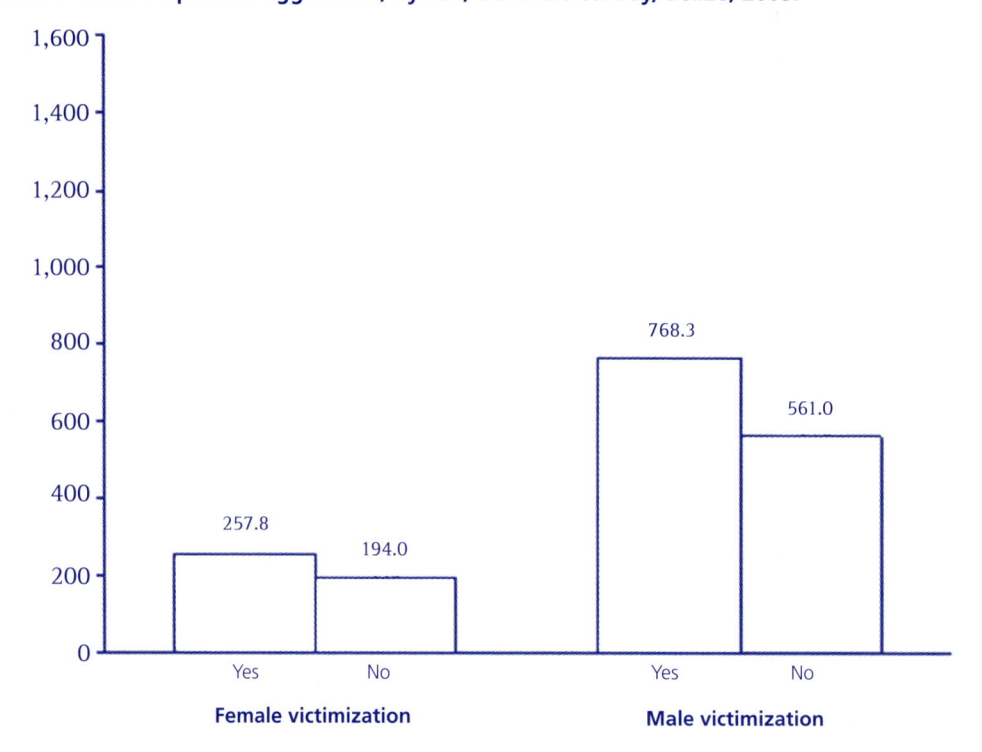

Female victimization: Yes 257.8, No 194.0
Male victimization: Yes 768.3, No 561.0

Discussion

Although the Domestic Violence Surveillance System provides valuable information regarding victims of partner violence in Belize, the current study provides additional insight by exploring partner aggression that does not necessarily come to the attention of authorities and by allowing comparisons of individuals who experienced partner aggression to those who did not report aggression. As noted by Johnson (2002), it is likely that many cases of domestic violence go unreported, so the current survey approach allows a broader view of domestic violence than that obtained through the government surveillance system.

One difference that emerged between the results from this household survey and that of the surveillance system is that although significantly more female than male survey respondents reported aggression by a partner, the gender difference in partner aggression was not large, with 4.4% of females and 3.1% of males reporting partner aggression, compared to 90% of victims of partner aggression in the surveillance system being female. There are a number of possible reasons for the difference between the relative proportions of males and females who reported being victims in the survey compared to the surveillance system data. First, the higher proportion of female victims found in the surveillance system may be because more severe incidents or incidents in which the victim needs protection are more likely to come to the attention of agencies such as the police. This is consistent with findings from the survey that ratings of severity of partner's aggression and how scared the victim felt were significantly higher for female respondents than for male respondents.

A second explanation for the more comparable rates of partner aggression by male and female respondents in the survey may relate to the way the survey question was worded (i.e., respondents were asked about acts of physical aggression rather than about violence or abuse) and the fact that the survey excluded questions regarding sexual aggression, which would be higher for females than for males. In addition, this was the first survey of its kind in Belize in which questions on drinking and aggression were addressed at the same time. Thus, although the interviewers were experienced and confidentiality was assured, respondents might not have felt comfortable revealing personal information of this type, resulting in possible underreporting of both partner aggression and alcohol consumption.

Third, the extent to which females used physical aggression toward a male partner in self-defense is unknown from the current survey data. That is, for at least some males who reported physical aggression by a partner, this aggression may have occurred in reaction to even more serious aggression done by the respondent. In these cases where more severe aggression was done by the male partner, even if the female partner had used physical aggression, she would likely have been classified as the victim if the incident had been recorded as part of the surveillance system.

As noted above, ratings of severity of aggression and fear were higher for female victims than for male victims. Moreover, females were much more likely than males to report severe aggression, such as being beaten up. Thus, although there was not a large difference in rates of partner aggression between males and females, the importance of violence against women is evident in the greater severity of aggression experienced by women. Therefore, it remains critical that public policy and education focus on gender issues and on preventing violence against women. At the same time, there is a growing need to develop approaches that prevent aggression by both male and female partners.

The survey also found a different pattern related to the age of victims than was evident from the surveillance system. The average age of victims in the surveillance system was 30.1 years for females and 36.9 years for males; in the GENACIS survey, on the other hand, the average age of victims was about 34 years for females and 39 years for males. This difference between the survey results and those of the surveillance system, taken together with the results shown in Figure 2 that the highest rate of partner aggression among females in the survey was for those in the 35–44-year-old age group, suggests that partner aggression is less likely to come to the attention of the authorities for women in older age groups (i.e., as part of the surveillance system), possibly because aggression is less severe or because older women have more strategies or resources for managing partner aggression. However, it should be noted that the age pattern observed in the Belize sample differs from that found in other countries participating in the GENACIS study. In particular, in the majority of other countries included in this book (see the chapter "Comparison of Partner Physical Aggression across Ten Countries"), partner aggression tends to be more likely among females who are under 35 years of age. Thus, the current findings suggest a need for further investigation of the relationship between age and risk of partner aggression among Belizean women.

Among both males and females in the survey, the highest rates of partner aggression were among those who were cohabiting or divorced/separated. This high risk of partner aggression among cohabiting couples was also reflected in the surveillance system, with about 50% of cases involving a common-law relationship between the victim and the aggressor.

Perhaps the most important finding from the survey is the extent to which partner aggression is linked with alcohol. Aggression was significantly more likely to occur among current drinkers than among abstainers. Moreover, despite the fact that approximately 50% of male respondents and more than 80% of female respondents reported that they were nondrinkers, more than 50% of female victims and 40% of male victims of partner aggression reported that one or both partners had been drinking at the time the incident of aggression occurred. While most aggression involved drinking only by the male, the female was drinking in 12.4% of incidents reported by female victims, and the female partner was drinking in 17.8% of incidents reported by male victims. Among drinkers, there was evidence that partner aggression was associated with a pattern of heavier drinking (i.e., drinking five or more drinks per occasion) and more frequent drinking occasions, although these relationships did not meet the criterion for statistical significance when controlling for age.

These results confirm the high rate of alcohol involvement found in incidents reported as part of the surveillance system and reinforce the importance of understanding the role of alcohol in partner aggression. In a culture in which a large proportion of the population abstains and in which drinking is relatively infrequent, the finding of a link between alcohol consumption and partner aggression is particularly noteworthy and suggests that the relevant authorities (e.g., the Ministry of Health, Ministry of Human Development and Social Transformation, Belize Police Department) need to invest additional resources in preventative strategies addressing the issue of alcohol problems and its relationship to partner violence.

Acknowledgments

We are grateful to Dr. Maristela Monteiro, PAHO Senior Advisor on Tobacco Control, Alcohol, and Substance Abuse, for the opportunity she and PAHO provided for Belize to be included in the GENACIS multicentric survey. We also wish to thank all those who made the survey possible in Belize and who assisted with its implementation. These include the PAHO/WHO Country Office in Belize, the Central Statistical Office, and the Ministry of Health. We likewise express our sincere thanks to the staff of the Women's Department of the Ministry of Human Development who were very kind in allowing us to use their library, learn more about their programs, and review the material developed in the struggle against domestic violence in Belize. PAHO played an important role in supporting the implementation of the survey and provided technical support to the Ministry of Health and all the relevant stakeholders. Finally, we are grateful to Englebert Emmanuel and Ethan Gough for their assistance with statistics from the Ministry of Health's Epidemiology Unit.

References

Belize, Central Statistical Office. Major Findings Belize Census 2000. Belmopan: CSO; 2002.

Belize, Ministry of Health; Pan American Health Organization. Health Sector Domestic Violence Management Protocol, 2001. Belmopan: Ministry of Health; 2001.

-----. Integrated model of care for family violence: state and civil society response—the Belize experience, 1998–2002. Belmopan: Ministry of Health; 2002.

Fonseca C, Humes I, Pate K, Dominguez C, Johnson L, Irving M, et al. 2006 Annual Report, Women's Department. Belmopan: Ministry of Human Development; 2007.

Johnson R. Belize National Gender Policy 2002. Report for the National Women's Commission. Belmopan: 2002

UNHAPPY HOURS:

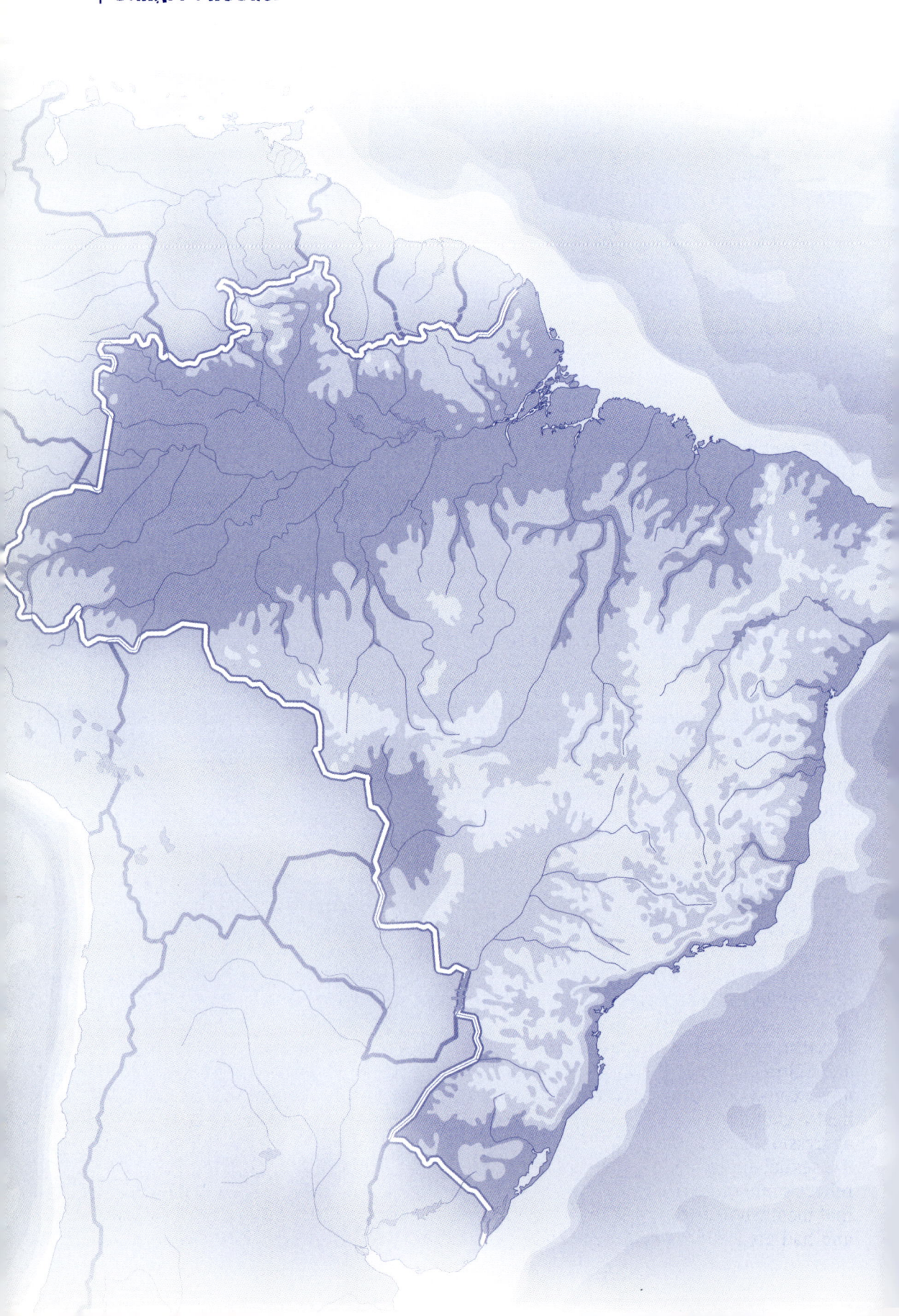

Brazil: Alcohol and Partner Physical Aggression in Metropolitan São Paulo

—Florence Kerr–Corrêa, Janaina Barbosa de Oliveira, Maria Cristina Pereira Lima, Adriana Marcassa Tucci, Maria Odete Simão, Mariana Braga Cavariani, and Miriam Malacize Fantazia

Introduction

Women are more likely than men to be the victims of physical aggression by someone they know or with whom they have an intimate relationship, often in their own home, while men, especially younger men, are more likely to be subjected to violence in public places, particularly homicide committed by strangers or acquaintances (Lima and Ximenes, 1998; Rechtman and Phebo, 2000; Schraiber et al., 2002; Day et al. 2003; Galvão and Andrade, 2004). Thus, although males may also experience aggression from their female partners, partner aggression is an especially important problem for women. Women who suffer domestic violence are more likely to experience psychological problems such as nervousness; forgetfulness; feelings of insecurity; sleep and eating disorders; permanent injuries; chronic problems such as headaches, abdominal pain, and vaginal infections; delayed-onset diseases such as arthritis, hypertension, and cardiac disease; substance abuse; obesity; disability; gastrointestinal and gynecological disorders; fibromyalgia; and miscarriage (Grossi, 1996; Coker et al., 2002; Day et al., 2003; Galvão and Andrade, 2004). Trauma-related effects are accentuated when the aggressor is an intimate partner, which increases sensations of vulnerability, betrayal of confidence, and loss of hope (Giffin, 1994).

A recent multinational study of violence against females (García–Moreno et al., 2006) included a sample of women from São Paulo and Zona da Mata (in the northeastern state of Pernambuco). Of the women in São Paulo, 8.3% of those who were currently or had ever been married had experienced physical violence from a partner in the past 12 months and 2.8% had experienced sexual violence. For women from Zona de Mata, 12.9% had experienced physical violence and 5.6% sexual violence. In an earlier study comparing all forms of violence reported by respondents from cities in Latin America and Spain, Orpinas (1999) found that 10.0% of men and 10.2% of women from Salvador, Bahia, reported hitting their partner (with 3.2% and 5.3%, respectively, hitting with an object) while 5.0% of men and 5.4% of women from Rio de Janeiro reported hitting their partner (with 0.2% and 0.5%, respectively, hitting with an object).

Based on an analysis of reports from the Brazilian civil state police, Soares (1999) and Schraiber et al. (2002) found that the partner or ex-partner was the aggressor in approximately 77.6% of the reported cases of domestic violence. Data from a primary health care unit in Porto Alegre in South Brazil found that of those reporting partner aggression, 55% reported psychological abuse, 38% reported physical aggression, and 8% sexual aggression (Kronbauer and Meneghel, 2005). However, these statistics may reflect some underreporting, given that a study by Schraiber et al. (2003) concluded that most women who reported aggression did not consider they had suffered violence and had great difficulty in reporting and recognizing the act as a violent one.

To address the inadequate response by the criminal justice system to violence against women, Brazil was the first country in the world to establish all-female police stations (Thomas, 1994). These stations were intended to deal more effectively with partner aggression and were rapidly implemented throughout Brazil. While they have raised public awareness of violence against women, they have not necessarily been successful as a deterrent (Thomas, 1994). In 2006, Law 11.340, also known as the "Maria da Penha" law, was approved by the Brazilian National Congress. Named after a victim of domestic violence, this law strengthens the country's legislation regarding partner aggression by including preventive detention and arrest of perpetrators caught in the act, incarceration for up to three years when found guilty, and the provision of social and psychological support to victims (Brasil, 2006). To date, no evaluation has been conducted to determine the impact of this law.

The Role of Alcohol

Although there are many possible contributing factors to partner aggression, alcohol is the psychoactive drug most frequently associated with violence (Minayo and Deslandes, 1998), including partner aggression (O'Leary and Schumacher, 2003), and its consumption has been identified as an important contributing factor (Poldrugo, 1998; Baltieri, 2003). One study of violence against women (Adeodato et al., 2005) found that 70% of aggressive partners had consumed alcohol and 11% had consumed illicit drugs before the incident.

The objective of the current research was to evaluate partner physical aggression and its relationship to patterns of alcohol use in Metropolitan São Paulo, Brazil.

Methods

The Setting

Metropolitan São Paulo includes São Paulo city—Brazil's most important city from a social, economic, and political point of view, as well as being the capital of São Paulo state—plus 38 other municipalities. In July 2005, the Institute of Geography and Statistics[1] estimated the population of metropolitan São Paulo to be 19,616,060.

The Sample

A stratified sample, representative of all socioeconomic and educational levels, was drawn from urban metropolitan São Paulo[2] and included residents over 18 years old. Those over 60 years old were over-sampled because this is the fastest growing population segment in São Paulo, and there is little information about this group in Brazil. Sample size was calculated, and the following age ranges were established for both sexes: 18 to 34 years, 35 to 59 years, and 60 years or older. Each stratum was composed by sector census (Instituto Brasileiro de Geografia e Estatística, 2000) and respondents were selected using cluster-sampling schemes. The sampling unit was

---

[1] This entity, known as the Instituto Brasileiro de Geografia e Estatística in Portuguese, is the agency responsible for collecting and recording statistical, geographic, cartographic, geodetic, and environmental information about the country.
[2] Formally known as the São Paulo Metropolitian Region and including the municipalities of Arujá, Barueri, Biritiba-Mirim, Cajamar, Caieiras, Carapicuíba, Cotia, Diadema, Embu, Embu-Guaçu, Ferraz de Vasconcelos, Francisco Morato, Franco da Rocha, Guararema, Guarulhos, Itapevi, Itaquaquecetuba, Itapecerica da Serra, Jandira, Juquitiba, Mairiporã, Mauá, Mogi das Cruzes, Osasco, Pirapora do Bom Jesus, Poá, Ribeirão Pires, Rio Grande da Serra, Salesópolis, Santa Isabel, Santana de Parnaíba, Santo André, São Bernardo do Campo, São Caetano do Sul, São Lourenço da Serra, São Paulo, Suzano, Taboão da Serra, and Vargem Grande Paulista.

family households, including condominiums and single dwellings; student housing and institutional and commercial buildings were not included. All individuals in the household sample who were over 18 years old could be interviewed. The sample size was increased to accommodate a possible nonresponse rate of 20%. The interviews were completed with 2,083 individuals, a response rate of 75.5%. Most refusals were from men and those living in more upper class neighborhoods. General characteristics of the male and female participants in the survey are presented in Table 1.

TABLE 1: Age, marital status, employment status, and drinking pattern of respondents in the 12 months preceding the survey, for male and female respondents, GENACIS survey, Brazil, 2006–2007.

	Males (weighted N=867)		Females (weighted N=1,216)	
	Number	Percent or mean	Number	Percent or mean
Age		39.8 years		41.3 years
18–24 years	164	18.1%	197	16.7%
25–34 years	254	28.1%	275	23.4%
35–44 years	174	19.2%	261	22.2%
45–54 years	148	16.3%	183	15.6%
55–64 years	91	10.1%	139	11.8%
65 years and older	73	8.1%	122	10.4%
Marital status				
Married	436	48.2%	491	41.6%
Cohibiting/Living with partner	152	16.8%	194	16.5%
Divorced	43	4.8%	97	8.2%
Never married	254	28.1%	282	23.9%
Widowed	19	2.1%	114	9.7%
Employment status				
In labor force (working full– or part–time, not working due to illness, on maternity leave, informal work)	682	75.5%	575	48.9%
Involuntarily unemployed	67	7.4%	81	6.9%
Not in labor force (voluntarily unemployed, housewife)	11	1.2%	404	34.2%
Student	15	1.6%	28	2.3%
Retired	129	14.3%	91	7.7%
Drinking pattern (past 12 months)				
Drank any alcohol during past 12 months	543	60.1%	352	30.0%
Average number of drinking days (drinkers only)		86.3 days		33.7 days
Average number of drinks per occasion (drinkers only)		4.3 drinks		2.5 drinks
Average annual volume (drinkers only)		589.6 drinks		117.9 drinks
Drank five or more drinks on one or more occasions (drinkers only)	259	48.0%	63	18.0%

The Survey Procedure

Face-to-face interviews were conducted in the households by trained interviewers who had been chosen based on their past experience participating in community surveys. This group was given advanced training on the Gender, Alcohol, and Culture: An International Study (GENACIS) questionnaire that included specific information on alcohol and drinking behaviors (e.g., antecedents and consequences, problematic behavior, and binge drinking). More female than male interviewers were selected due to the belief that females would more easily be able to gain access to the family home and that respondents would feel more comfortable in their presence, especially when intimate questions are asked. Letters were sent to the selected households informing them of the study's objectives, its methodology and international nature, and the importance of their contribution. Access to additional information about the project for those who desired it was provided via a special Web site. Interviewers carried identification badges and booked appointments in advance. Privacy was guaranteed. Several different approaches were attempted when a refusal occurred. One was to mail a more detailed letter about the project at a later time, followed by a telephone call. Several telephone numbers in São Paulo City, including three mobile cell numbers of interviewer-coordinators, were also available to potential respondents.

Ethical Considerations

A research ethics committee of the University of São Paulo's Botucatu Medical School approved this project on 13 September 2004.

Results[3]

Figure 1 shows the percent of male and female respondents reporting physical aggression by whether respondent was the victim or aggressor. A larger percentage of females than males reported being victims (although this difference was not statistically significant). A larger percentage of females reported being victims than males reported being aggressors ($p < .05$). No other differences between percentages of male and female victims and aggressors were statistically significant. Among those who reported any partner physical aggression, 38.4% of males and 37.8% of females were involved in both aggression by a partner and aggression toward a partner, 39.0% of females and 36.3% of males reported being a victim only, and 23.3% of females and 25.3% of males reported being a perpetrator only.

---

[3] Weights were applied to the analysis in this section to adjust for over-sampling in some geographic areas of respondents over age 60.

FIGURE 1. Percent of respondents who reported having been a victim or aggressor, by sex, GENACIS survey, Brazil, 2006–2007.

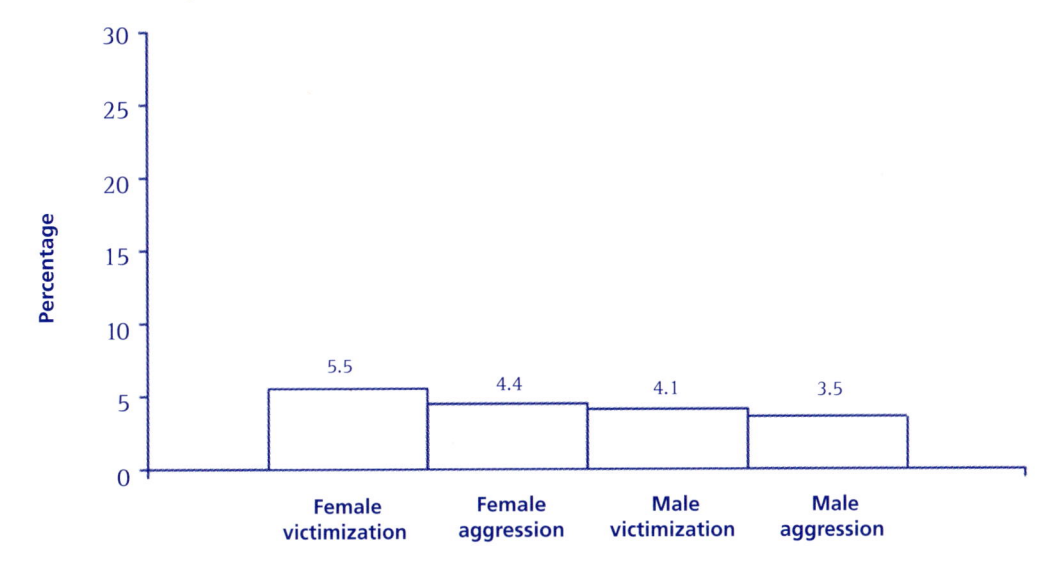

	Female victimization	Female aggression	Male victimization	Male aggression
Percentage	5.5	4.4	4.1	3.5

The average age of respondents in each of the four groups was as follows: female victims, 35.8 years; male victims, 33.0 years; female aggressors, 31.1 years; and male aggressors, 30.9 years. As shown in Figure 2, the percent who reported aggression by a partner and aggression toward a partner tended to decline with age for both males and females, but with some exceptions. Female victims and aggressors in the 25–34-year-old age group were more likely than those in the 18–24-year-old age group to report partner aggression, while male aggressors in the 25–34-year-old age group were less likely than those in the 35–44-year-old age group to report partner aggression.

FIGURE 2. Percent of respondents who reported having been a victim or aggressor, by age group and sex, GENACIS survey, Brazil, 2006-2007.

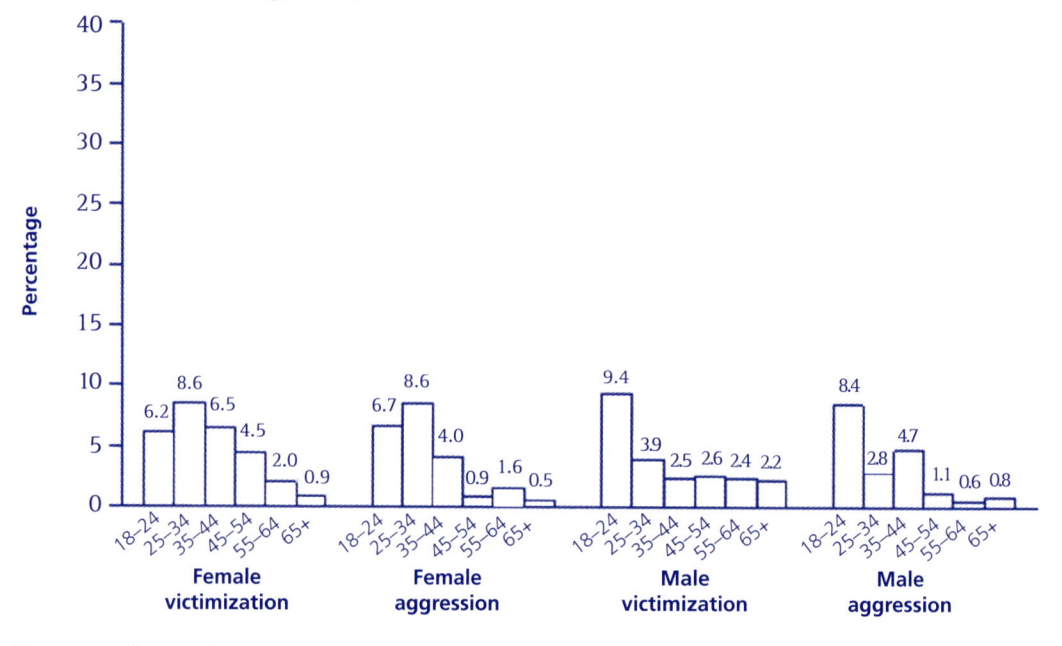

Figure 3 shows the percent of males and females reporting aggression by a partner and aggression toward a partner by marital status. Those who were cohabiting were more likely than those in other marital status groupings to report partner aggression for males and females and victims and aggressors (this relationship was significant only for cohabiting male victims, compared to married male victims (p < .01). No other significant differences were found between marital status groups for male or female victims or aggressors.

FIGURE 3. Percent of respondents who reported having been a victim or aggressor, by marital status and sex, GENACIS survey, Brazil, 2006-2007.

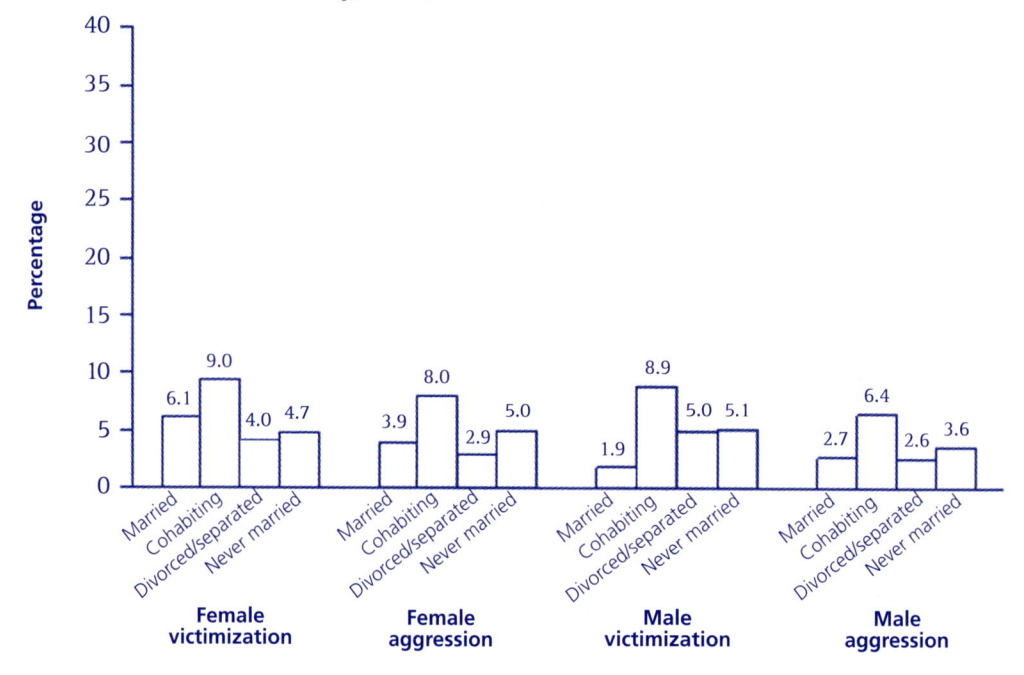

As shown in Figure 4, the most common form of aggression was being pushed, shaken, or grabbed. Female victims were more likely than male victims to report being punched, kicked, or hit and were more likely to report being the victim of these acts, compared with the percent of male aggressors who reported using this type of aggression (although these differences did not meet the criterion for significance of ($p < .01$). Male victims were more likely than female victims to report being slapped ($p < .01$). No other differences between male victims and aggressors and female victims and aggressors in the type of aggression used were found to be significant.

FIGURE 4. Type of aggressive act against females as reported by female victims and male aggressors, and against males as reported by male victims and female aggressors, GENACIS survey, Brazil, 2006–2007.

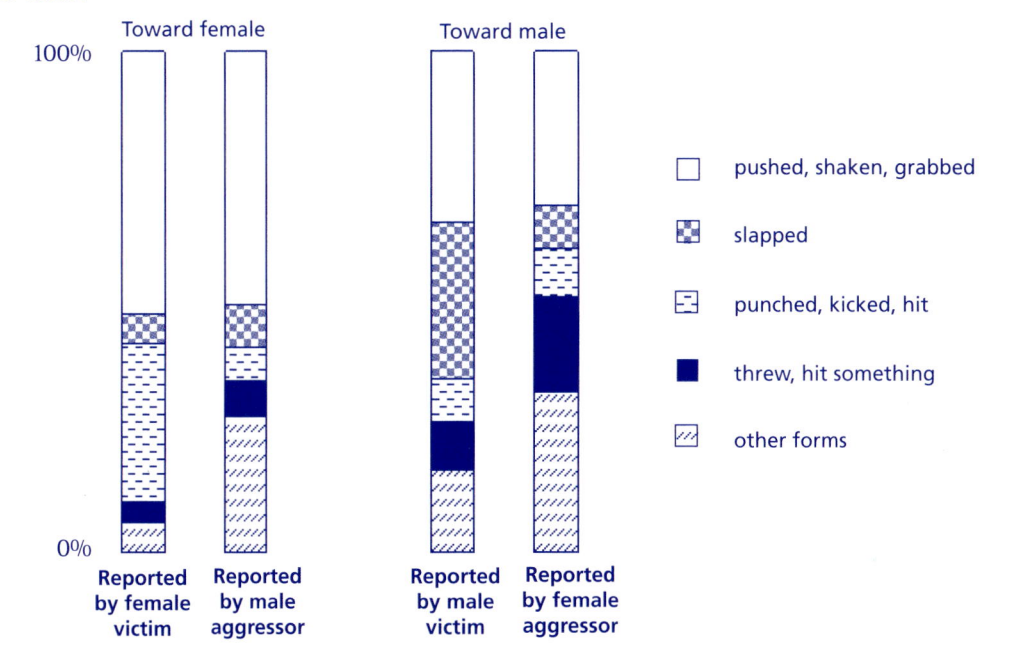

Figure 5 shows mean ratings of the level of severity of aggression, as well as how scared, upset, and angry the respondent felt at the time of the incident. Overall, there was a general pattern for female victims to rate their partner's aggression as being more severe and themselves as being more afraid, upset, and angry, compared to the ratings given by female aggressors and male victims and aggressors, while male victims gave the lowest ratings for all four measures. Significant differences were found between male and female victims for severity ($p < .01$), upset ($p < .001$), and anger ($p < .001$) after controlling for age. There were no significant differences found between the ratings of male and female aggressors (after controlling for age). Female victims reported being more upset and angry, compared with male aggressors ($p < .05$ for both), but the two groups were not significantly different in their ratings of severity and fear (after controlling for age). The ratings by female aggressors were higher than those by male victims for all four measures (even though this difference was significant only for ratings of anger ($p < .01$)). In addition to higher severity ratings, a larger percentage of female victims (19.6%) than male victims (4.5%) reported seeking medical attention immediately after the incident or the following day (however, this difference did not meet the criterion of $p < .05$ for statistical significance).

FIGURE 5. Mean ratings of severity of aggression, fear, upset, and anger by male and female victims and aggressors, GENACIS survey, Brazil, 2006–2007.

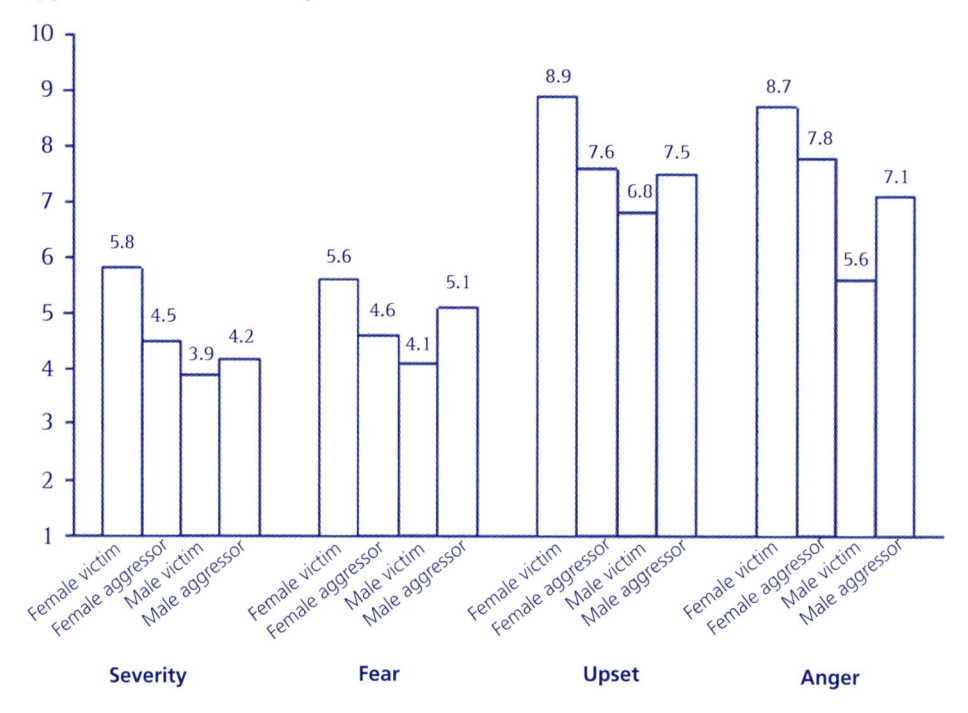

As shown in Figure 6, a larger percentage of females (57.1% of victims, 49.9% of aggressors) than males (27.6% of victims, 27.3% of aggressors) reported that one or both partners were drinking alcohol at the time of the incident. Female victims and aggressors and male victims were more likely to report that the male was the only partner drinking, compared to the female only or both drinking. The following significant relationships were found. A larger percentage of female victims than male victims reported the aggressor was the only partner drinking (p < .01). A larger percentage of female aggressors than male aggressors reported that the victim was the only partner drinking (p < .01), while a larger percentage of male aggressors than female aggressors reported that they (the respondent) had been drinking at the time (p < .01). A larger percentage of female aggressors than male victims reported that the male was the only partner drinking (p < .001). Female victims were more likely than male aggressors to report that only the male aggressor had been drinking (p < .01). No other significant pair-wise relationships were found between the four groups of respondents.

FIGURE 6. Percent of incidents in which no partner had been drinking, both partners had been drinking, only the male partner had been drinking, or only the female partner had been drinking, as reported by male and female victims and aggressors, GENACIS survey, Brazil, 2006–2007.

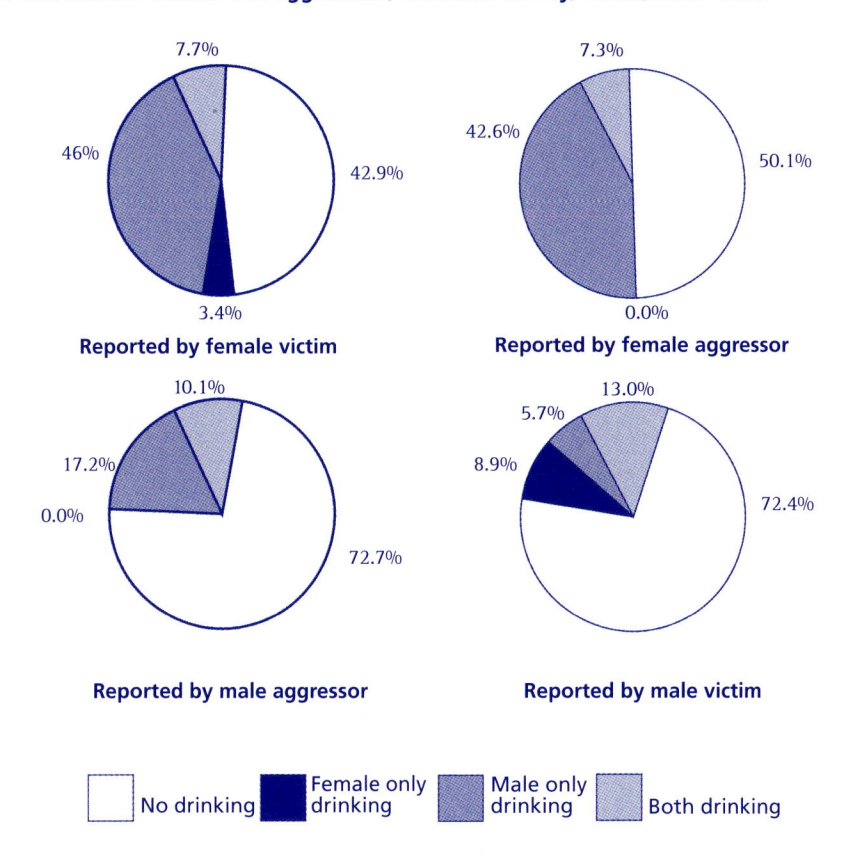

Reported by female victim: 7.7%, 46%, 42.9%, 3.4%

Reported by female aggressor: 7.3%, 42.6%, 50.1%, 0.0%

Reported by male aggressor: 10.1%, 17.2%, 0.0%, 72.7%

Reported by male victim: 13.0%, 5.7%, 8.9%, 72.4%

No drinking | Female only drinking | Male only drinking | Both drinking

Female victims who reported that one or both of the partners were drinking during the incident rated the severity of the aggression higher than did female victims in incidents that did not involve alcohol (6.4 versus 4.9); however, this difference was not significant after controlling for age. Among female aggressors, average severity ratings were lower for incidents that involved alcohol than for incidents in which neither of the partners was drinking (4.8 versus 5.7), although this difference was also not significant. The number of male victims and aggressors who reported that someone was drinking during the incident was too small to permit an analysis comparing incidents involving alcohol to those not involving alcohol similar to that done for female victims and aggressors.

The Relationship between Alcohol Consumption and Partner Aggression

Among respondents who consumed alcohol in the year before the survey, the percentage reporting partner physical aggression was higher than among those who abstained from alcohol. In particular, 8.4% of females who drank alcohol reported being the victim of partner physical aggression, compared to 4.3% of females who abstained (odds ratio 1.8, $p < .05$ after controlling for age); 7.5% of female drinkers, compared to 3.1% of female abstainers, reported being aggressive (odds ratio 2.2, $p < .05$ controlling for age); 5.3% of males who drank, versus 2.3% of males who abstained, reported being a victim (not significant after controlling for age); and 4.9% of male drinkers, versus 1.4% of male abstainers, reported being aggressive (not significant after controlling for age).

Respondents' Drinking Pattern and Partner Aggression

As shown in Figure 7, the percent of female victims and aggressors and male victims was higher for those who drank five or more drinks in the past year compared to those who never drank as much as five drinks (odds ratios significant after controlling for age for female victims and female aggressors ($p < .05$) but not for male victims). The percent of

FIGURE 7. Percent of respondents who reported victimization (aggression by a partner) or aggression (aggression toward a partner) by whether respondent had consumed five or more drinks on an occasion or had never consumed five drinks on an occasion, by sex, GENACIS survey, Brazil, 2006–2007.

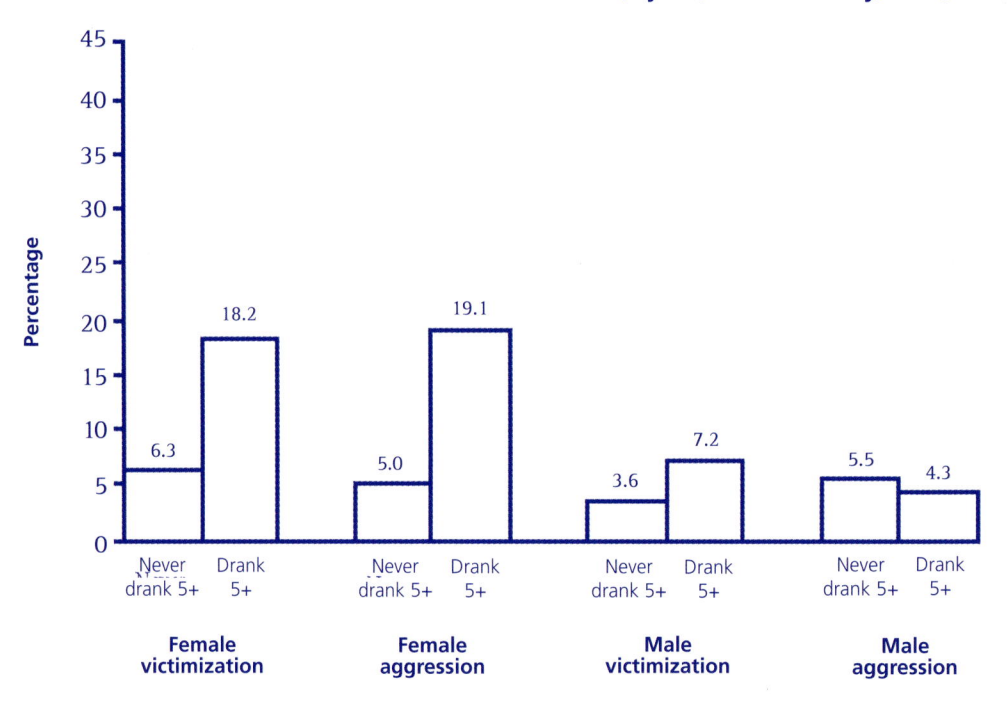

male aggressors was higher (but not significantly different) among males who never drank as much as five drinks than among those who did.

As shown in Figures 8 and 10, the number of days on which alcohol was consumed and the total number of drinks consumed in the year preceding the survey were higher for female victims and female aggressors than for females who were not victims and aggressors, respectively, and for male victims compared to males who were not victims (none of these differences reached the $p < .05$ criterion for statistical significance). However, these two measures were lower (albeit not significantly) for male aggressors than for males who reported not being aggressive.

As shown in Figure 9, the number of drinks consumed per occasion was higher for female victims compared to females who were not victims, and for female aggressors, compared to females who were not aggressors ($p < .01$ for both after controlling for age). Similarly, the number of drinks was higher for male victims and aggressors than for males who reported no partner physical aggression (differences among male respondents, however, were not significant after controlling for age).

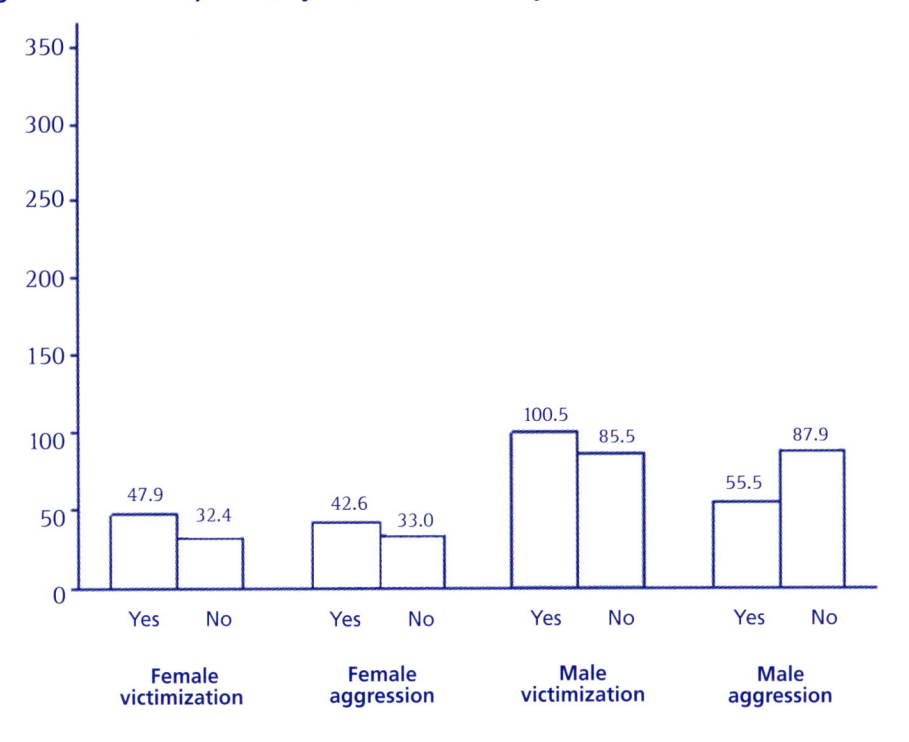

FIGURE 8. Mean number of drinking days in the year preceding the survey by whether the respondent had been the victim of partner aggression and whether the respondent had been aggressive toward a partner, by sex, GENACIS survey, Brazil, 2006–2007.

FIGURE 9. Mean number of drinks consumed on usual drinking occasions by whether the respondent had been the victim of partner aggression and whether the respondent had been aggressive toward a partner, by sex, GENACIS survey, Brazil, 2006–2007.

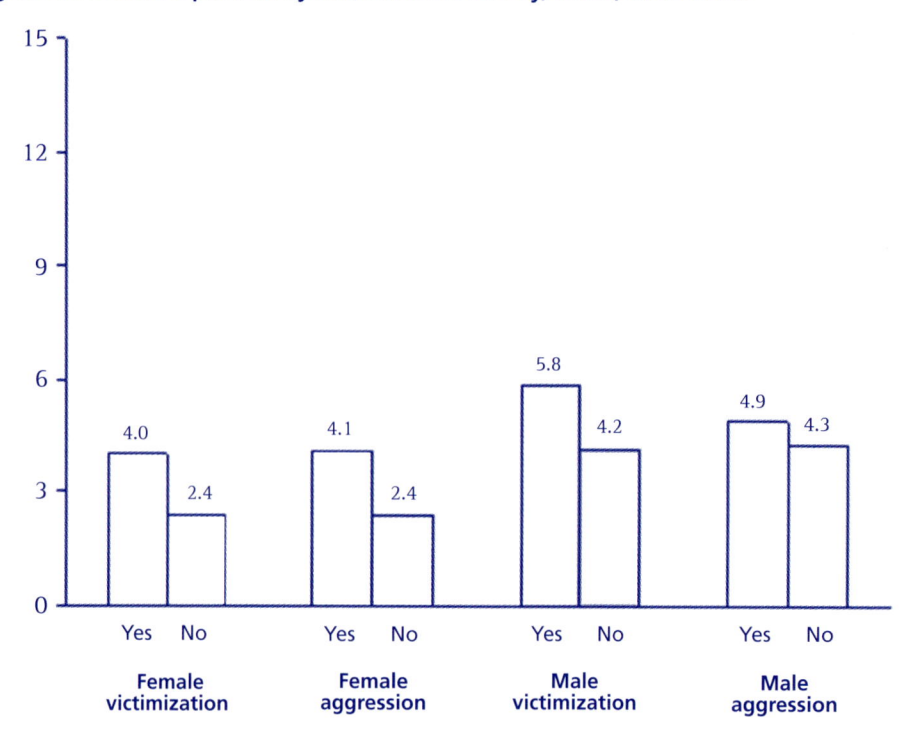

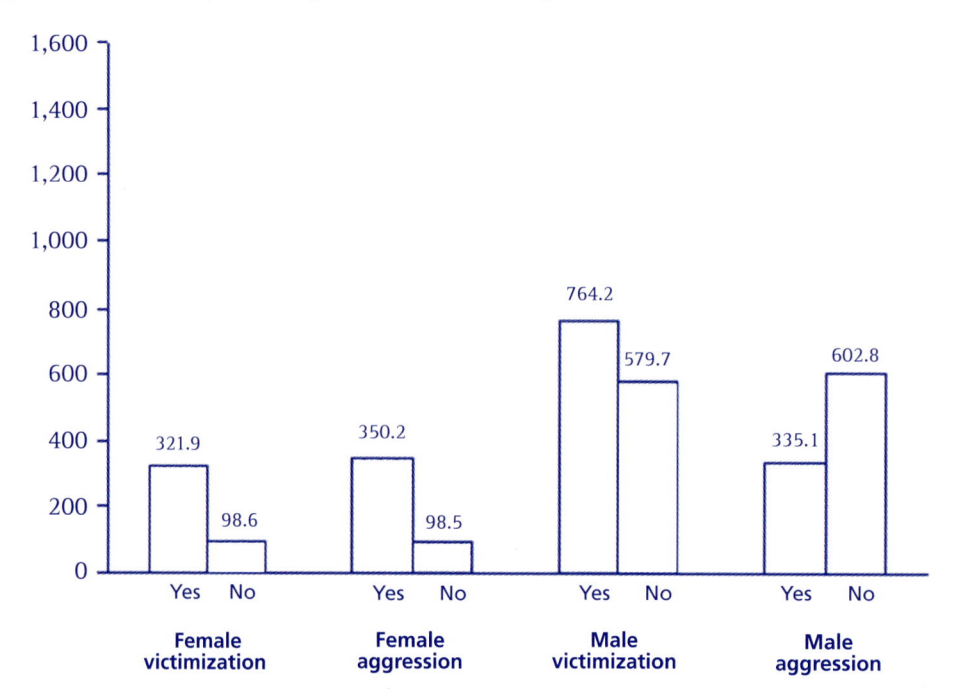

FIGURE 10. Overall mean number of drinks consumed annually by respondents by whether the respondent had been the victim of partner aggression and whether the respondent had been aggressive toward a partner, by sex, GENACIS survey, Brazil, 2006–2007.

Discussion

Consistent with previous findings for Brazil, the results showed that partner physical aggression in the last two years was a fairly frequent event (6.7%). Violence occurred mostly among younger couples, with females (victims and aggressors) tending to be slightly older than males (victims and aggressors). There was a trend for aggression to be reported more frequently by cohabiting couples than by married ones, as has been found in other research (Brownridge and Halli, 2002). Females reported more severe aggression than did males, including the need for medical care (four times as often for females), as well as feeling angrier and more upset than males in these situations. While over half of female victims and approximately half of female aggressors reported that one or both partners (usually only the male partner) had been drinking at the time of the incident, only about one-quarter of male victims and aggressors reported drinking at the time of the incident, and males were more likely to report that both partners or only the female (for male victims) had been drinking. In terms of usual drinking pattern, males and females who had consumed alcohol in the past year were more likely than those who had not drunk in the past year to be involved in partner physical aggression, although this relationship was significant only for females. Similarly, females who reported drinking five or more drinks per occasion were significantly more likely than those who never drank as much as five drinks to report partner aggression. This pattern was similar but not significant for male victims and was not evident for male aggressors.

In this study, only physical aggression was assessed. Gender differences in reporting aggression are similar to those found in other studies in which females report higher rates of victimization and aggression toward a partner, whereas males report lower rates, especially in terms of their own aggression toward female partners (Kimmel, 2001; Hamby, 2005; Krahé and Berger, 2005). In this sample, a similar trend was found, with more female victims than males reporting being aggressive toward a partner, which might reflect a response bias. The lower rate of reporting by males might be caused by forgetting, concealing information, and other reasons leading to underreporting. Alternatively, the discrepancy may be due to the fact that many incidents are ambiguous as violence is not a clear-cut phenomenon. These issues can pose a significant problem for partner violence research as in other research dealing with interpersonal relationships and sensitive topics.

The fact that violence was more frequent among younger couples is in accordance with findings from other surveys. Perhaps, tolerance develops with maturity, and younger couples are more likely than older couples to use maladaptive strategies to resolve disagreements, such as engaging in physical fights (Bookwalla, Sobin, and Zdaniuk, 2005). As expected, aggression severity (as reflected by the need for medical care) and emotional impact (as expressed through level of fear, upset, and anger) were higher for female than for male victims (although not all differences were significant), as found in previous research (Graham and Wells, 2002a and 2002b).

When using the cutoff of five or more drinks per occasion or "binge" drinking (Wechsler et al., 1994; Plant and Plant, 2006), female respondents who reported drinking five or more drinks per occasion in the past year had a significantly higher risk of partner aggression compared to females who did not drink as much as five drinks per occasion, while this association was not found for males. However, when drinking was measured as usual number of drinks per drinking occasion, there was evidence that partner aggression was associated with drinking more drinks per occasion for both males and females, although not all results met the criterion for statistical significance. These results suggest a possible link between drinking pattern and partner aggression. Future analyses examining the relationship between victimization and drinking by the partner would shed more light on this potential link.

In general, acute consequences are clearly associated with heavy alcohol consumption per occasion, and this is a rising problem in Brazil (Hamby, 2005; Kerr-Corrêa et al., 2005; Silveira et al., 2007). The relationship between violent behavior and alcohol intoxication is a common finding, both for victim and perpetrator, and is also described in other studies (Wechsler et al., 1994; Rossow, 1996; Gianini, Litvoc, and Neto, 1999; O'Leary and Schumacher, 2003; Rehm et al., 2003; Wells and Graham, 2003; Lipsky et al., 2005).

A possible limitation of this study was the refusal rate of 25.5%, which was higher amongst males than females. Refusers were mainly from the middle and upper socio-economic classes and resided in high-rise condominiums featuring centralized security services, possibly due to the desire to protect themselves from urban violence and assaults. The refusal rate is similar or lower than that found in other international studies and expected in big cities, especially those with a high incidence of urban violence (Cryer et al., 2001; Laranjeira et al. 2007). It is possible that a selection bias occurred since the refusal rate was higher among males. There was a high rate of abstainers (28% of males and 72% of females), a frequent finding in Brazil, especially among less-educated populations (Kerr-Corrêa et al., 2005; Laranjeira et al., 2007; Silveira et al., 2007). Because the sample was from metropolitan São Paulo, the results would apply to other large urban centers but might not reflect patterns in more rural areas of Brazil.

In summary, these results show the importance of alcohol involvement in partner aggression, highlight the association between alcohol use and victimization risk, and point out the necessity for the formulation of specific public health policies regarding this issue.

Acknowledgments

The research presented in this chapter emanated from a grant received from the Fundação de Amparo Pesquisa do Estado de São Paulo (FAPESP 04/11729-2). Janaina Barbosa de Oliveira was the recipient of a Coordenação de Aperfeiçoamento de Pessoal de Nível Superior (CAPES) master's degree fellowship. Mariana Braga Cavariani is the recipient of a FAPESP fellowship. Comments and suggestions during different phases of the project from Albina Rodrigues Torres, Arlinda Kristjanson, Maristela Monteiro, and Sharon Wilsnack were greatly appreciated.

References

Adeodato VG, Carvalho RR, Siqueira VR, Souza FGM. (2005). Qualidade de vida e depressão em mulheres vítimas de seus parceiros. (Quality of life and depression in women victims of their partners). *Revista de Saúde Pública*, 39, 108–113.

Baltieri DA. (2003). Álcool e crime. (Alcohol and crime.) In: Rigonatti SP, Serafim AP, Barros EL (eds.) *Temas em Psiquiatria Forense e Psicologia Jurídica*. São Paulo: Vetor, pp.151–163.

Bookwala J, Sobin J, Zdaniuk B. (2005). Gender and aggression in marital relationships: A life-span perspective. *Sex Roles*, 52, 797-806.

Brownridge DA, Halli SS. (2002). Understanding male partner violence against cohabiting and married women: an empirical investigation with a synthesized model. *Journal of Family Violence*, 17, 341-161.

Brasil. Lei nº 11.340, de 7 de agosto de 2006. Cria mecanismos para coibir a violência doméstica e familiar contra a mulher. (Law nº 11.340, August 7th, 2006. Creates mechanisms to curb domestic and familiar violence against woman). Internet: *https://www.planalto.gov.br/ccivil_03/_Ato2004-2006/2006/Lei/L11340.htm*

Coker AL, Davis KE, Arias I, Desai S, Sanderson M, Brandt HM, Smith PH. (2002). Physical and mental health effects of intimate partner violence for men and women. *American Journal of Preventive Medicine*, 24, 260-268.

Cryer PC, Saunders J, Jenkins LM, Neale H, Cook AC, Peters TJ. (2001). Clusters within a general adult population of alcohol abstainers. *International Journal of Epidemiology*, 30, 756-765.

Day VP, Telles LEB, Zoratto PH, Azambuja MRF, Machado DA, Silveira MB, Debiaggi M, Reis MG, Cardoso RG, Blank P. (2003). Violência doméstica e suas diferentes manifestações. *Revista de Psiquiatria do Rio Grande do Sul*, 25, 9-21.

Galvão EF, Andrade SM. (2004). Violência contra a mulher: análise de casos atendidos em serviços de atenção à mulher em município do Sul do Brasil. (Violence against women: analysis of cases seem in women health services in a southern town of Brazil) *Saúde e Sociedade*, 13, 89-99.

García-Moreno C, Jansen HA, Ellsberg M, Heise L, Watts C. *on behalf of the WHO multi-country study on women's health and domestic violence against women study team* (2006), Prevalence of intimate partner violence: findings from the WHO multi-country study on women's health and domestic violence. Lancet, 368: 1260-69.

Gianini RJ, Litvoc, J, Neto JN (1999). Agressão física e classe social. (Physical aggression and. social class.) *Revista de Saúde Pública*, 33, 180-186.

Giffin K. (1994). Violência de gênero, sexualidade e saúde. (Gender violence, sexuality and health). *Cadernos de Saúde Pública*, 10, 146-155.

Graham K, Wells S. (2002a). Mutual versus one-sided physical aggression: findings from a general population survey of aggression among adults. In: Shohov, S.P. (ed.) *Advances in Psychology Research*, vol. 16. New York: Nova Science Publishers, pp. 95-111.

Graham K, Wells S. (2002b). The two world of aggression for men and women. *Sex Roles*, 45, 595-622.

Grossi K. (1996). Violência contra a mulher: implicações para os profissionais de saúde. (Violence against women: implicatins for the health professionals). In: Lopes, M.J.M., Meyer, D.E., Waldow, V.R. (orgs.) *Gênero e saúde*. Porto Alegre: Artes Médicas, pp.133-149.

Hamby S. (2005). Measuring gender differences in partner violence: implications from research on other forms of violent and socially undesirable behaviour. *Sex Roles*, 52, 725-742.

IBGE. Instituto Brasileiro de Geografia e Estatística (2000). Internet: *http://www.ibge.gov.br/home/estatistica/populacao/censo2000/universo.php?tipo=31&paginaatual=1&uf=35&letra=S*

Kimmel MS. (2001). Male Victims of domestic violence: a substantive and methodological research review. Report to the Equality Committee of the Department of Education and Science, Ireland, 2001. Internet: *http://www.xyonline.net/downloads/malevictims.pdf*

Kerr-Corrêa F, Hegedus AM, Sanches AF, Trinca LA, Kerr-Pontes LRS, Tucci AM, Floripes TMF. (2005). Differences in drinking patterns between men and women in Brazil (Chapter 3). In: Obot, I., Room, R. (eds.) *Alcohol, gender and drinking problems: perspectives from low and middle-income countries and drinking problems.* Geneva: World Health Organization, Department of Mental Health and Substance Abuse, pp.49-68.

Krahé B, Berger A. (2005). Sex Differences in Relationship Aggression among Young Adults in Germany. *Sex Roles*, 52, 829-838.

Kronbauer JFD, Meneghel SN. (2005). Perfil da violência de gênero perpetrada por companheiro. (Gender violence profile perpetrated against partner). *Revista de Saúde Pública*, 39, 695-701.

Laranjeira R, Pinsky I, Zaleski M, Caetano R. (2007). I Levantamento Nacional sobre os padrões de consumo de álcool na população brasileira. (I National survey on patterns of alcohol use by the Brazilian population). Centro brasileiro de Informações sobre Drogas Psicotrópicas, Escola Paulista de Medicina, São Paulo, Brazil.

Lima MLC, Ximenes R. (1998). Violência e morte: diferenciais da mortalidade por causas externas no espaço urbano do Recife, 1991. (Violence and death: mortality differenctials by external causes in the urban space in Recife, 1991). *Cadernos de Saúde Pública*, 14, 829-840.

Lipsky S, Caetano R, Field CA, Larkin GL. (2005). Psychosocial and substance-use risk factors for intimate partner violence. *Drug and Alcohol Dependence*, 78, 39-47.

Minayo MCS, Deslandes SF. Complexidade das relações entre drogas, álcool e violência. (Complexity in the relationship among drugs, alcohol and violence). *Cadernos de Saúde Pública*, 14, 35-42.

O'Leary KD, Schumacher JA. (2003). The association between alcohol use and intimate partner violence: Linear effect, threshold effect, or both? *Addictive Behaviors*, 23, 1575-1585.

Orpinas P. (1999). Who is violent? Factors associated with aggressive behaviors in Latin America and Spain. *Revista Panamericana de Salud Pública*, 5, 232-244.

Plant M, Plant M. (2006). Binge Britain: alcohol and the national response. Oxford: Oxford University Press.

Poldrugo F. (1998). Alcohol and criminal behaviour. *Alcohol & Alcoholism*, 33, 12-15.

Rechtman M, Phebo L. (2000).Violência contra a mulher. Relatórios 1 a 5 do Centro de Atenção à mulher Vítima de Violência (CEAMVV). (Violence against woman. Reports 1 to 5 from the Center on attention to the woman victim of violence). Rio de Janeiro: CEAMVV.

Rehm J, Room R, Graham K, Monteiro M, Gmel G, Sempos CT. (2003). The relationship of average volume of alcohol consumption and patterns of drinking to burden of disease: an overview. *Addiction*, 98, 1209-1228.

Rossow I. (1996). Alcohol-related violence: the impact of drinking pattern and drinking context. *Addiction*, 91, 1651-1661.

Schraiber LB, D'oliveira AFPL, França-Junior I, Pinho AA. (2002). Violência contra a mulher: estudo em uma unidade de atenção primaria à saúde. (Violence against woman: study in a primary care health center). *Revista de Saúde Pública*, 36, 470-477.

Schraiber LB; D'Oliveira AFLP. (1999). Violência contra mulheres: interfaces contra a Saúde. (Violence against women: interfaces against health). Interface - Comunicação, Saúde e Educação, 3, 11-26.

Silveira CM, Wang Y-P, Andrade AG, Andrade LH. (2007). Heavy episodic drinking in the São Paulo Epidemiologic Catchments Area Study in Brazil: gender and sociodemographics correlates. *Journal of Studies on Alcohol and Drugs*, 68, 18-27.

Soares BS. Mulheres invisíveis: violência conjugal e novas políticas de segurança. Rio de Janeiro: Civilização Brasileira; 1999.

Thomas DQ. (1994). In search of solutions: women's police stations in Brazil In: Davies, M. (ed.) *Women and violence. Realities and responses worldwide.* London: Zed Books, pp. 32-43.

Wechsler H, Davenport A, Dowdall G, Moeykens, B., Castillo, S. (1994). Health and behavioral consequences of binge drinking in college. *Journal of the American Medical Association*, 272, 1672-1677.

Wells S, Graham K. (2003). Aggression involving alcohol: relationship to drinking patterns and social context. *Addiction*, 98, 33-42.

UNHAPPY HOURS:

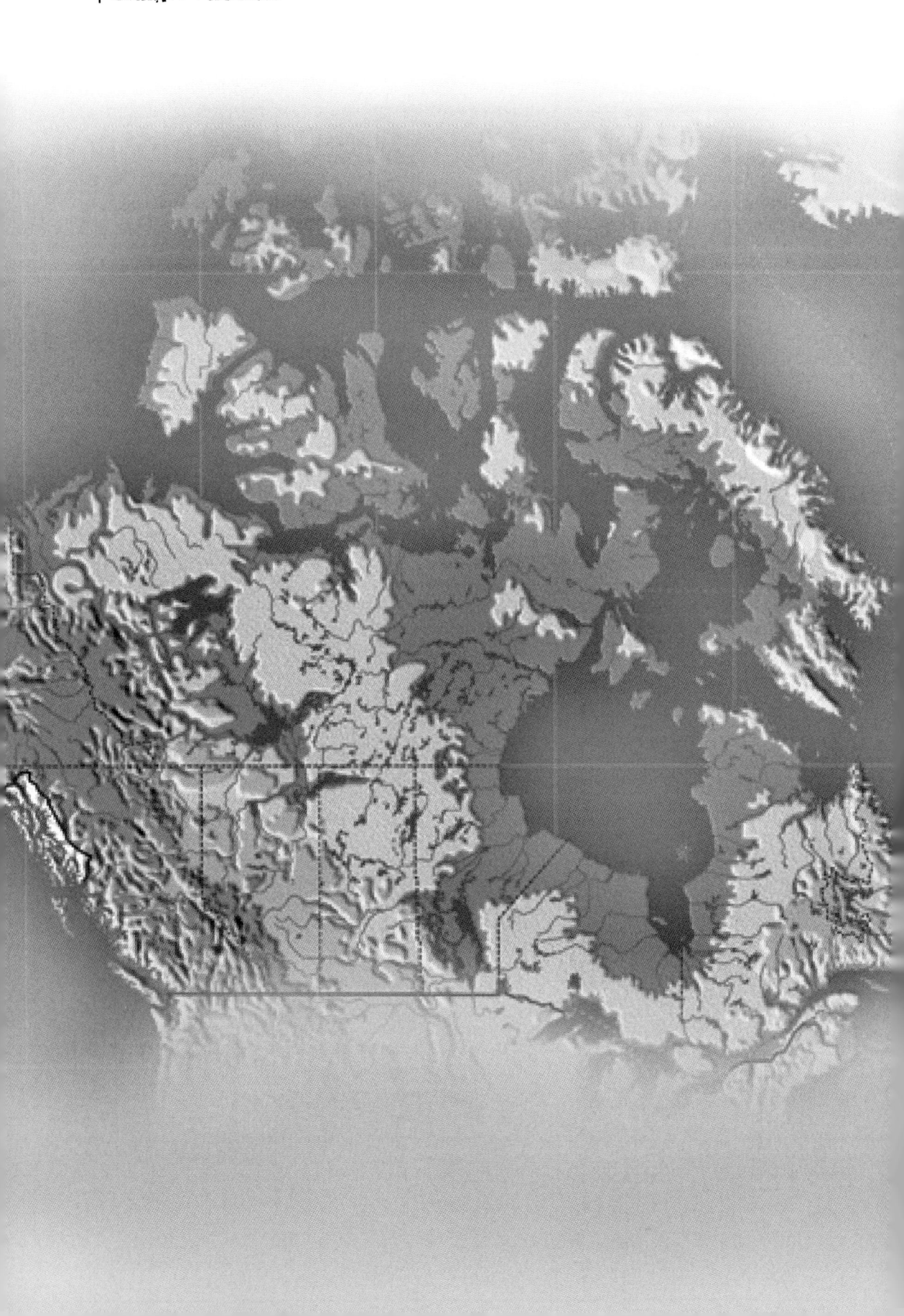

Canada: Alcohol and Partner Physical Aggression in the 10 Provinces

—*Kathryn Graham and Sharon Bernards*

Introduction

The first major research initiative explicitly focusing on intimate partner violence in Canada was the 1993 Violence against Women (VAW) Survey. This study found that 3% of those who had ever been married or were living in a common-law relationship reported violence by a male partner or ex-partner in the year before the survey (Johnson and Sacco, 1995) and that an additional 2% of Canadian women aged 18 and older reported having been the victim of threats of physical or sexual aggression by a male date or boyfriend. More recently, the 1999 and 2004 General Social Surveys (GSS) of Canadian residents aged 15 or older (Bunge and Locke, 2000; AuCoin, 2005) found similar past-year rates of physical or sexual assault by a current or former partner for women who were married, living in a common-law relationship, or had had contact with a partner during the previous five years (3% in 1999 and 2% in 2004); however, the percent reporting partner violence over the previous five years had decreased from 12% in 1993 to 8% in 1999 and 7% in 2004 (Johnson, 2006). About 2% of male GSS respondents reported physical aggression by a partner in the year prior to the surveys, while 7% in 1999 and 6% in 2004 reported violence by a partner during the past 5 years. In general, partner violence (Johnson, 2006), including spousal homicides against women (Wilson, Johnson, and Daly, 1995), has been found to decrease with age.

Results from the 2004 GSS indicate that females were more likely than males to report severe acts of aggression (receiving threats of violence, being beaten or choked, or having a gun or knife used against them) and ongoing incidents of violence by their partner (Mihorean, 2005). In addition, women were three times more likely than men to have suffered physical injuries and five times more likely to report fearing for their lives.

Women are also more likely than men to be killed by an intimate partner. The rate of spousal homicides against women has been about four to five times higher than the rate of spousal homicides against men, with 2,178 women and 638 men killed by a spouse between 1975 and 2004 (Johnson, 2006); in addition, women were more likely than men to kill in self-defense (Johnson, 2006).

Women in 2004 also were more likely than men to have reported using the services of community agencies (e.g., counselors, crisis lines, shelters), to have taken time off from paid or unpaid work as a direct result of partner violence, to have spent time in the hospital, and to have sought police protection from a spouse (Mihorean, 2005). In 2000, women accounted for 85% of all victims of spousal violence reported to a sample of police agencies in Canada (Trainor, 2002).

The Role of Alcohol

Intimate partner aggression in Canada has been found to be related to the drinking pattern of the offender, with more frequent consumption of five or more drinks per occasion (Bunge 2000; Johnson, 2000; Brownridge, 2002; Mihorean, 2005) associated with increased odds of being violent toward a female partner. In addition, a substantial proportion of violence against women occurred when the male partner had been drinking. About one-half of the respondents to the 1993 VAW survey who had ever been assaulted by their husbands or ex-husbands reported that the husband was usually drinking at the time of the violence (Rodgers, 1994). Of the incidents of violence by a partner reported to have occurred during the five years prior to the 2004 GSS, 44% of female victims and 24% of male victims reported that their partner had been drinking at the time (Mihorean, 2005).

Data from the 1999 GSS also indicated that alcohol use at the time of the incident was associated with more severe violence, including higher risk of injury and associated fear (Desjardins and Hotton, 2004). In incidents of spousal homicide between 1979 and 1998 (394 committed by women and 1,338 committed by men), alcohol or both alcohol and drugs were known to have been consumed by 59% of accused wives and 30% of accused husbands (Locke, 2000).

The Response of the Criminal Justice System

In 1996, the *Toronto Star* published a series of news articles on the outcomes of charges of spousal abuse which revealed major weaknesses in the response by the legal system. For eight months, the newspaper staff tracked 133 cases of spousal abuse that appeared before the courts in metropolitan Toronto during one week in July of 1995. The victims included 127 women and 6 men with almost all accused offenders being male. A third of the cases occurred after the relationship had ended and usually involved stalking by the offender. In addition, 32% of those charged during the week under study were already facing charges from a previous domestic assault incident. The newspaper noted that alcohol and drugs were involved in over half of the cases.

The *Star's* 9 March 1996 edition (p.A1-A4) reported the following highlights of the criminal justice process:
- While 60% of cases resulted in conviction, in most cases the men pled guilty to a lesser crime and received no jail time.
- Thirty-seven percent of the cases were not prosecuted because the victim failed to show up in court or recanted.
- In cases where the victim recanted her testimony, the court dropped the charges rather than use other forms of evidence, such as injury photographs, taped emergency calls, or statements from other witnesses.
- Eighty-five percent of offenders were released on bail, and almost half violated bail conditions by harassing, stalking, or moving back in with victims;
- After 8 months, 25% of cases were still awaiting trial;
- At 12 months following the original case, 35 of the 133 had committed new offenses; 85% of these occurred with the same victim (3 November 1996, p.B1).

The newspaper further indicated that many victims were intimidated by the partner and afraid to testify, while others did not want the offender to be incarcerated because he was the family's primary wage earner. Probably at least in part as a result of the exposé by the *Toronto Star*, special courts were set up in Ontario to deal specifically with domestic violence cases, based on the example of a similar court established in Winnipeg, Manitoba, in 1990. These courts now exist in other provinces and are structured to provide better support to victims and a greater focus on early intervention and prevention (for further information, see chapter 5 in Johnson and AuCoin, 2003); however, to date, there has been no rigorous evaluation of their effectiveness.

As in other countries, the criminal justice system in Canada has struggled to deal effectively with violence between intimate partners (see Johnson, 2007). Despite policies across Canada for the mandatory arrest of perpetrators of intimate partner violence, statistics from the 2004 GSS indicated that the police used their discretion in dealing with domestic violence cases. According to victim reports, 62% of police responding to domestic violence calls gave the abuser a warning, 44% removed the abuser from the home, and only about one-third made an arrest (Mihorean 2005). In 2002, violence involving spouses resulted in a prison sentence less often than violence involving non-spouses (19% versus 29%).

Other Programs for Partner Aggression

In terms of other programs and services addressing intimate partner aggression in Canada, the number of shelters for women has risen dramatically over the past 30 years from 18 in 1975 to 543 in 2004, as have treatment programs for abusive men (Johnson, 2006). Transition houses and shelters for abused women, services and programs for abused men, and treatment programs for abusive men are provided by government, police, or community organizations in all provinces and territories, including in large and small cities. In addition, 24-hour telephone helplines for victims are provided in many jurisdictions throughout the country. However, the majority of victims tend to turn to family (67% of women, 44% of men) or friends (63% of women, 41% of men) for assistance following partner aggression (Mihorean, 2005).

Methods
Survey and Sample
The GENACIS Canada survey included a representative sample of 14,063 Canadian residents (6,009 men and 8,054 women) aged 18 to 76 years from all 10 provinces. The survey was conducted between January 2004 and March 2005 as part of the GENACIS international collaboration (Gender, Alcohol, and Culture: An International Study). A random sample was selected using a two-stage sampling design: (1) households were selected using random digit dialing (RDD) of residential telephone numbers; and (2) within a household, the adult whose birthday most closely followed the interview date was selected as the survey respondent. Interviews were conducted using computer-assisted telephone interviewing (CATI). The response rate was 52.8% of all estimated eligible households. However, most refusals were made at the time of the initial household contact, and the participation rate among contacted eligible respondents was 85.4%. Weights were applied to adjust for under-sampling of persons in multi-adult households and slight over-sampling of smaller provinces.

General characteristics of male and female participants in the survey are shown in Table 1. Female respondents were overrepresented compared to the proportions of men and women in Canada based on 2006 national census data (50.2% women, 49.8% men aged 15–79). More than 80% of men and almost 75% of women in the sample reported drinking alcohol in the past 12 months. Men drank more frequently and in larger quantities per occasion than women, and a larger percentage of men (67.2%) than women (36.3%) drank heavily (five or more drinks) on at least one occasion during the past year.

TABLE 1. Age, marital status, employment status, and drinking pattern in the 12 months preceding the survey, for male and female respondents, by sex, GENACIS survey, Canada, 2004–2005.

	Males (weighted N=5,991)		Females (weighted N=8,072)	
	Number[a]	Percent or mean	Number[a]	Percent or mean
Age		44.4 years		45.6 years
18–24 years	609	10.3%	698	8.9%
25–34 years	1,102	18.6%	1,315	16.7%
35–44 years	1,341	22.6%	1,807	22.9%
45–54 years	1,293	21.8%	1,776	22.5%
55–64 years	938	15.8%	1,286	16.3%
65–76 years	641	10.8%	1,006	12.8%
Marital status				
Married	2,925	48.9%	3,857	48.0%
Cohabiting/Living with partner	750	12.6%	970	12.1%
Divorced or separated	487	9.8%	1,101	13.7%
Never married	1,588	26.6%	1,549	19.3%
Widowed	126	2.1%	553	6.9%
Employment status				
In the labor force	4,334	72.7%	4,892	60.9%
Caring for family	18	0.3%	543	6.8%
Unemployed	240	4.0%	445	5.5%
Long–term illness or disability	172	2.9%	249	3.1%
Student	353	5.9%	497	6.2%
Retired	843	14.1%	1,410	17.5%
Drinking pattern (past 12 months)				
Drank any alcohol during past 12 months	4,890	81.7%	6,023	74.6%
Average number of drinking days (drinkers only)		103.5 days		67.0 days
Average number of drinks per occasion (drinkers only)		3.2 drinks		2.1 drinks
Average annual volume (drinkers only)		431.6 drinks		182.6 drinks
Drank five or more drinks on at least one occasion (drinkers only)	3,050	63.2%	2167	36.3%

[a] Note that total numbers within each category vary due to missing responses.

Measures that Differed from the Core Questions

The sex of the respondent was determined by the interviewer at the beginning of the interview, and the interviewer was prompted to confirm this judgment later in the interview. Responses to the questions regarding the most severe physical act that was done by and toward a partner were open-ended, and interviewers were not explicitly instructed to either exclude or include sexual aggression. When the response fit into one of the preset categories provided to the interviewer, the response was coded by the interviewer using this option; otherwise, the interviewer recorded the response verbatim, and these open-ended responses were subsequently coded according to the guidelines described in the chapter "Common Survey Method and Analysis Conducted for Each Country Chapter". Respondents who had same-sex partners were excluded from these analyses. In addition to victims being asked whether they sought medical attention after the incident, respondents who indicated they had been aggressive toward a partner were also asked if *their partner* sought medical attention after the incident. Whether the respondent consumed five or more drinks on any occasion in the past year was based on the item regarding how often the respondent drank five or more drinks, as described in the aforementioned chapter on methods.

Results

As shown in Figure 1, men were significantly more likely than women to report aggression by an opposite sex partner in the previous two years (7.2% vs. 5.3%, $p < .001$), and, conversely, women were more likely than men to report being physically aggressive *toward* a partner (5.7% vs. 3.4%, $p < .001$). For both men and women, the proportion that reported having been the victim of physical aggression was higher than the proportion of the opposite sex who reported being the aggressor (7.2% of men reported being the victim, while 5.7% of women reported being the aggressor, $p = .002$; 5.3% of women reported being the victim, while 3.4% of men reported being the aggressor, $p < .001$). Of those who reported any partner physical aggression, a similar percentage of men and women reported being both a victim and an aggressor (27.6% of men, 25.4% of women). However, a larger percentage of men than women reported being a victim only (60.1% versus 36.5%), while a larger proportion of women than men reported only aggression toward a partner (38.1% versus 12.3%).

The average age of female and male victims was 35.6 years and 34.9 years, respectively. Female aggressors were 35.7 years on average, and male aggressors were 33.2 years. As shown in Figure 2, aggression tended to be most prevalent among younger adults and to decrease with age.

As shown in Figure 3, for all groups, the lowest rate of partner aggression was reported by those who were currently married, and the difference between being married versus all other marital status groups was significant ($p < .001$) for female and male victims, and being married versus cohabiting and never having been married for female and male aggressors. It is notable that victimization was especially high for respondents who were divorced/separated, especially for female respondents, while this pattern was less apparent for aggressors. In fact, 9.1% of divorced/separated female respondents reported having been the victim of partner aggression, while only 3.7% of divorced/separated male respondents reported being aggressive toward a female partner.

FIGURE 1. Percent of respondents who reported having been a victim or aggressor, by sex, GENACIS survey, Canada, 2004–2005.

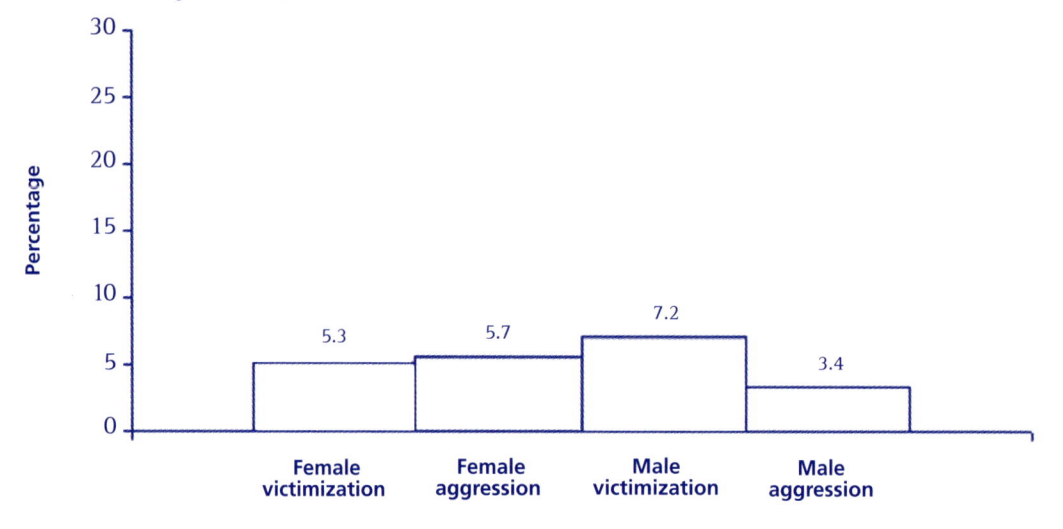

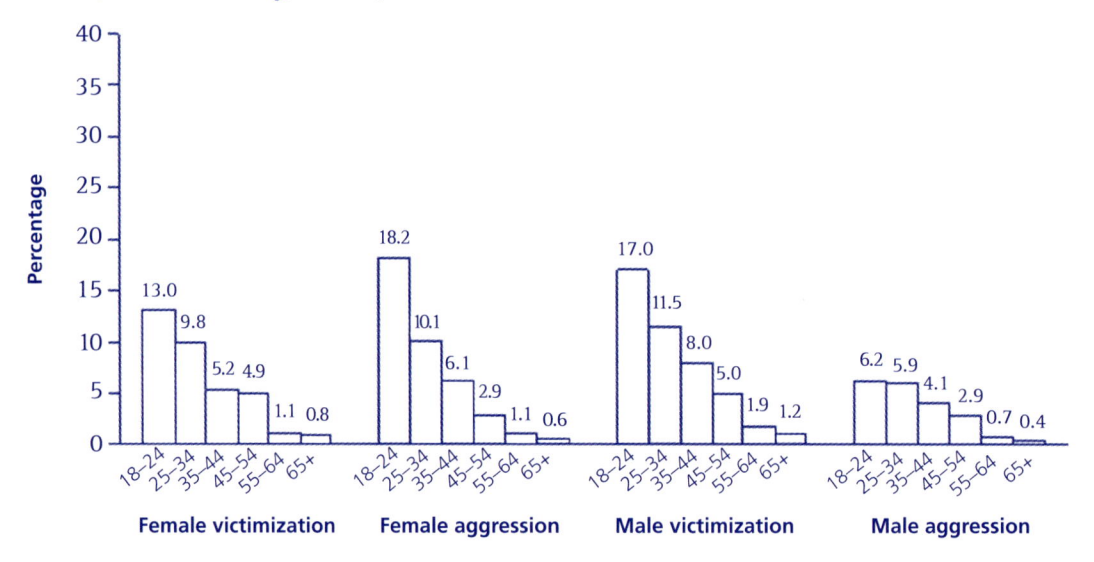

FIGURE 2. Percent of respondents who reported having been a victim or aggressor, by age group and sex, GENACIS survey, Canada, 2004–2005.

FIGURE 3. Percent of respondents who reported having been a victim or aggressor, by marital status and sex, GENACIS survey, Canada, 2004–2005.

	Married	Cohabiting	Divorced/separated	Never married
Female victimization	2.7	6.7	9.1	9.8
Female aggression	3.6	9.1	5.6	10.3
Male victimization	4.3	10.8	8.9	10.9
Male aggression	2.5	5.2	3.7	4.7

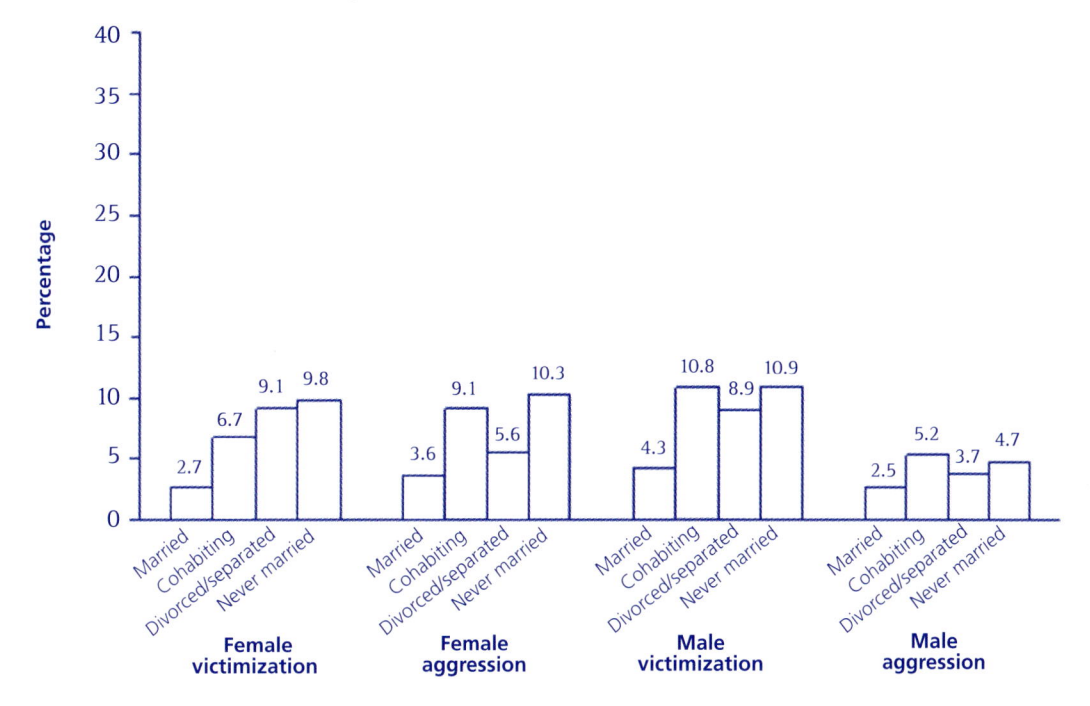

Figure 4 shows the type of aggressive act done to and by respondents. These graphs are set up to visually compare reports of aggression toward females (i.e., as reported by female victims and male aggressors) versus reports of aggression toward males (i.e., as reported by male victims and female aggressors). As is evident in this figure, male victims were significantly more likely than female victims to report being slapped, while female victims were more likely than male victims to report being pushed and grabbed ($p < .01$). Female victims also were more likely than male victims to report being beaten and punched, but this difference did not meet the criterion for statistical significance of $p < .01$.

Among respondents who reported being aggressive toward a partner, male aggressors were more likely than female aggressors to report pushing and grabbing, while females were more likely to report slapping and throwing something at the partner ($p < .01$). Female aggressors were also more likely than male aggressors to report punching ($p < .01$).

In terms of differences in whether the act was reported by a victim or aggressor, male aggressors were less likely than female victims to report punching and beating up, and female aggressors were less likely than male victims to report punching, but none of these differences was significant.

FIGURE 4. Type of aggressive act against females as reported by female victims and male aggressors, and against males as reported by male victims and female aggressors, GENACIS survey, Canada, 2004–2005.

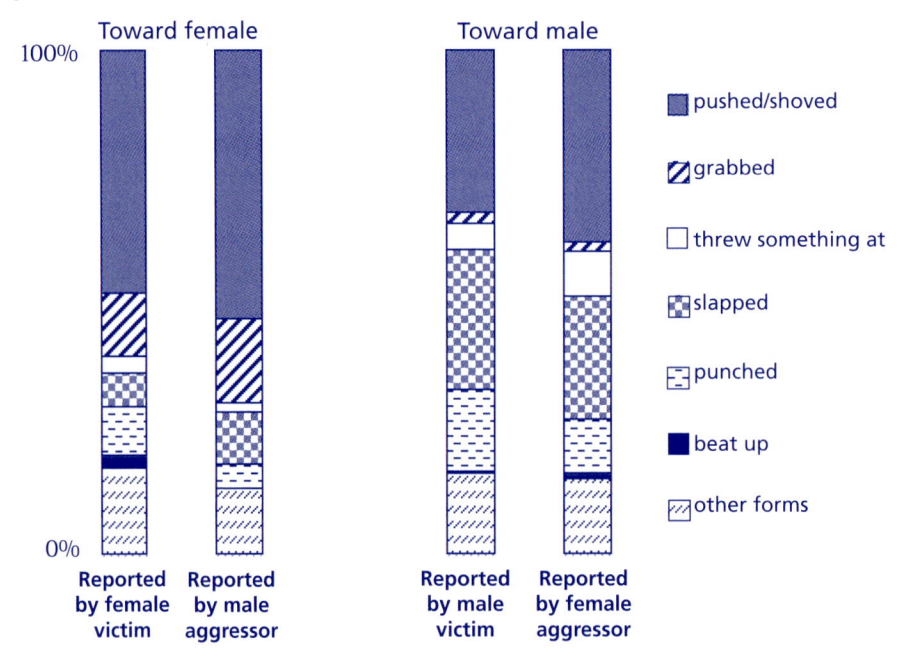

Figure 5 shows the respondent's ratings of severity of aggression by partner (for victims) and of the respondent's own aggression (for aggressors), as well as how scared, upset, and angry the respondent felt at the time of the aggression (all rated on a scale of 1–10). As shown in this figure, overall, female victims rated the partner's aggression as being more severe and themselves as more scared, upset, and angry, compared with ratings of aggression by female aggressors and male victims and aggressors. Male victims, on the other hand, gave lower ratings of fear, upset, and anger, compared to ratings by male aggressors and female victims and aggressors.

Among respondents who reported being the victim of partner aggression, female victims rated the aggression as being more severe than did male victims (p < .001), and female victims reported being significantly more afraid (p < .001), more upset (p < .001), and more angry (p < .001). Among aggressors, females rated themselves as significantly more upset (p = .028) and angry (p = .003), compared with ratings by male aggressors, but did not differ significantly on ratings of aggression severity or fear.

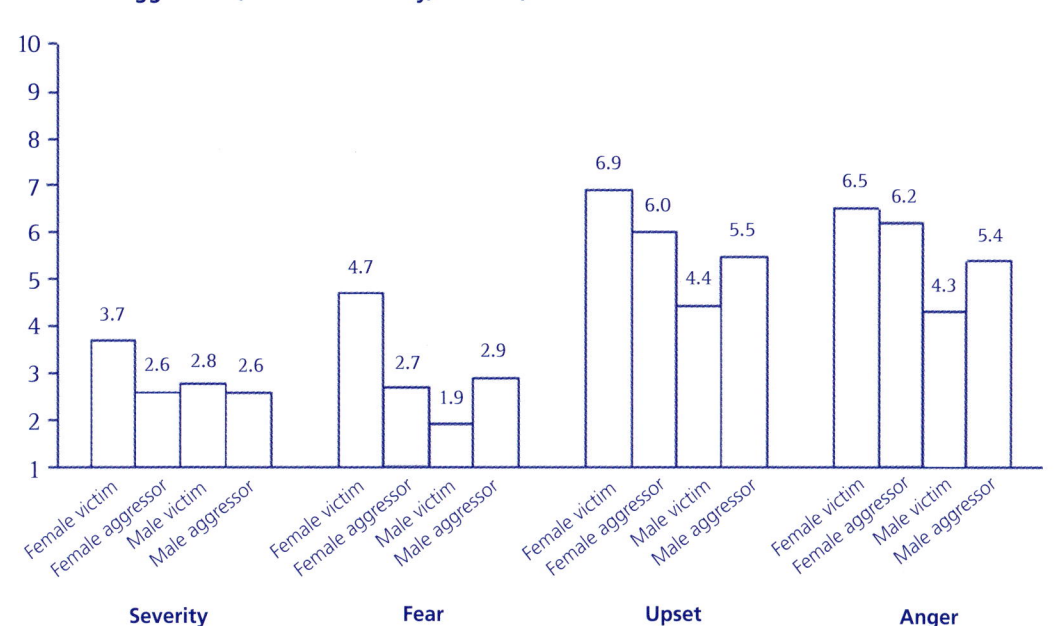

FIGURE 5. Mean ratings of severity of aggression, fear, upset, and anger by male and female victims and aggressors, GENACIS survey, Canada, 2004–2005.

Category	Female victim	Female aggressor	Male victim	Male aggressor
Severity	3.7	2.6	2.8	2.6
Fear	4.7	2.7	1.9	2.9
Upset	6.9	6.0	4.4	5.5
Anger	6.5	6.2	4.3	5.4

Comparing female victims to male aggressors, females rated the aggression by the male partner as significantly more severe and themselves as being more afraid, upset, and angry (all comparisons p < .001), compared with ratings made by male respondents who were aggressive toward a female partner. Male victims did not differ significantly from female aggressor in terms of their rating of aggression severity; however, ratings of fear, upset, and anger were significantly lower for male victims, compared with ratings made by female aggressors (all comparisons p < .001).

In addition to higher ratings of severity and fear, female victims were more likely than male victims to seek medical attention following the incident. Specifically, a significantly larger percentage of female victims (11.2%) than male victims (3.4%) sought medical attention after the incident (p < .001), and a larger percentage of male aggressors (5.4%) than female aggressors (1.7%) reported that their partner sought medical attention after the respondent's aggression (although this difference was not significant).

Figure 6 shows the extent to which alcohol was involved in incidents reported by female and male victims and female and male aggressors. As is evident in this figure, most incidents did not involve alcohol; this proportion ranged from 69.0% of incidents reported by female victims to 82.4% of those reported by male victims. Male victims were significantly less likely than female victims to report that at least one person had been drinking prior to the incident (p < .001), while there was no significant difference between male and female aggressors in terms of their reporting of whether anyone was drinking.

FIGURE 6. Percent of incidents in which no partner had been drinking, both partners had been drinking, only the male partner had been drinking, or only the female partner had been drinking, as reported by male and female victims and aggressors, GENACIS survey, Canada, 2004–2005.

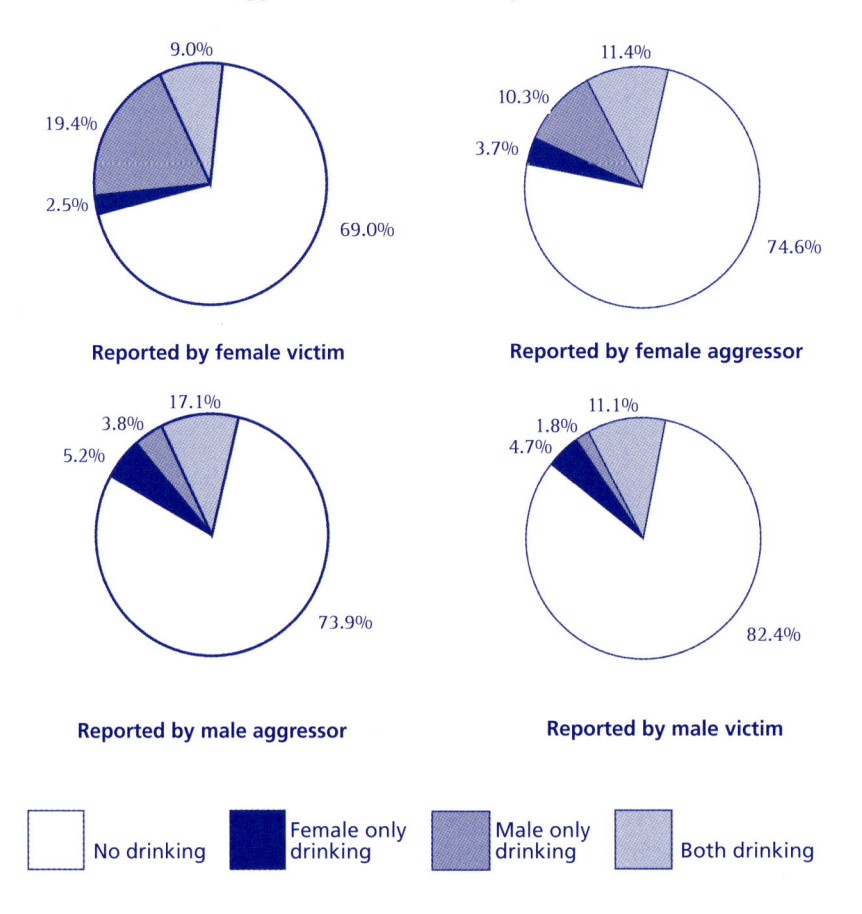

Reported by female victim: 69.0%, 2.5%, 19.4%, 9.0%

Reported by female aggressor: 74.6%, 3.7%, 10.3%, 11.4%

Reported by male aggressor: 73.9%, 5.2%, 3.8%, 17.1%

Reported by male victim: 82.4%, 4.7%, 1.8%, 11.1%

Legend: No drinking | Female only drinking | Male only drinking | Both drinking

Female victims were significantly more likely than male victims to report that only the aggressor had been drinking (p < .001), and female aggressors were more likely than male aggressors to report that only the victim had been drinking (p = .046). That is, female respondents were more likely to report that the male partner had been drinking than male respondents were to report that the female partner had been drinking. There were no significant differences between male and female victims regarding whether they reported that they themselves had been drinking or that both had been drinking.

For female victims compared to male aggressors (the two pie charts in Figure 6 on the left), female victims were significantly more likely than male aggressors to report that only the male was drinking (p < .001) and were less likely to report that both were drinking (p = .011). For male victims and female aggressors (the two pie charts in

Figure 6 on the right), female aggressors were significantly more likely (p < .001) than male victims to report that only the male was drinking.

Finally, incidents involving alcohol were rated as being more severe than were incidents that did not involve alcohol, regardless of whether the respondent was male or female or the victim or the aggressor. This difference was significant overall (p < .001) and when alcohol incidents were compared to incidents without alcohol for each of the four groups (p < .001 for female victims and aggressors and for male victims, and p = .001 for male aggressors), controlling for age in all analyses.

The Relationship between Alcohol Consumption and Partner Aggression

The percent of victims and aggressors was higher among those who drank alcohol in the year before the survey than among those who abstained, with 5.8% of female drinkers reporting being the victim of partner aggression and 6.5% reporting aggression toward a partner, versus 4.0% and 3.4%, respectively, for female abstainers. Among male drinkers, 8.0% reported being the victim of partner aggression and 3.8% reported aggression toward a partner, versus 3.6% and 1.9%, respectively, for male abstainers. Logistic regression of partner physical aggression (yes/no) on whether respondent was a past-year drinker (yes/no) controlling for age resulted in odds ratios that were significantly greater than one for male and female aggressors (p < .05) and male victims (p = .001), but not for female victims.

The analyses in the following section are limited to respondents who consumed alcohol during the year preceding the survey.

Respondents' Drinking Pattern and Partner Aggression

As shown in Figure 7, respondents who consumed five or more drinks on an occasion in the past year were more likely to report partner physical aggression, compared with respondents who reported never consuming as much as five drinks on an occasion. Multinomial logistic regression models were used to examine the relationship of consuming five or more drinks on an occasion with: (1) partner aggression without alcohol, (2) partner aggression with alcohol, and (3) no partner aggression (comparison category) controlling for age, and with separate models for female and male victims and aggressors. Respondents who consumed five or more drinks were significantly more likely than those who never consumed as much as five drinks in the past year to report partner aggression in which one or both partners had been drinking (versus no aggression) (female victims and aggressors: p < .001; male victims: p = .003; male aggressors: p = .002). Interestingly, respondents who consumed five or more drinks per occasion were also more likely than were respondents who did not consume as much as five drinks to report aggression that did not involve alcohol; however, this difference was significant (p = .007) only for reporting of victimization by female respondents.

FIGURE 7. Percent of respondents who reported victimization (aggression by a partner) or aggression (aggression toward a partner) when one or both partners had been drinking or neither had been drinking by whether respondents had consumed five or more drinks on an occasion or never had consumed five drinks on an occasion, by sex, GENACIS survey, Canada, 2004–2005.

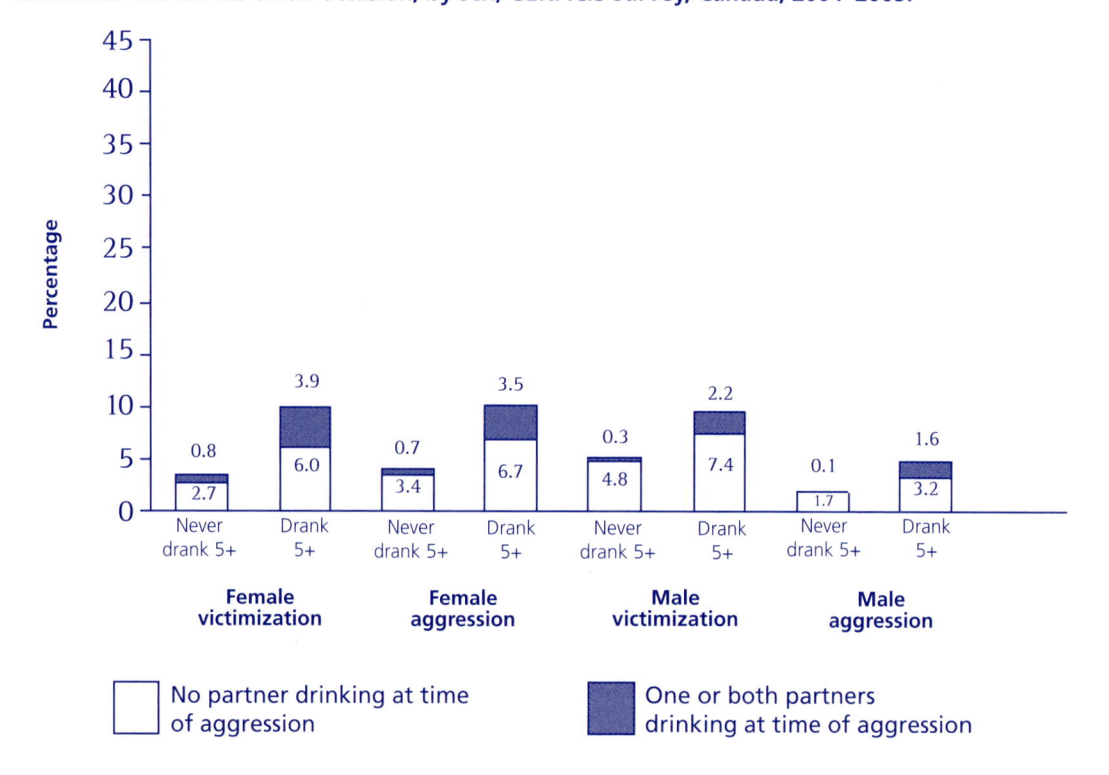

Figures 8, 9, and 10 show the mean level of alcohol consumption (frequency of drinking in number of days per year, usual number of drinks consumed per occasion, and total number of drinks consumed annually) among those who reported (1) an aggressive incident in which one or both had been drinking, (2) an incident in which no one had been drinking, or (3) no aggression relating to male and female victimization and aggression. Multinomial logistic regression was used to compare the two groups who had experienced aggression (with alcohol, no alcohol) to those who reported no aggression in separate models for male and female victimization and aggression using each of the three alcohol consumption measures as predictors and controlling for age. These analyses indicated that all measures of alcohol consumption were significant predictors of aggression involving alcohol compared to no aggression for male and female victimization and male and female aggression (all comparisons $p \leq .001$). Usual level of alcohol consumption by those who reported an incident of aggression that did not involve alcohol tended to be higher compared with consumption by those who reported no aggression, but this difference did not meet the significance criterion of $p < .05$ except for usual quantity consumed by female victims ($p = .001$).

FIGURE 8. Mean number of drinking days in the year preceding the survey for respondents who had been victims or aggressors in incidents involving alcohol, in incidents not involving alcohol, or who reported no victimization or aggression, by sex, GENACIS survey, Canada, 2004–2005.

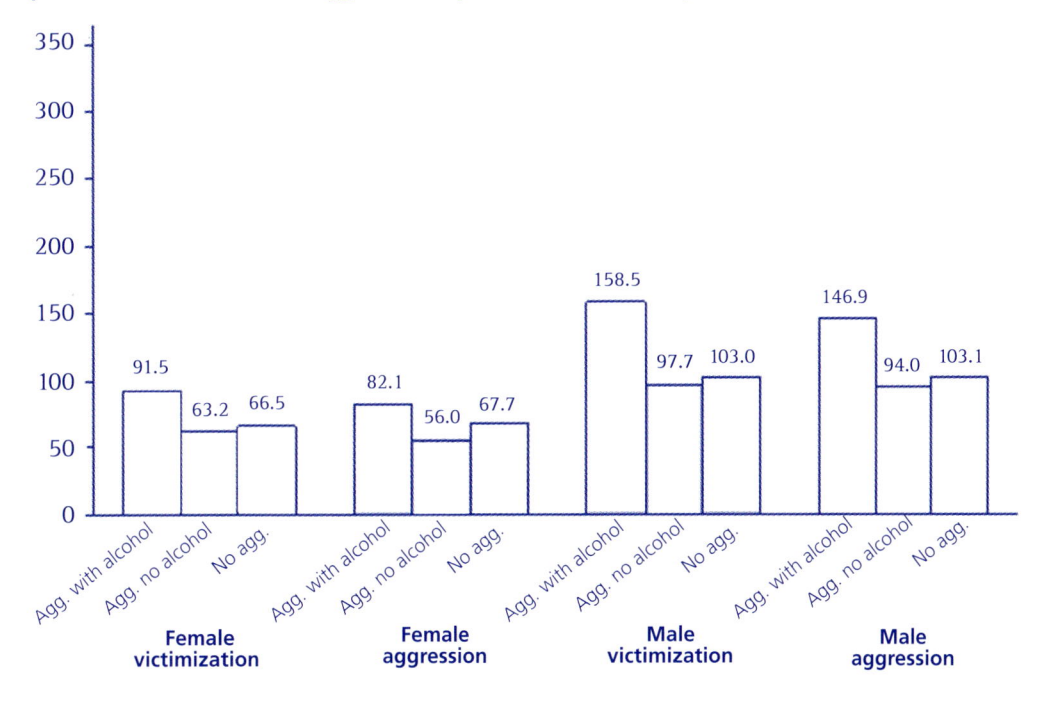

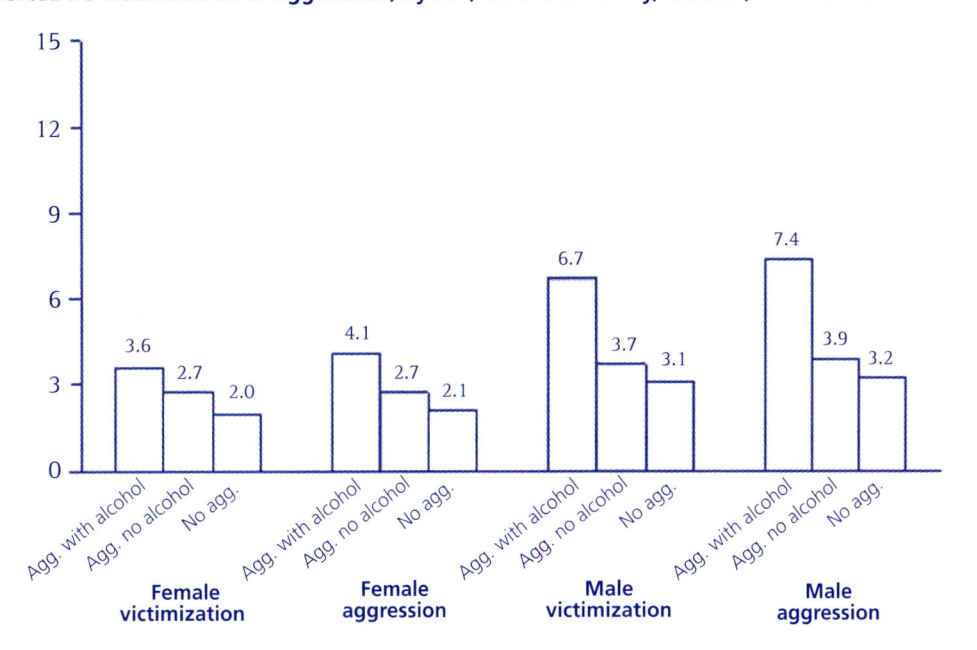

	Agg. with alcohol	Agg. no alcohol	No agg.
Female victimization	91.5	63.2	66.5
Female aggression	82.1	56.0	67.7
Male victimization	158.5	97.7	103.0
Male aggression	146.9	94.0	103.1

FIGURE 9. Mean number of drinks consumed on usual drinking occasions by respondents who had been victims or aggressors in incidents involving alcohol, in incidents not involving alcohol, or who reported no victimization or aggression, by sex, GENACIS survey, Canada, 2004–2005.

	Agg. with alcohol	Agg. no alcohol	No agg.
Female victimization	3.6	2.7	2.0
Female aggression	4.1	2.7	2.1
Male victimization	6.7	3.7	3.1
Male aggression	7.4	3.9	3.2

FIGURE 10. Overall mean number of drinks consumed annually by respondents who had been victims or aggressors in incidents involving alcohol, in incidents not involving alcohol, or who reported no victimization or aggression, by sex, GENACIS survey, Canada, 2004–2005.

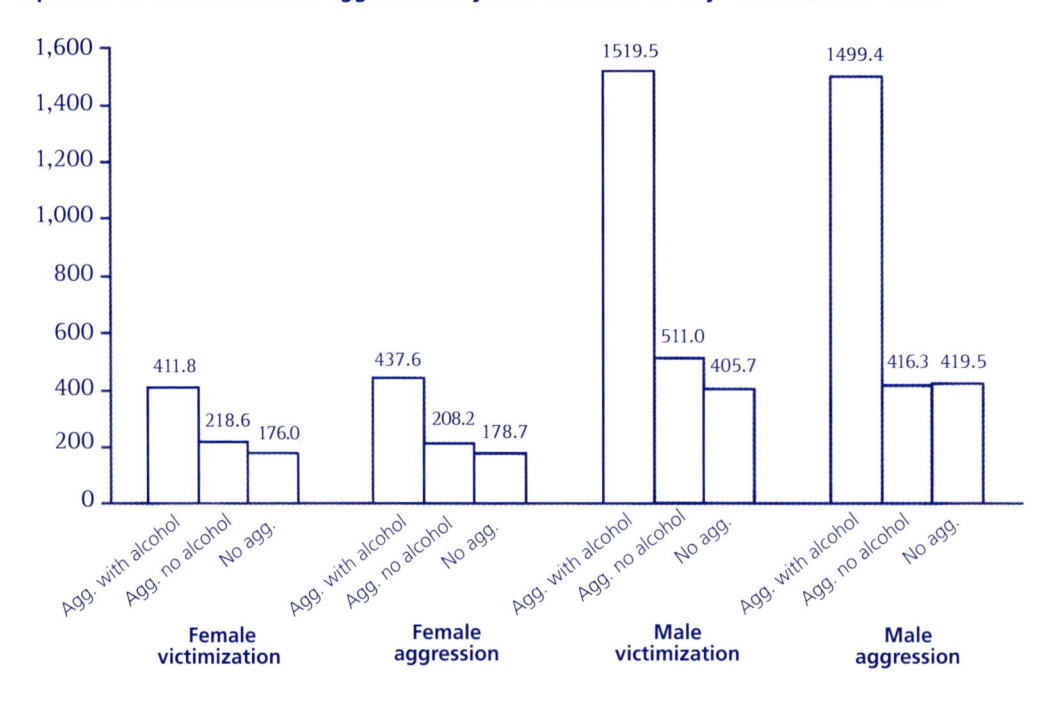

When the drinking pattern of those who reported an incident involving alcohol versus those who reported an incident that did not involve alcohol (i.e., excluding respondents who reported no aggression) was compared using logistic regression (controlling for age), those who reported that the incident involved alcohol were significantly heavier drinkers compared to those who reported that the incident did not involve alcohol on all three measures of alcohol consumption (p values < .01 for all comparisons).

Discussion

Rates of partner aggression in the GENACIS Canada survey were slightly higher than those found in previous Canadian national surveys (Johnson, 2006), possibly because of the two-year rather than one-year time frame, possibly because the sample was limited to persons aged 76 and younger or because the definition of physical aggression included even minor aggression and did not specify whether the aggression occurred within the context of conflict. Although the decrease in partner aggression with age is similar to previous findings (Wilson, Johnson, and Daly, 1995; Johnson, 2006), a notable difference of the GENACIS results, compared to those of previous surveys, is that a higher proportion of male than female respondents reported being the victim of partner aggression. Part of this difference may be attributable to earlier surveys explicitly asking about sexual aggression (Johnson, 2006), while the GENACIS survey used an open-ended approach that did not preclude sexual aggression but did not specifically remind respondents to include it. Thus, rates of partner aggression may be underestimated, especially for female respondents, because forced sex was not listed explicitly in the examples of types of physical aggression.

An interesting pattern of partner aggression emerged relating to marital status; specifically, that married persons reported the lowest rate of partner aggression compared to cohabiting partners, divorced/separated, and never married. Surveys including questions on partner aggression, such as the GSS (Bunge and Locke, 2000; AuCoin, 2005), often include only persons who are currently married or were previously involved in a relationship. These results suggest the importance of also examining aggression between intimate partners who are not married or living together (i.e., the never-married group). In addition, this study confirms previous research of the increased risk of victimization for women who are divorced/separated (Dekeseredy, Rogness, and Schwartz 2004; AuCoin, 2005).

The current study adds to knowledge on partner aggression in Canada by allowing gender comparisons involving victimization by one gender and aggression by the other. For example, the higher rate of men than women reporting aggression by a partner is mirrored by the higher rate of women than men reporting aggression *toward* a partner. Thus, although we did not collect reports from both the male and female partners of the same couple, reports from men and women on both perpetration and victimization allow comparison that may identify important gender differences in how partner aggression is perceived or measured.

One such gender difference emerged regarding the severity ratings. Although female victims rated aggression against them as being more severe than did male victims (consistent with gender differences in severity found in previous research—see Johnson, 2006), male aggressors did not rate their own aggression toward female partners at the same level of severity as did female victims—that is, female victims perceived acts of aggression against them as being more severe than male aggressors rated their own acts toward female victims. This difference in rating of severity was not found between male victims and female aggressors.

A similar difference between victim and aggressor reports was apparent in reporting of type of aggressive act. While both male and female respondents reported that men were more likely to push, shove, and grab, while females were more likely than males to slap (which is consistent with gender differences in acts of aggression found in previous studies—see Johnson, 2006), female victims were more likely than male aggressors to report that the male partner punched or beat them up. Consistent with the victim's perspective, female victims were also more likely than male victims to seek medical attention following the incident.

Unfortunately, we do not know from the current study whether these victim/aggressor differences are due to underrepresentation in the survey of men who perpetrate more severe acts of violence or because men underestimate or underreport the severity of their own violence. The relatively low rate of aggression toward a partner reported by divorced/separated men, compared to the high rate of victimization reported by divorced/separated women, also suggests either reporting bias by some aggressive men or underrepresentation of some types of aggressive men, such as those who are divorced/separated.

In terms of gender differences in being afraid, upset, or angry, female victims gave the highest ratings (which would be expected, given that this group perceived the aggressive act as having been more severe than did other groups); however, the next highest ratings for upset and angry were by female aggressors, suggesting possibly a gender factor in either experiencing or reporting aggression. Interestingly, of the four groups, male victims rated themselves as the least afraid, upset, and angry. Thus, even though the current study did not explicitly include sexual aggression and did not include items regarding other aspects of emotional or psychological abuse, these findings reinforce results from previous studies suggesting that not only are women more likely than men to suffer physical injury from aggression, the emotional and psychological experience of aggression may be quite different for women than for men (Graham and Wells, 2001), as well.

Gender and victim/aggressor differences also emerged relating to which of the partners was drinking at the time of the incident. In particular, for female-to-male aggression, male victims were more likely than female aggressors to report that no one was drinking, while female aggressors were more likely to report that only the male victim was drinking. With regard to reporting of alcohol involvement for female victims versus male aggressors, there was a significant pattern for female victims to be more likely to report that only the male aggressor was drinking, while male aggressors were more likely to report that both or only the female was drinking. This is similar to findings from the 1999 GSS that female victims were more likely than male victims to report that the aggressor had been drinking (Bunge, 2000).

The results linking greater severity of aggression with drinking by one or both partners at the time of the incident confirm findings from previous research in Canada (Desjardins and Hotton, 2004). In the current study, despite gender and role differences in reporting who was drinking, there was a consistent pattern across male and female victims and aggressors for aggression to be rated as more severe in incidents in which one or both partners had been drinking, compared to incidents in which no one had been drinking. This suggests that alcohol may play an important role in the escalation of aggression or in the aggressor being unable to control the forcefulness of his or her aggression.

Previous studies of intimate partner aggression have identified a relationship between drinking pattern of the male partner and higher risk of violence against women (Johnson, 2000, 2006). In the present study, we analyzed the drinking pattern of the respondent, not the partner, but were able to examine this relationship for both victimization and aggression toward a partner, and for respondents whose most severe incident involved alcohol versus respondents whose most severe incident did not involve alcohol. A clear pattern emerged across all alcohol consumption measures; namely, that men and women who reported that their most severe incident involved one or both partners drinking, drank more frequently, more drinks per occasion, and more overall, compared with both respondents who reported no aggression and with respondents who reported that the most severe incident did not involve alcohol.

Although previous studies linking drinking and partner aggression have not tested whether the link is limited to aggression involving alcohol, the findings from the present study are consistent with previous research based on Canadian respondents that drinking pattern is linked to those reporting aggression involving alcohol but less related to aggression that does not involve alcohol (Wells and Graham, 2003). However in the current analyses, there was a trend (significant only for female victims) for drinking more drinks per occasion to be higher for those who reported aggression that did not involve drinking, compared with those who reported no aggression. While the relationship between whether aggression involved drinking and respondent's frequency of drinking may simply reflect exposure or criterion contamination rather than an actual relationship between drinking and aggression (i.e., people who drink more often are more likely to have been drinking at the time of an aggressive incident purely by chance), the strong relationship with usual quantity consumed per occasion (even after controlling for age), taken together with the greater severity of aggression when alcohol is involved, suggests that other mechanisms may be involved. For example, the effects of alcohol on emotions, problem-solving, and risk-taking (Graham, West, and Wells, 2000) may influence the escalation of conflict to make aggression both more likely and more severe. There may, of course, be other factors linking drinking with violence, including risk factors for partner aggression being greater among heavier drinkers (Johnson, 2001), situational influences associated with drinking occasions (Wilkinson and Hamerschlag, 2005), and heavier drinking being a consequence rather than a cause of partner aggression (Martino, Collins, and Ellickson, 2005).

Some limitations are noteworthy in the present analyses. First, some partner violence would have been missed because the questions focused only on physical aggression and did not include verbal threats or emotional or psychological abuse or explicitly ask about sexual aggression. On the other hand, as was evident from the kinds of acts described and the severity ratings, the question was able to elicit even minor aggression, in that many respondents were describing very minor acts of aggression that would not necessarily constitute "abuse." Including even minor aggression may be an important aspect of this approach because existing research suggests that the majority of homicides between intimate couples in Canada were preceded by a history of violence between the victim and the accused (Johnson, 2006).

Acknowledgments

Funding for this research was provided through an operations grant from the Canadian Institutes of Health Research. Kathryn Graham was Principal Investigator and Andrée Demers was Co-Principal Investigator. Sharon Bernards was Project Coordinator. Co-Investigators were Louise Nadeau, Jürgen Rehm, Sylvia Kairouz, Colleen Ann Dell, Christiane Poulin, Anne George, and Samantha Wells. We are grateful to the staff at the Institute for Social Research at York University and to Jolicoeur and Associates for their assistance in implementing the survey. This research was conducted in Canada as part of the GENACIS initiative, a collaborative multinational project led by Sharon Wilsnack and affiliated with the Kettil Bruun Society for Social and Epidemiological Research on Alcohol.

References

AuCoin K. (Ed.) (2005). *Family violence in Canada: A statistical profile.* Ottawa, Canada: Canadian Centre for Justice Statistics , Statistics Canada. www.statcan.ca. Catalogue no. 85-224-XIE

Brownridge D. (2002). Cultural variation in male partner violence against women: A comparison of Quebec with the rest of Canada. *Violence against Women*, 8(1), 87–115.

Bunge VP. (2000). Spousal violence (pp. 11–26). In V. P. Bunge & D. Locke (Eds.), *Family violence in Canada: A statistical profile*. Ottawa, Canada: Canadian Centre for Justice Statistics, Statistics Canada. www.statcan.ca. Catalogue no. 85-224-XIE

Bunge VP, Locke D. (eds.) (2000). *Family violence in Canada: A statistical profile*. Ottawa, Canada: Canadian Centre for Justice Statistics, Statistics Canada. www.statcan.ca. Catalogue no. 85-224-XIE

Dekeseredy WS, Rogness, M. and Schwartz, M.D. (2004). Separation/divorce sexual assault: The current state of social scientific knowledge. *Aggression and Violent Behavior*, 9, 675–691.

Desjardins N, Hotton T. (2004). Trends in drug offences and the role of alcohol and drugs in crime. Juristat (Statistics Canada – Catalogue no. 85-002-XPE, Vol. 24, no. 1), Canadian Centre for Justice Statistics.

Graham K, West P, Wells S. (2000). Evaluating theories of alcohol-related aggression using observations of young adults in bars. *Addiction*, 95(6), 847–863.

Graham K, Wells S. (2001). The two worlds of aggression for men and women. *Sex Roles. A Journal of Research*, 45, 595–622.

Johnson H. (2000) The role of alcohol in male partners' assaults on wives. *Journal of Drug Issues*, 30, 725–740.

Johnson H. (2006) *Measuring violence against women. Statistical trends 2006*. Ottawa, Canada: Canadian Centre for Justice Statistics, Statistics, Canada.

Johnson H. (2007) Preventing violence against women: Progress and challenges. *Institute for the Prevention of Crime Review*, 1, 69–88.

Johnson H, AuCoin KA. (Eds.) (2003) *Family violence in Canada. A statistical profile*. Ottawa, Canada: Canadian Centre for Justice Statistics, Statistics, Canada.

Locke D. (2000). Family homicide (pp. 39–44). In V. P. Bunge & D. Locke (Eds.), *Family violence in Canada: A statistical profile*. Ottawa, Canada: Canadian Centre for Justice Statistics, Statistics Canada. *www.statcan.ca*. Catalogue no. 85-224-XIE

Martino SC, Collins RL, Ellickson PL. (2005). Cross-lagged relationships between substance use and intimate partner violence among a sample of young adult women. *Journal of Studies on Alcohol*, 66, 139–148.

Mihorean K. (2005). Trends in self-reported spousal violence. In K. AuCoin (Ed.) *Family violence in Canada: A statistical profile*. Ottawa, Canada: Canadian Centre for Justice Statistics, Statistics Canada. *www.statcan.ca*. Catalogue no. 85-224-XIE

Statistics Canada. Overview 2006. Population by sex and age group. *http://www40.statcan.ca/l01/ind01/l2_3867.htm*

Trainor C. (Ed.) (2002). *Family violence in Canada: A statistical profile*. Ottawa, Canada: Canadian Centre for Justice Statistics , Statistics Canada. www.statcan.ca. Catalogue no. 85-224-XIE

Wells S, Graham K. (2003). Aggression involving alcohol: Relationship to drinking patterns and social context. *Addiction*, 98(1), 33–42.

Wilkinson DL, Hamerschlag SJ. (2005). Situational determinants in intimate partner violence. *Aggression and Violent Behavior*, 10, 333–361.

Wilson M, Johnson H, Daly M. (1995). Lethal and nonlethal violence against wives. *Canadian Journal of Criminology*, 37(3), 331–361.

UNHAPPY HOURS:

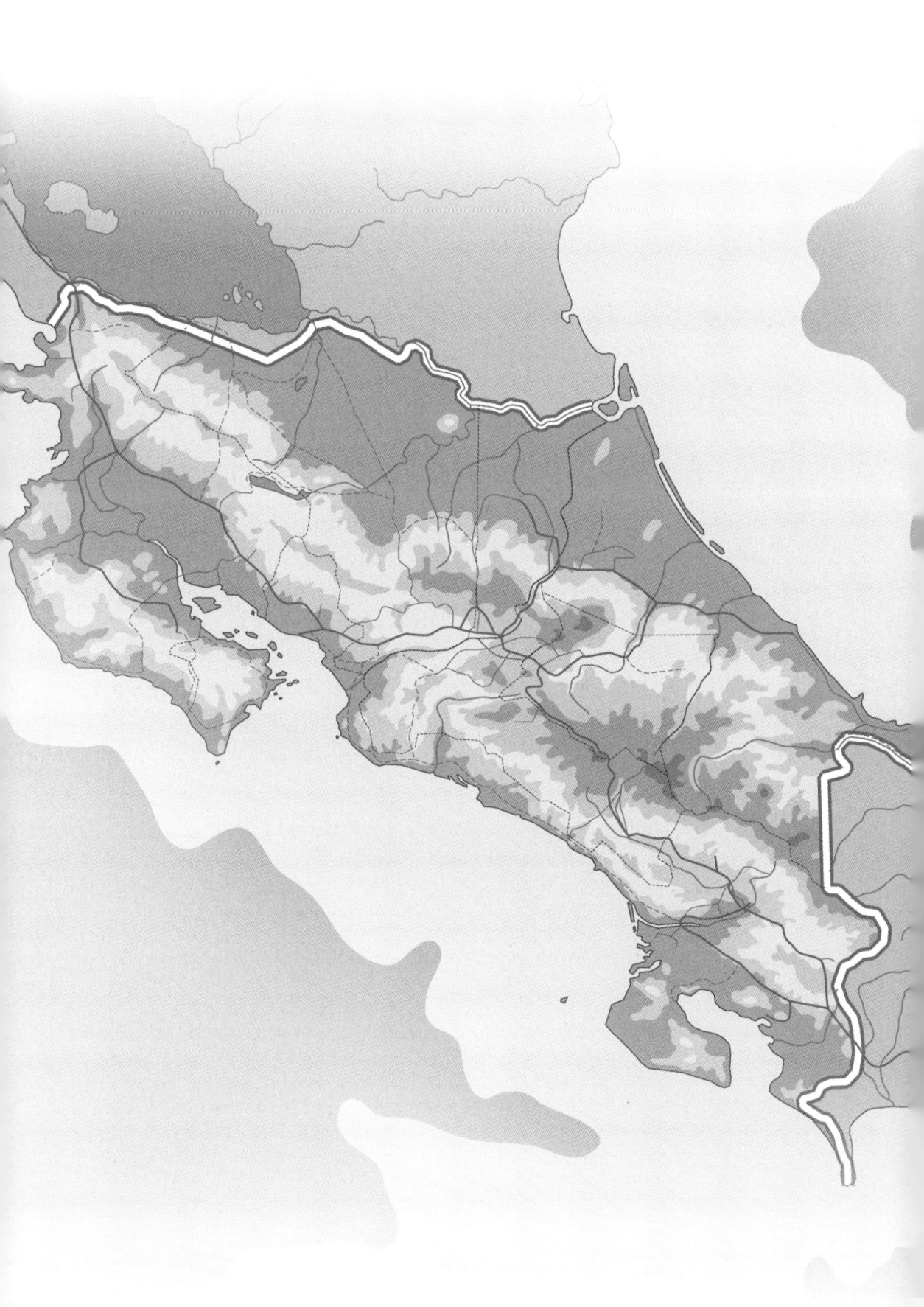

Costa Rica: Alcohol and Partner Physical Aggression in the Greater Metropolitan Area of San José —Julio Bejarano

Introduction

According to the Inter-American Development Bank, 2% of the gross national product of Latin America is spent on addressing the effects of domestic violence. Women who are victims of domestic violence undergo more surgical interventions and medical and pharmacological treatment and spend more days in hospitals and in mental health sessions, compared with women who have not been the victims of violence (Creel, 2001).

A survey on domestic violence conducted in 2002 (González, 2003) determined that 67% of Costa Rican women experienced at least one type of physical or psychological violence during their lifetime. Four out of 10 of these victims experienced physical aggression, and 15% experienced sexual violence. The most common acts of physical aggression were hair-pulling, arm-twisting, pushing, hitting, kicking and biting, and, less frequently, being strangled, asphyxiated, burned, or attacked by any kind of weapon.

An examination of 6,000 medical postmortem evaluations carried out over a five-year period in the province of Cartago (located next to San José province and the capital city) established that domestic violence had occurred in 12% of the cases, yielding a ratio of 5.5 female victims for each male victim (Uribe, 2001). However, during the study period, the percentage of male victims increased from 15% to 22%. Homicide cases involving female victims also provide information about domestic violence. During the 1990s, there were 315 female homicide victims, with 58% of these being attributed to domestic or sexual violence. In 2005 alone, there were 60 cases, with half of these being attributed to domestic violence and 20% being related to problems of a sexual or passionate nature (Costa Rica, Poder Judicial, 2006).

A law against domestic violence was enacted in Costa Rica in 1996 to regulate and enforce protective measures towards the life, integrity, and dignity of victims of domestic, or intra-family, violence. Domestic violence was defined as an action or the lack of action taken by a family member that directly or indirectly puts at risk or diminishes the physical, sexual, or psychological integrity of a person. The offices of the public prosecutor, the police, and the ombudsman have special units devoted to domestic violence issues. The law requires training for police personnel on the handling of domestic violence situations, and for public hospitals to report cases of domestic violence. Nineteen measures may be taken by the courts, including relocating the victim into a new household; forcing aggressors to leave their current home and prohibiting future access; not allowing aggressors to continue serving as the primary caregiver, educator, and protector of their children; and issuing protective orders for the neighborhood police. The victim also may carry a copy of the protective order so that she or he can obtain assistance from the nearest authority if the partner makes a threat away from the home. These measures usually remain in effect for no less than a month and not more than six months, but may be altered if needed. (Costa Rica, Asamblea Legislativa, 1996). Law 8589, enacted in 2006, increases the penalties for cases in which a woman is abused or killed by an intimate partner or by sexual violence. Criminal penalties range from 10 to 100 days in prison for aggravated threats and up to 35 years in prison for aggravated homicide.

It is estimated that between 5,000 and 6,000 complaints of domestic violence are brought to the attention of the Costa Rican police each year. However, only one in every four of these cases will be forwarded by the law enforcement system to the courts (Rojas, 2002). During 2000–2001, 11,286 new violence protective order applications were filed (Rojas, Jiménez, and Cruz, 2004), with 90% of these involving petitions by women against their partners. Some have argued that although reporting of domestic violence has been on the rise since the time the 1996 law was enacted, this number may start to decrease as more individuals become aware of the legal penalties for committing acts of domestic violence and curb their violent behavior in order to avoid these penalties (Solana, 2006).

In 1999, the Women's National Institute provided services to 5,188 women; this figure rose to 5,404 in 2002 and stood at 5,934 in 2005. This government institution also administers three shelters in the country; however, these facilities have only limited occupancy given the increasing demand for their services (Rojas, Jiménez, and Cruz, 2004). For instance, while approximately 80 women received services from the shelters in 1995, 749 women and children received services in 2000, and by 2005 this number had risen to 340 women and 693 children.

Alcohol Consumption and Partner Aggression

In terms of the relationship between partner violence and alcohol consumption in Costa Rica, the available research is very scarce. Per capita consumption of alcohol in the country is about 2 liters of absolute alcohol, which is below the average of 5.45 liters for the population aged 15 years and older in the Region of the Americas (WHO, 2004). Although this consumption level is low compared to that of industrialized nations, heavy episodic drinking (i.e., drinking large amounts per occasion) is common. Household surveys conducted during the 1990s indicated that males drank more frequently and more drinks per occasion than did females within all age groups (Bejarano and Ugalde, 2003). However, this gender difference seems to be narrowing as the drinking patterns of young educated females become increasingly similar to those of their male counterparts (Bejarano, Ugalde, and Fonseca, 2004)

A number of sources suggest that males in Costa Rica are much more likely than females to be physically aggressive toward an intimate partner (González, 2003; Rojas, Jiménez, and Cruz, 2004; Sagot and Guzmán, 2004). Males also produce greater injury and are more able to generate fear and terror in their partners. While women may also engage in aggressive acts toward a partner, this aggression is more likely to be minor, and females are more likely than males to end up more seriously injured (Bland and Orne, 1986; Arias, Samios, and O'Leary, 1987; Archer, 2002).

Methods
Survey and Sample
The sample framework for this research was obtained from the National Institute of Statistics and Census of Costa Rica. The study used a multi-stage cluster design in a household survey of persons 18 years of age or older residing temporarily or permanently in the Greater Metropolitan Area of San José. This region consists of the national capital of San José as well as the capital cities of the country's other three principal provinces (Alajuela, Cartago, and Heredia) which, together, contain nearly one-half of the country's population and households. The primary unit for sampling was a geographic area with an arbitrary delimitation of streets and approximately 70 households each. The selection of each of these segments was proportional to the current number of households. The second sampling stage was the household, which was selected systematically from an initial random start. To facilitate this task, the interviewers used current, detailed maps of the study area. The last unit of sampling was the individual per household. Each subject was randomly selected through a route page.

The survey was conducted as part of the GENACIS collaboration (Gender, Alcohol, and Culture: An International Study).The data were collected between July and November 2003 utilizing face-to-face interviews carried out by nine senior-level university students, most of whom had previous interviewing experience. As is usual in this type of study, the sample did not include persons in hospitals and detention centers. Table 1 shows the general characteristics of the male and female respondents.

Measures that Differed from the Core Questions
Respondents who indicated that their current partner was the same sex and was also the partner involved in the aggression were excluded from these analyses (15 males and 10 females for victimization and 15 males and 10 females for aggression by the respondent). This group included some respondents for whom the most severe aggression involved their current same sex partner, but the type of aggression was subsequently considered to not be physical (e.g., verbal threats). Whether the respondent drank five or more drinks during the past year was based on a graduated frequency approach described in the chapter "Common Survey Method and Analyses Conducted for Each Country Chapter."

Results
As shown in Figure 1, similar rates of males and females reported aggressive acts toward a partner as well as being victims of aggression. Both males and females were more likely to report being victims than aggressors (but none of these differences reached the criterion for statistical significance). Males and females who reported being involved in partner physical aggression were also similar in terms of those who reported being both a victim and an aggressor (21.1% and 23.5%, respectively), a victim only (47.4% and 47.1%, respectively) and an aggressor only (31.6% and 29.4%, respectively).

TABLE 1. Age, marital status, employment status, and drinking pattern in the 12 months preceding the survey, for male and female respondents, GENACIS survey, Costa Rica, 2003.

	Males (N=416)		Females (N=857)	
	Number	Percent or mean	Number	Percent or mean
Age		38.4 years		40.0 years
18–24 years	98	23.6%	175	20.4%
25–34 years	96	23.1%	170	19.8%
35–44 years	80	19.2%	204	23.8%
45–54 years	71	17.1%	160	18.7%
55 years and older	71	17.0%	148	17.3%
Marital status				
Married	181	43.5%	400	46.7%
Cohabiting/Living with partner	56	13.5%	108	12.6%
Divorced or separated	23	5.5%	90	10.5%
Never married	148	35.6%	206	24.0%
Widowed	8	1.9%	53	6.2%
Employment status				
In labor force (working for pay or temporarily not working due to illness or parental leave)	300	72.1%	298	34.7%
Voluntarily unemployed (homemaker or other reasons)	6	1.4%	444	51.8%
Involuntarily unemployed	24	5.8%	22	2.6%
Student	44	10.6%	51	6.0%
Retired	42	10.1%	40	4.7%
Drinking pattern (past 12 months)				
Drank any alcohol during past 12 months	285	68.5%	367	42.8%
Average number of drinking days (drinkers only)		54.1 days		28.4 days
Average number of drinks per occasion (drinkers only)		5.0 drinks		2.7 drinks
Average annual volume (drinker only)[a]		349.0 drinks		97.6 drinks
Drank five or more drinks on at least one occasion (drinkers only)	153	53.7%	95	25.9%

Costa Rica

FIGURE 1. Percent of respondents who reported having been a victim or aggressor, by sex, GENACIS survey, Costa Rica, 2003.

Category	Percentage
Female victimization	7.1
Female aggression	5.3
Male victimization	6.5
Male aggression	5.0

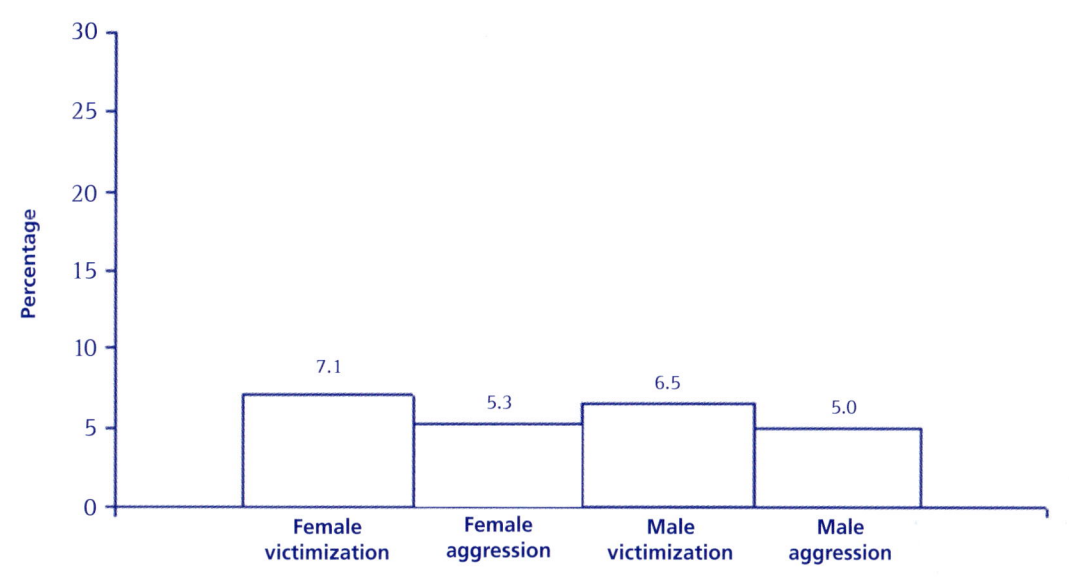

Female victims were 33.4 years of age on average, while the mean age of male aggressors was 28.9 years. The average age of male victims was 29.8 years and of female aggressors, 30.7 years. As shown in Figure 2, in general terms, physical aggression by a partner and toward a partner was higher for the younger age groups than for the oldest age group; however, there was no consistent decline with age, except for female aggressors. These results should be interpreted with caution, however, given the low number of reported cases in each age group, particularly among males.

FIGURE 2. Percent of respondents who reported having been a victim or aggressor, by age group and sex, GENACIS survey, Costa Rica, 2003.

Age group	Female victimization	Female aggression	Male victimization	Male aggression
18–24	10.4	8.7	7.4	9.5
25–34	9.5	8.9	13.8	5.3
35–44	5.5	5.9	4.0	6.6
45–54	8.4	1.3	4.4	1.5
55+	1.4	0.7	0.0	0.0

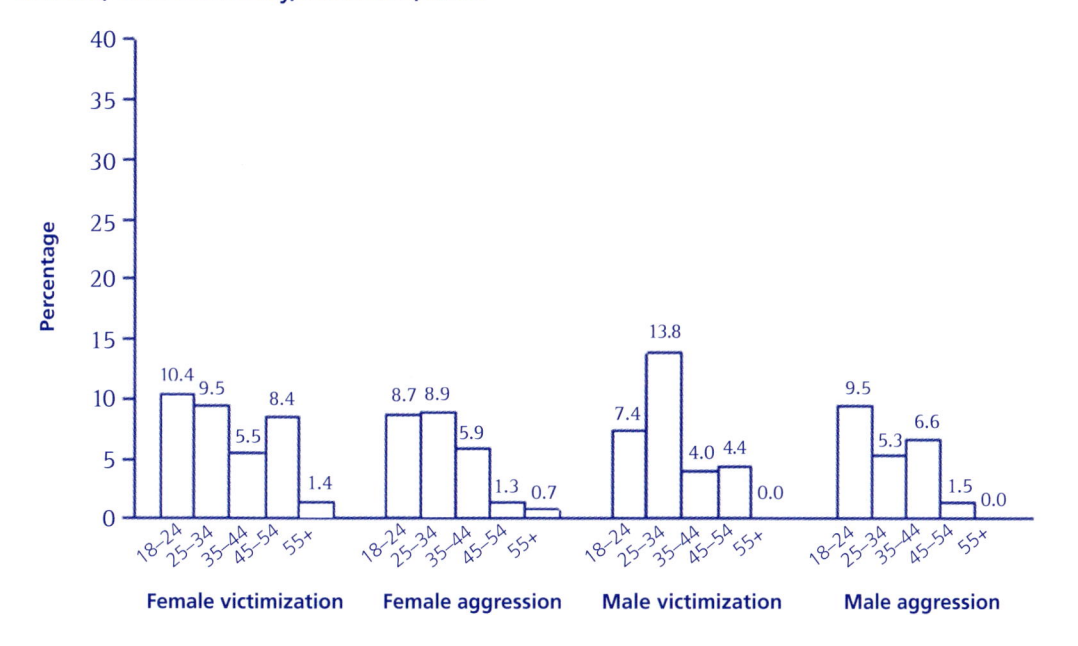

As shown in Figure 3, the percent reporting partner physical aggression varied by marital status (although these results, likewise, should be regarded with caution, due to the low number of reported cases, particularly for male victims and aggressors). Females who were cohabiting were more likely to report aggression by a partner, compared with females in other marital status groups, with the lowest percent of aggression by a partner being reported among never-married females. The percent of females reporting aggression toward a partner was similar across marital status groups, but tended to be highest among divorced or separated females and lowest among married females. Among male victims, never-married males reported the highest percent of physical aggression by a partner and cohabiting males reported the lowest. Never-married and cohabiting males reported the highest rates of being physically aggressive toward a partner, while none of the males who were divorced or separated reported aggression toward a partner. Using a p < .01 criterion for significance because of the number of comparisons, only the differences for cohabiting versus married female victims and cohabiting versus never married female victims were significant (p < .001 for both).

FIGURE 3. Percent of respondents who reported having been a victim or aggressor, by marital status and sex, GENACIS survey, Costa Rica, 2003.

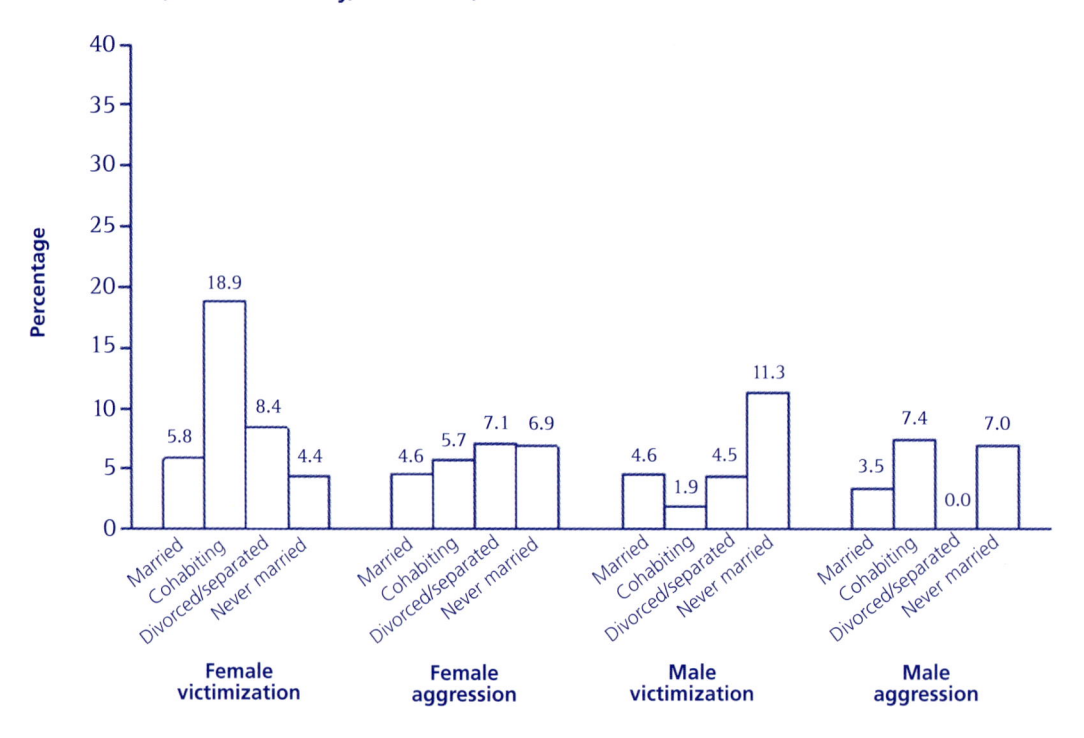

Category	Married	Cohabiting	Divorced/separated	Never married
Female victimization	5.8	18.9	8.4	4.4
Female aggression	4.6	5.7	7.1	6.9
Male victimization	4.6	1.9	4.5	11.3
Male aggression	3.5	7.4	0.0	7.0

Figure 4 shows the frequency of each type of aggression by sex and by whether the respondent was the victim or the aggressor. As shown in this figure, male aggressors were more likely than female aggressors to push ($p < .001$) or grab ($p < .01$), while male victims were more likely than female victims to report having an object thrown at them by an intimate partner ($p = .001$). Although the differences did not reach statistical significance, 18.3% of female victims reported being punched and 13% reported being beaten up while none of the male aggressors reported using these forms of aggression toward a female partner, and no male victims reported being beaten up. No other types of aggressive acts used by aggressors or reported by victims were significantly different between males and females.

FIGURE 4. Type of aggressive act against females as reported by female victims and male aggressors, and against males as reported by male victims and female aggressors, GENACIS survey, Costa Rica, 2003.

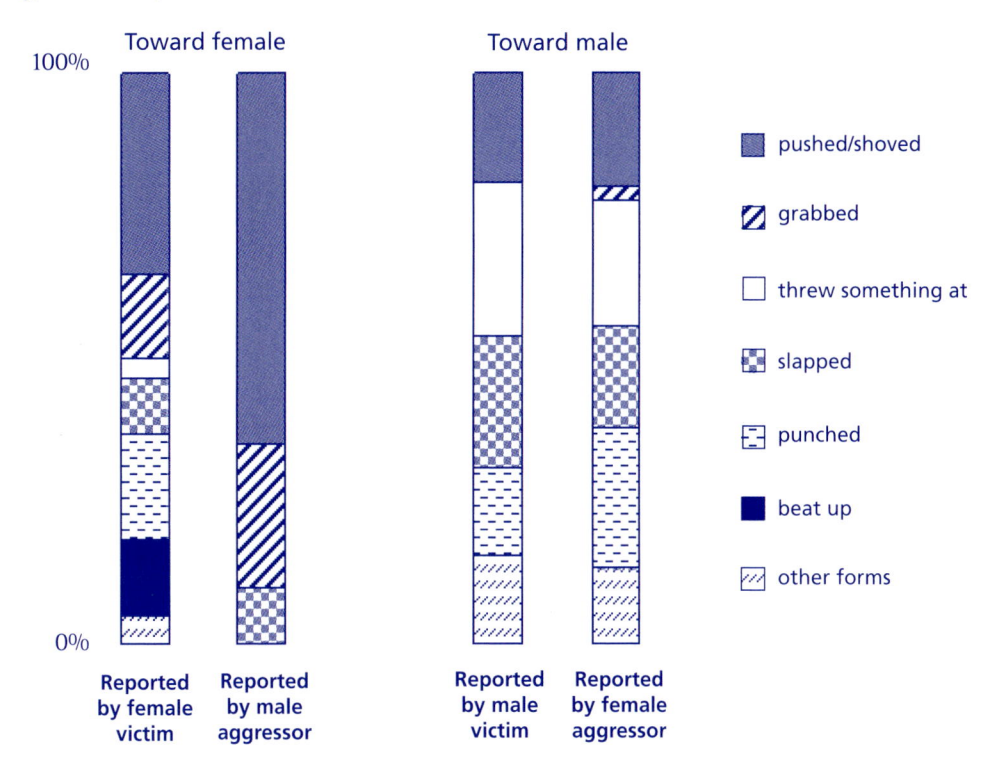

Figure 5 shows average ratings of the severity of aggression, as well as how scared, upset, and angry male and female victims and aggressors felt at the time of the aggressive incident. Analyses of variance controlling for age were used to test for significant differences between male and female victims, male and female aggressors, and for comparing male and female victims with aggressors of the opposite sex. Female victims rated the severity of the aggression used against them higher than did male victims ($p < .001$), and ratings by female victims were higher than ratings of male victims for the level of fear, upset (both $p < .001$), and anger ($p < .01$) felt. Ratings by male and female aggressors were significantly different only for anger, with female aggressors reporting higher levels of anger ($p < .05$) than their male counterparts. The levels of severity, upset, and fear reported by female victims were significantly higher than those reported by male aggressors ($p < 0.01$ for severity, $p < .001$ for upset and fear). A significant difference was also found between the level of severity ($p < .05$) and anger ($p < .001$) reported by female aggressors versus male victims. In addition to reporting that aggression was more severe, female victims were more likely than male victims to report seeking medical attention as a result of physical aggression by their partner (11.7% for female victims versus 0% for male victims, although this difference was not statistically significant.

FIGURE 5. Mean ratings of severity of aggression, fear, upset, and anger by male and female victims and aggressors, GENACIS survey, Costa Rica, 2003.

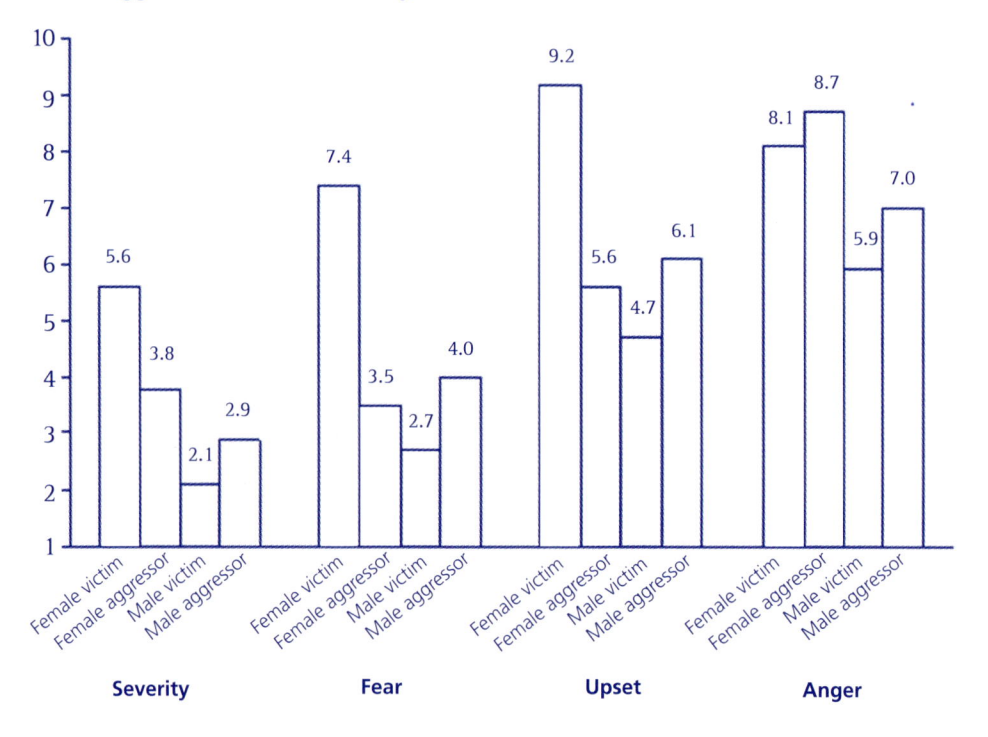

As shown in Figure 6, nearly 40% of female victims reported that one or both partners had been drinking (33% said only the male partner had been drinking), compared with 25% of male aggressors who reported that one or both had been drinking (20% male only drinking). About the same proportion (slightly under 27%) of male victims and female aggressors reported that one or both partners had been drinking; however, male victims were more likely to report that both partners had been drinking (11.5% male only, 11.5% both drinking), while female aggressors were more likely to report that only the male partner had been drinking (17.8% male only, 4.4% both drinking). None of these differences reached the criterion for statistical significance; moreover, all results should be interpreted with caution, once again due to low number of cases, particularly for males.

FIGURE 6. Percent of incidents in which no partner had been drinking, both partners had been drinking, only the male partner had been drinking, or only the female partner had been drinking, as reported by male and female victims and aggressors, GENACIS survey, Costa Rica, 2003.

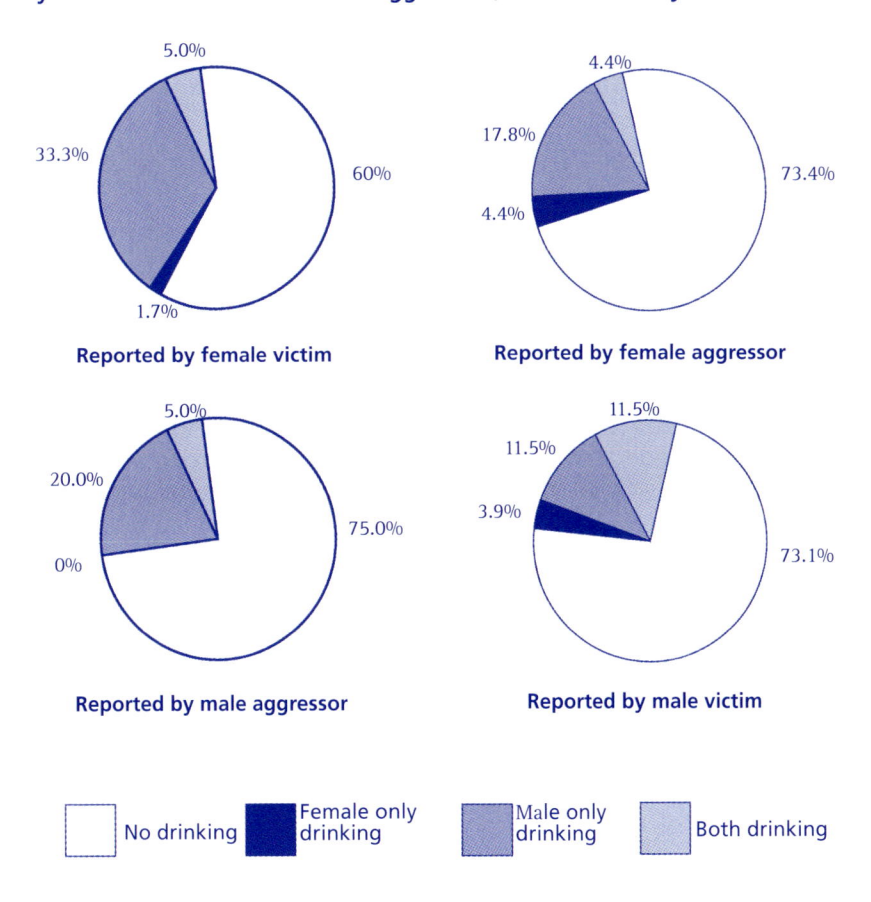

Reported by female victim: 60% No drinking, 1.7% Female only drinking, 33.3% Male only drinking, 5.0% Both drinking

Reported by female aggressor: 73.4% No drinking, 4.4% Female only drinking, 17.8% Male only drinking, 4.4% Both drinking

Reported by male aggressor: 75.0% No drinking, 0% Female only drinking, 20.0% Male only drinking, 5.0% Both drinking

Reported by male victim: 73.1% No drinking, 3.9% Female only drinking, 11.5% Male only drinking, 11.5% Both drinking

Legend: No drinking | Female only drinking | Male only drinking | Both drinking

Female victims who reported that one or both partners had been drinking rated the severity of the partner's aggression significantly higher (mean rating of 6.8 out of 10), compared to ratings by female victims who reported no drinking at the time of the incident (mean rating of 4.8) ($p < .05$). It was not possible to compare ratings of severity for incidents in which one or both partners were drinking to incidents in which no one had been drinking for female aggressors and for male victims and aggressors because of the low number of cases.

The Relationship between Alcohol Consumption and Partner Aggression

The percentage of males and females who reported partner physical aggression was higher for those who drank alcohol in the past year than for those who abstained: among males, 8.4% of drinkers versus 2.4% of abstainers reported being victims, and 7.3% of drinkers versus 0.0% of abstainers reported being aggressors; among females, 8.2% of drinkers versus 6.2% of abstainers reported being victims, and 8.2% of drinkers versus 3.1% of abstainers reported being aggressors. Logistic regression analysis of victimization or aggression on drinker status indicated a significant relationship only for female aggression after controlling for age (odds ratio = 2.27, $p = .013$). It was not possible to perform logistic regression for aggression by male respondents due to the small cell sizes.

Respondents' Drinking Pattern and Partner Aggression

The analysis in this section will be limited to current drinkers, i.e., respondents who consumed alcohol during the year preceding the survey.

As shown in Figure 7, the percentage of respondents reporting partner physical aggression was higher among those who consumed five or more drinks on at least one occasion during the past year, compared to those who did not drink five or more drinks (significant for both female and male aggressors controlling for age [$p < .05$ for both] but not for victims of either sex).

FIGURE 7. Percent of male and female respondents who reported victimization (aggression by a partner) and aggression (aggression toward a partner) by whether respondent had consumed five or more drinks on an occasion or had never consumed five drinks on an occasion, by sex, GENACIS survey, Costa Rica, 2003.

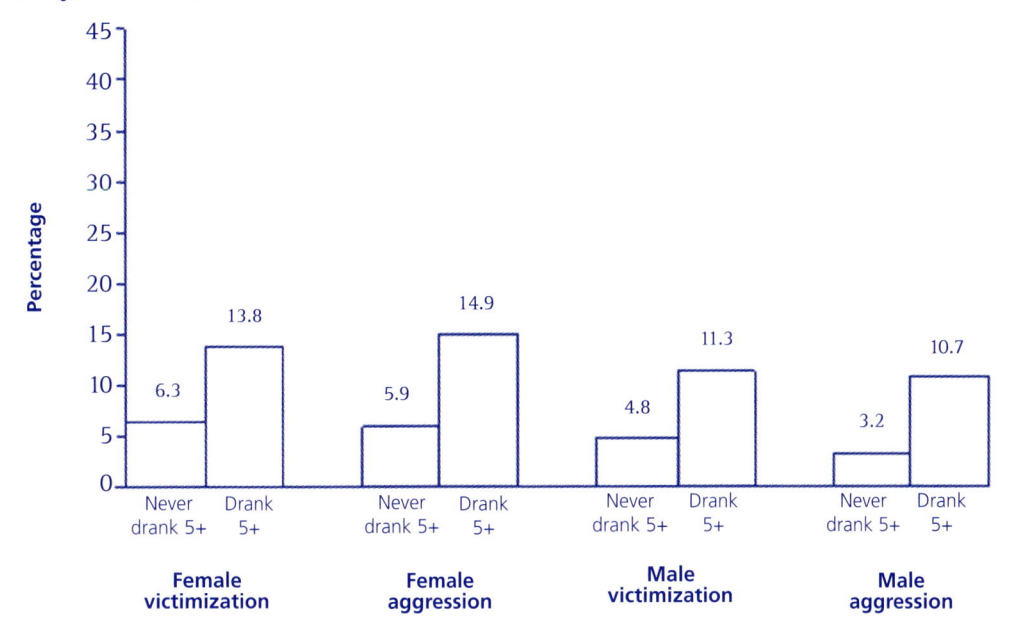

	Never drank 5+	Drank 5+
Female victimization	6.3	13.8
Female aggression	5.9	14.9
Male victimization	4.8	11.3
Male aggression	3.2	10.7

Female victims and male aggressors reported more frequent drinking than did female and male respondents who reported no partner aggression, and the number of drinks per occasion and total number of drinks in the past year were higher for those who reported partner physical aggression compared to those who reported no aggression among female victims and aggressors and male victims and aggressors (see Figures 8, 9, and 10). Differences between those who reported aggression and those who reported no aggression were significant (controlling for age) only for male aggressors for number of drinking days (i.e., frequency of drinking) and total number of drinks (both $p < .05$), and for female aggressors for usual number of drinks per occasion ($p < .01$).

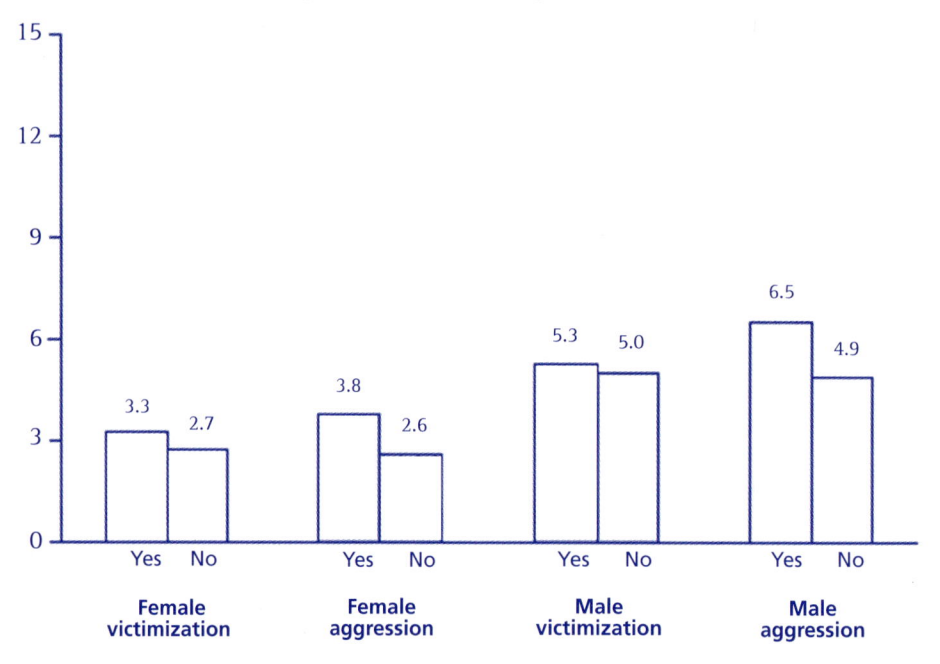

FIGURE 8. Mean number of drinking days in the year preceding the survey by whether the respondent had been a victim of partner aggression and whether the respondent had been aggressive toward a partner, by sex, GENACIS survey, Costa Rica, 2003.

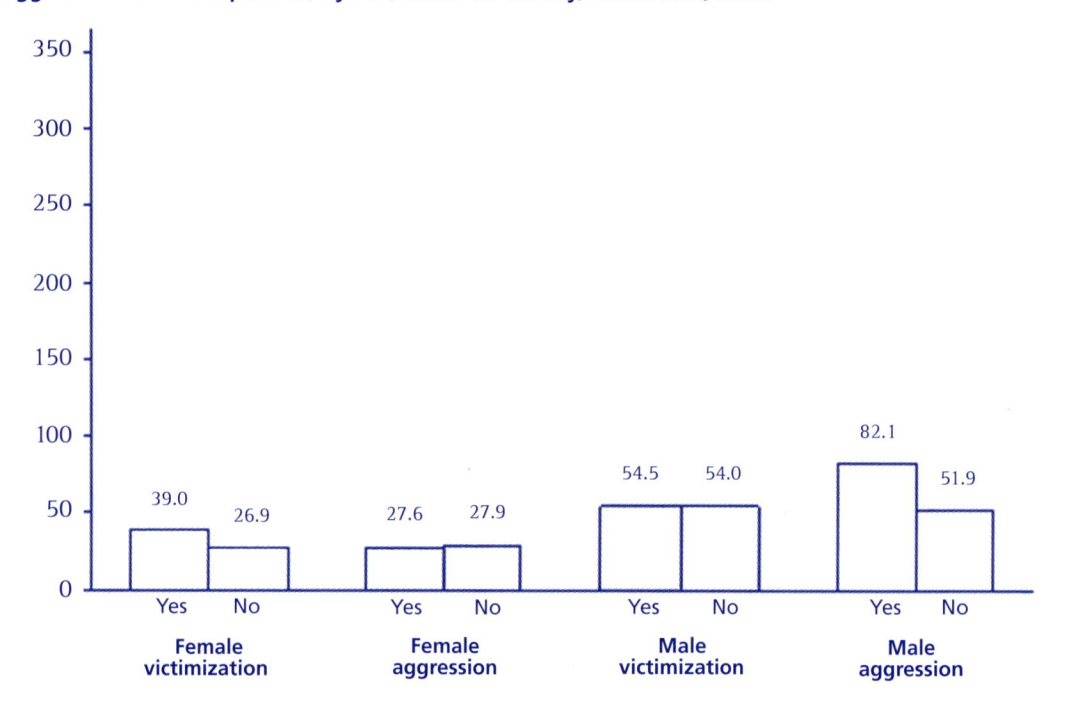

	Yes	No
Female victimization	39.0	26.9
Female aggression	27.6	27.9
Male victimization	54.5	54.0
Male aggression	82.1	51.9

FIGURE 9. Mean number of drinks consumed on usual drinking occasions by whether the respondent had been a victim of partner aggression and whether the respondent had been aggressive toward a partner, by sex, GENACIS survey, Costa Rica, 2003.

	Yes	No
Female victimization	3.3	2.7
Female aggression	3.8	2.6
Male victimization	5.3	5.0
Male aggression	6.5	4.9

FIGURE 10. Overall mean number of drinks consumed annually by whether the respondent had been a victim of partner aggression and whether the respondent had been aggressive toward a partner, by sex, GENACIS survey, Costa Rica, 2003.

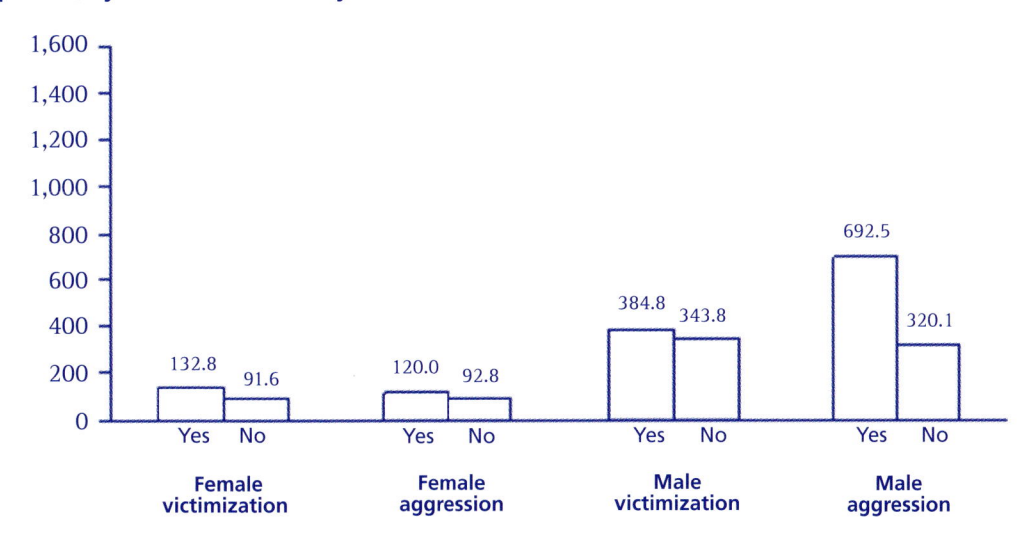

	Yes	No
Female victimization	132.8	91.6
Female aggression	120.0	92.8
Male victimization	384.8	343.8
Male aggression	692.5	320.1

Discussion

Although this study shows that about the same percentage of males and females reported physical aggression by and toward a partner within a two-year time frame consistent with previous research, female victims rated the severity of the physical aggression and their feelings of fear, anger, and upset higher than did male victims. Female aggressors also rated the severity of their own aggression and their level of anger higher than did male victims and male aggressors. In addition to higher ratings of severity, female victims were more likely to report experiencing more severe types of aggression, such as being beaten up or punched, although no male aggressors reported using these types of aggression against their female partners. Female victims were also more likely than male victims to have sought medical attention (although this difference was not significant).

The fact that partner aggression is more prevalent among younger age groups may be partly related to the fact that younger people drink more and show higher alcohol-related risk behaviors than those in older age groups. Local research carried out in the 25–59-year-old age group (Bejarano, Ugalde, and Fonseca, 2006) and in the age group of 60 years and older (Bejarano and Sáenz, 2004) confirm the riskier drinking behavior of younger adults. A previous study carried out in Costa Rica showed that physical aggression toward the partner was higher among younger respondents than among older adults and in those who reported binge drinking one or more times during the month prior to the survey (Orpinas, 1999). These findings have several implications for prevention. Prevention should focus on managing conflict and aggression for young people of both sexes. Each needs to understand the role both play, while still putting a differential responsibility on males, since this group can and often does inflict greater injury.

Reports by men and women with respect to alcohol consumption at the time of the incident were inconsistent, in that female victims were more likely than male aggressors to report that if any of the partners was drinking during the incident, it was only the male who drank. Similarly, female aggressors tended to report that the male only was drinking, while more male victims reported that both partners or only the female were drinking than that only the male was drinking. These analyses, however, as already noted, were limited by the small number of cases, and the findings should be treated with caution. Nevertheless, other findings related to respondents' usual drinking habits suggest that a relationship does exist between alcohol consumption in general and partner aggression. Men and women who drank five or more drinks on at least one occasion during the past year were more likely than those who did not drink five drinks to report aggression by a partner and aggression toward a partner. The mean number of drinks consumed per occasion and the total number of drinks per year were higher for all four groups of those reporting aggression (female and male victims, female and male aggressors) than for males and females who reported no aggression, and female victims and male aggressors reported a higher number of drinking days in the past year than did females who were not victims and males who were not aggressors. In addition, female victims rated the severity of the aggression higher when one or both the partners were drinking during the incident compared to incidents in which no one was drinking.

Thus, the findings of this study add to the current state of knowledge about the relationship between alcohol, gender, and violence, which has been insufficient in Costa Rica, specifically, and in Latin America in a general sense. Moreover, risks associated with alcohol consumption have, to date, been viewed more from a medical model perspective in terms of health consequences, with insufficient attention being accorded to the social consequences of drinking, such as partner physical aggression.

The status of women in Costa Rica is in transition, with women increasingly tending to have a higher educational level, work outside the home, and be a principal family wage-earner, within a social environment characterized by laws that promote gender equity within the educational system and workplace and legislation that protects them against domestic violence. It is difficult to know whether this change in status will place women at greater risk of other types of partner aggression (i.e., more psychological than physical) because men feel threatened by these changes or whether the improved status of women will result in greater empowerment and lower risk of partner aggression. A national survey carried out in 2003 established that women who had attained higher levels of education (high school [64%] or some university [63.1%]) reported the highest incidence of violence, although this finding may be related to their greater capacity, compared to women with lower educational levels, to identify and recognize violence against them. Women with income (particularly if earned while working outside the home) reported more violence (61.1%) than the national average and also reported a higher level of violence than women without income (52.6%). One interpretation of these findings is that women with income are more confident about their capacity to effectively deal with violent situations and in their ability to denounce the situation to the justice system (Sagot and Guzman, 2004), although these findings may reflect the fact that better educated women who are working outside the home tend to be younger than women who are less educated and work in the home.

It is important to acknowledge some limitations of the study. Males in the sample were underrepresented because it was more likely to find a woman at home during the fieldwork. Therefore, results should be treated with caution due to the small number of cases, particularly for men. Also, as discussed above, women who were employed outside the home may be more likely than those in the home to have reported a higher rate of aggression both by and toward a partner, and this might explain in part why the rates of violence against women found in the current sample were lower than those found in other studies. Similarly, given that it is normative for men to work outside the home, men who participated in the survey (i.e., those who were found at home during the daytime) may also not have been representative of males generally in terms of partner aggression. Another possible explanation for the lower rates of aggression found in the current study is related to the household face-to-face interview methodology, which may have increased the tendency of respondents to give socially desirable responses and thus lead to underreporting of aggression.

Despite these limitations, this study sheds important new light on the nature of partner physical aggression by both males and females; the greater physical and emotional impact of partner aggression felt by females versus males; and the relationship between partner aggression, age, marital and employment status, and, especially, alcohol consumption.

References

Archer J. (2002). Sex differences in physically aggressive acts between heterosexual partners: A meta-analytic review. Aggression and Violent Behavior. 7, 213-351.

Arias I, Samios M, O'Leary K. (1987). Prevalence and correlates of physical aggression during courtship. *Journal of Interpersonal Violence.* 2, 82-90.

Costa Rica, Asamblea Legislativa. (1996). Ley 7586. Ley contra la violencia doméstica. Publicación 02/05/1996.

Costa Rica, Poder Judicial. (2006). Police Annuary 2005. Department of Publications and Prints.

Bejarano J, Ugalde F, Fonseca S. (2006). El consumo de drogas in hombres y mujeres costarricenses. Análisis de una década en personas de 25 a 59 años de la población general. Costarricense de Salud Pública. 15(28), 29-43.

Bejarano J, Sáenz M. (2004). El consumo de drogas en personas costarricenses mayores de 60 años. Estudio de tres cohortes. Psicoactiva. 18(22), 25-46

Bejarano J, Ugalde F. (2003). Drug consumption in Costa Rica. Results from the National Househol Survey on Drug Abuse of 2000-2001. San José.: I.A.F.A.

Bejarano J, Ugalde F, Fonseca S. (2004). Drug consumption among youth in Costa Rica. An examination of ten years of research. *Psychiatric Act and Psychological in Latin America.* 50(3), 203-217.

Bland R, Orne H. (1986). Family violence and psychiatric disorder. Canadian Journal of Psychiatry. 31, 129-137.

Creel L. (2001). Domestic violence: An ongoing threat to women in Latin America and the Caribbean. Obtenido de Internet el 04 de abril de 2007: *http://www.prb.org/Template.cfm?Section=PRB&template/ContentManagement/ContentDisplay.cfm&ContentID=4744*

González R. (2003). Domestic Violence affects 67% of Costa Rican women. University Presence. N° 78, (página 35).

Orpinas P. (1999). Who is violent?: Factors associated with aggressive behaviors in Latin America and Spain. *Rev Panam Salud Publica.* vol.5 n.4-5 Washington April/May 1999

Rojas J. (2002) Domestic violence and cautious measures. *Legal Medicine of Costa Rica.* 19(1), 17-38.

Rojas M, Jiménez S, Cruz M. (2004). The social violence in Costa Rica. Organización Panamericana de la Salud. Ministerio de Salud, San José, C.R

Sagot M, Guzman L. (2004). Research Final Report. Program N° 824-A1-908. Prevention of violence against women in Costa Rica". Project N° 824-A1-545 National survey on violence against women. San José: Research Center on Women Studies. University of Costa Rica.

Solana E. (2006). Justice Administration Twelve Debrief on the sustainability of human development on the nation state. San José: Project of the Nation State.

Uribe S. (2001). Domestic Violence. A comparative study of *casuística*. Medical Legal Unit of Cartago. 1996 y 2000. *Legal Medicine of Costa Rica.* 18(2), 28-33.

WHO (2004). Global Status Report: Alcohol Policy. Geneva: World Health Organization.

UNHAPPY HOURS:

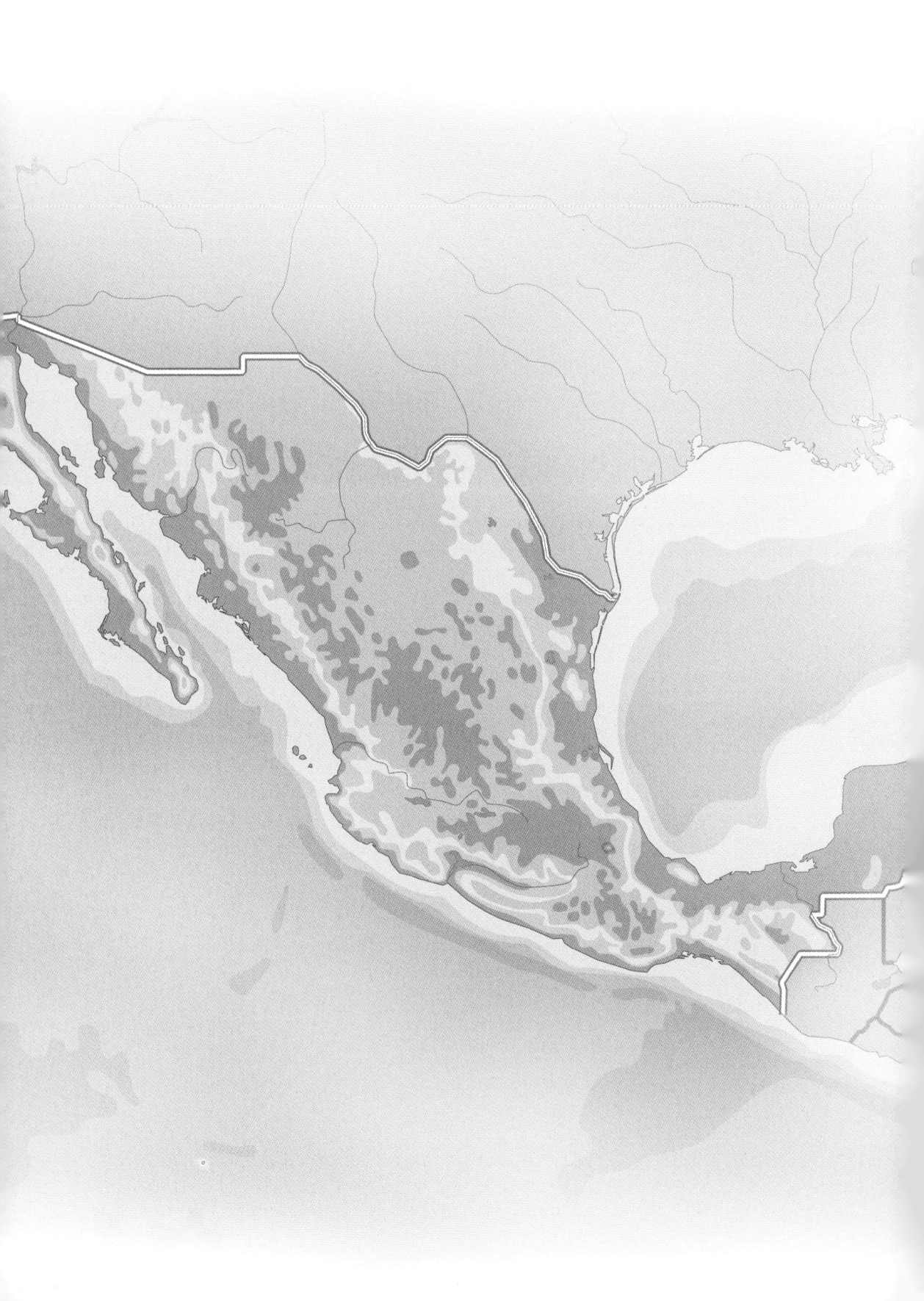

Mexico: Alcohol and Partner Physical Aggression in Ciudad Juárez, Monterrey, Querétaro, and Tijuana
—*Martha Romero Mendoza, María Elena Medina-Mora, Jorge Villatoro Velázquez, Clara Fleiz, Leticia Casanova, and Francisco Juárez*

Introduction

In Mexico, partner violence continues to be a social and cultural problem that is often regarded as "normal," even by the women who have been mistreated, and is often "invisible" to other people around them. Until recent years, the issue's invisibility and normality has led to an inadequate response. The elements that contribute to this denial and acceptance are manifold as well as involve personal factors, including those linked to individual couples' relationships, as well as institutional, social, and cultural characteristics of Mexican society (Agoff, Rajsbaum, Herrera, 2006).

Violence against women is a social practice that is understood to involve the exercise of power in asymmetrical social contexts that damage women's integrity and encourage their subordination and control by men. Such violence includes actions and failure to act that are both real and symbolic (Ramírez-Rodríguez, 2006). However, other aspects and issues related to physical aggression between intimate partners, including aggression by women toward male partners, are not yet well understood.

According to Valdez-Santiago (2004a), attempts to prevent and control domestic violence in Mexico increased significantly during 1976–2001, leading to the introduction of regulations in various sectors and giving rise to national programs, legal reforms in civil and penal codes, and even to the passage of specific laws.

Within the legal sphere, in 1996 the Law of Assistance and Prevention of Intra-familial Violence in the Federal District was approved, comprising 29 articles designed to lay the groundwork and establish procedures for preventing family violence (Mexico, Código Penal para el Distrito Federal, 2006).

In 2000, the Secretariat of Health invited several governmental and nongovernmental organizations to draw up the Mexican Official Norm NOM190-SSA1-199, entitled "Health Services Provision: Criteria for the Medical Care of Family Violence," which was published on 8 March 2000 in the *Diario Oficial*. In May of that year, state-by-state training regarding the norm began to be carried out.

On 8 March 2001, the National Women's Institute was created. Its work focuses on issues related to violence against women. Among other actions, it created a System of Indicators for Monitoring Women's Status, which includes a section that deals with violence against women by an intimate partner. At this writing, an interactive system for following up on the Convention for Eliminating All Forms of Discrimination against Women (SICEDAW) is being designed, the aims of which include widely disseminating the efforts currently under way at the national and regional level.

On 26 April 2006, the General Law for Women's Access to a Life Free of Violence was approved. This is the first law in Latin America that focuses on the different forms of violence from a gender and human rights perspective: family violence, community violence, labor violence, violence in educational settings, institutional violence, and feminicide[1], and it also establishes the mechanisms for the eradication of each (Mexico, Ley General de Acceso de las Mujeres a una Vida Libre de Violencia, 2006).

Partner Aggression Rates in Various Mexican Cities

According to Ramírez-Rodríguez (2006), studies that have sought to measure the scope of violence against women may be divided into two categories: those referring to the general population and those that study specific populations. Both types of studies display a high degree of heterogeneity in the methodology employed, in the criteria used in the selection and type of population studied, the instrument utilized, the structure of the questions and variables, and the indices for measuring the frequency and duration of the violence exercised by men.

Household Surveys

The 1998 National Survey on Addictions used a version of the Danger Assessment instrument, adapted and used in a previous study by Natera, Tiburcio, and Villatoro (1997), to evaluate partner violence among a sample of 1,149 urban women aged 18–65 who were currently living with a partner or who once lived as a couple. Overall, 45.7% of women reported that they had suffered some type of violence in their lifetime, with 13% reporting having experienced violence within the past year (Natera, Juárez García, Tiburcio, 2004).

Rivera-Rivera and colleagues. (2004) conducted a study to determine the prevalence of and risk factors for violence against women inflicted by their male partners in a representative sample of 1,535 women aged 15–49 years residing in the metropolitan area of Cuernavaca, Morelos state, Mexico. In response to questions from the Conflict Tactics Scale and the Index of Spousal Abuse, 35.8% of respondents reported low-to-moderate levels of violence (e.g., men exerting control over daily activities, not allowing women to hold a job outside the home, verbal insults), while 9.5% reported severe violence (e.g., being struck with an object, burned, or locked up). The main factors associated with violence were lower socioeconomic status, lower educational level, fewer years living with partner, alcohol use (OR = 2.56, 95% CI = 2.02–3.25), illegal drug abuse by partner, history of violence during childhood, and a history of rape.

A 2003 National Survey on the Dynamics of Household Relationships (Encuesta Nacional sobre la Dinámica de las Relaciones en los Hogares, or ENDIREH), and a second ENDIREH conducted in 2006, focused specifically on violence against women.

---

[1] A term generally used in Mexico to refer to the murders of more than 400 women in Ciudad Juárez, Chihuahua, Tijuana, and other areas, most of whom were employed in the maquiladora industry, that have occurred over the past decade and a half. Most of these crimes remain unsolved.

The ENDIREH 2003 included females aged 15-69 from 57,230 households who had a partner. Overall, 9.3% of the women reported experiencing an incident of physical violence during the past 12 months, including being pushed (7.1%), being beaten up (6.3%), being kicked (2.2%), having had an object thrown at them (2.8%), being strangled (0.9%), having had a knife (0.8%) or a gun (0.1%) used against them, and being tied up (0.2%) (Mexico, ENDIREH 2004). The ENDIREH 2006 included a sample of 128,000 females over the age of 15 who were married or living with a partner; of this group, 10.2% reported experiencing violence by a partner during the previous 12 months (Mexico, ENDIREH, 2007).

Of the 34% of respondents to a survey conducted in four cities in Mexico (Guadalajara, Hermosillo, Mérida, Oaxaca) who reported some kind of violence in their lifetime, females were significantly more likely than males to report experiences of violence in childhood, intimate partner violence, and family violence, whereas males most often reported violence perpetrated by friends, acquaintances, and strangers (Baker et al. 2005).

The National Survey on Psychiatric Epidemiology conducted in Mexico between 2001 and 2002 evaluated 28 different violent events using the World Health Organization Composite International Diagnostic Interview (WHO CIDI), in order to obtain the prevalence of these events and of post-traumatic stress disorder. Among other findings, 10.7% of females versus 0.8% of males reported "being beaten by one's partner" during their lifetime. Despite the fact that males and females were both exposed to violence, the proportion of females who developed post-traumatic stress disorder was significantly higher (4.73 females for every male).

Surveys with Special Populations

The National Survey on Violence against Women in Mexico conducted in 2003 found that among 26,042 females requiring treatment at primary- and secondary-level public health care facilities, 7.8% had experienced domestic partner violence (Olaiz et al., 2006).

Pregnant women have been found to be a high-risk group, due to the considerable harm that physical aggression poses for maternal and child health, for the burden that violent acts committed against pregnant women creates for health services, and for the high prevalence of pregnant women who are victims of violence (Castro, Peek-Asa, Ruiz 2003; Freyermuth 2004; Valdéz-Santiago 2004b, Cuevas et al., 2006).

In recent years, there has been growing interest in studying the extent of violence during courtship among young populations. Rivera-Rivera and colleagues (2006) conducted a baseline cohort study of a sample of 13,293 students aged 12-24, measuring violence using the 10 items of the Conflict Tactics Scale for the most recent courtship relationship. Alcohol abuse was defined as getting drunk to the extent of not being able to walk or stand on one's feet on one or more occasions every two weeks. The total prevalence of dating violence among females was 28%, and alcohol abuse (OR = 1.30, 95% CI 1.12-1.51) was found to be associated with this phenomenon as were depression, smoking tobacco, and poor academic performance.

Alcohol Involvement in Partner Aggression

In a household survey conducted in the southern part of Mexico (Natera, 1997), 544 women currently living with a partner were asked about lifetime violence experiences using the Danger Assessment Scale of 15 items, obtaining the number of violent acts and associated risks such as drunkenness of the partner. The latter was found to be significantly associated with violent acts and threats among the 38.4% of women who suffered some type of violence.

In a study of 717 women admitted to three emergency departments in the city of Pachuca, Hidalgo state, Ramos and colleagues (2002) found that 3.6% were admitted as a result of some form of interpersonal violence. All of these women lived with the aggressor, mainly in the form of common-law marriage, and reported lower educational attainment. Over one-half of the men in the study who physically mistreated their partners were heavy drinkers, with only one being an abstainer.

Recently, in an economic study of alcohol abuse and domestic violence in rural Mexico, Angelucci (2007) found that a "long-lasting 20 dollar monthly increase" in the wife's income was associated with a 15% decrease in the husband's alcohol abuse and a 21% decrease in aggressive behavior by the husband.

Methods
Survey and Sample

Data presented in this chapter were taken from the Household Survey on Addictions conducted between October and December 2005 in four Mexican cities: Ciudad Juárez, Monterrey, Querétaro, and Tijuana. The main objective of the survey was to evaluate alcohol, tobacco, and drug use prevalence; consumption trends; and related problems in a representative sample of each of the four cities. Information regarding violence and victimization, suicide, accidents, and diseases was also collected, as well as data on migration to the United States.

This was a cross-sectional epidemiological study based on a household survey. The sample design was probabilistic, multistage, stratified, and by conglomerates.

Sampling Units

During the first sampling stage, 210 Basic Geo-statistical Areas (BGSA) were selected in proportion to the number of dwellings in each, according to the 2000 census (60 BGSA were selected for the Metropolitan Area of Monterrey, and 50 each were selected for Ciudad Juárez, Querétaro, and Tijuana). During the second stage of the sampling, two blocks were chosen from each of the BGSA selected, in order to obtain approximately six dwellings per block (12 dwellings per BGSA), anticipating a nonresponse rate in the order of 17%. These blocks were selected using proportional probability to size (PPT) according to the number of dwellings in each block.

During the third stage, once the BGSA and blocks had been selected, the sampling was divided into segments of approximately six occupied dwellings (excluding businesses, land plots, unoccupied houses, etc.) and one segment was chosen (from the table of random numbers carried by each interviewer) to be analyzed at the same time as the survey was conducted. All household members between the ages of 12 and 65 living in the selected dwellings were eligible to be interviewed.

Finally, during the fourth stage of the sampling, one member of each household between the ages of 12 and 65 was selected using the last birthday technique (i.e., of all the members within that age range, the most suitable respondent would be the one with a birthday closest to the date of the interview). The only case in which a potential respondent to the individual questionnaire could be replaced was if the person was deemed to possess some mental disability that would prevent him or her from being able to adequately answer the interview questions. In these exceptional cases, the household member with the next closest birthday was selected. The household was excluded if there were no members aged 12-65 living in the dwelling. In the event that the selected respondent was not at home at the time of the interview visit, up to four follow-up visits were made on different dates and at different times.

Training Interviewers

Training for the field work took place 17-21 October 2005 on the premises of the Ramón de la Fuente Muñiz National Institute of Psychiatry (INP). INP personnel explained the project's scope and importance, the basic concepts contained in the survey, and the handling of the individual questionnaire. The field logistics, the methodology for selecting appropriate respondents, the instructions for completing the household survey, and the survey's administration were carried out by a private firm. Twenty-three interviewers, four supervisors, and a field coordinator participated in the training. The personnel who would be responsible for evaluating and encoding the questionnaires also participated.

The field work was carried out between 25 October and 10 December 2005, by the respective research teams, each of which was assigned a work route. Eighteen interviewers, four supervisors, and a general coordinator of operational logistics took part in the survey. The team supervisor was responsible for the organization and supervision of the listing and sampling activities, assigning the workload, and verifying the quality of the information collected.

During the operation, the field teams were supervised by INP personnel. During the field work, the following supervisory activities were carried out regarding the interviews.
- Direct or coincidental supervision: each of the interviewers were accompanied to ensure that they were correctly locating the areas within the sample and properly applying the field instruments. In the event of detecting a flaw, supervisors corrected it following the interview and continued to accompany the interviewer until they were satisfied with his or her performance.
- Subsequent supervision: during the field work, supervisors randomly selected questionnaires from each of the interviewers and revisited the dwellings. This technique allowed supervisors to verify that interviewers had indeed visited the dwelling and, after asking a few questions from the original questionnaire, to confirm that the interviewer had actually interviewed the preselected respondent.
- Supervision of all types of nonresponse.

One of the supervisors' routine tasks involved checking that the questionnaires not directly supervised in the field had been completed correctly, prior to their being sent to the INP central office to be encoded and captured.

As Table 1 shows, 36.4% of the total household interviews and 38.3% of the individual interviews were supervised in the field. These figures include both direct supervision (at the time of the interview) and subsequent supervision.

TABLE 1. Percentage of supervised interviews, by city and questionnaire type, Household Survey on Addictions, Mexico, 2005.

City	Type of Questionnaire	Direct	Subsequent	Total
Tijuana	Household	3.3	12.2	15.5
	Individual	12.3	17.0	29.3
Ciudad Juárez	Household	4.5	20.4	24.9
	Individual	6.9	20.3	27.2
Monterrey	Household	18.8	46.0	64.8
	Individual	20.9	38.5	59.4
Querétaro	Household	14.3	26.4	40.7
	Individual	13.8	20.1	33.9
Total	Household	10.1	26.3	36.4
	Individual	13.7	24.6	38.3

Survey Instrument

The questionnaire used in the study was specifically created for the 2005 Household Survey on Addictions for the cities of Ciudad Juárez, Monterrey, Querétaro, and Tijuana and targeted the population aged 12–65. It consisted of 45 pages and contained various areas that were covered in previous National Surveys on Addictions, including alcohol consumption patterns and legal and illegal psychoactive substances use and related problems (México, ENA, 1998; México, ENA, 2002).

The 2005 questionnaire included the following questions on violence:
(1) People can be physically aggressive in many ways, by pushing, hitting, or slapping. Has someone with whom you have or have had a romantic relationship, such as your spouse, partner, boy/girlfriend, *ever done* any things to you such as: push, grab, slap, punch, kick, slap, throw things, hit with an object, beat up, threaten with a pistol, or actually use a pistol on you?
(2) The interviewer then used a list to ask about each of these options, allowing the interviewee to add other forms of physical violence.
(3) The interviewee was then asked about the most violent act he or she had experienced over the past two years.
(4) On the subject of alcohol: during this event (i.e., the most aggressive act) was either of those involved drinking alcohol at the time? Who?
(5) Where did the incident take place?
(6) Did you seek medical assistance from a doctor, nurse, paramedic, or other type of health professional?
(7) Did you file a complaint?

Respondents were not asked about their own physical aggression toward a partner. In this chapter, only the results of the respondents aged 18 to 65 years are reported. Weights were applied to these analyses to adjust for the selection probability of each individual in the household. Table 2 presents the general characteristics of the population sample participating in the survey.

TABLE 2. Age, marital status, employment status, and drinking pattern in the 12 months preceding the survey, for male and female respondents, Household Survey on Addictions, Mexico, 2005.

	Males (weighted N=840)		Females (weighted N=896)	
	Number	Percent or mean	Number	Percent or mean
Age		31.4 years		35.2 years
18–24 years	198	23.6%	214	23.9%
25–34 years	271	32.3%	294	32.8%
35–44 years	182	21.7%	162	18.1%
45–54 years	109	12.9%	138	15.4%
55–65 years	80	9.5%	88	9.8%
Marital status				
Married	398	47.4%	461	51.5%
Cohabiting/Living with partner	129	15.4%	125	14.0%
Separated	26	3.1%	47	5.3%
Divorced	16	1.9%	25	2.8%
Never married	265	31.5%	210	23.5%
Widowed	6	0.7%	27	3.1%
Employment status				
Working for pay	538	71.5%	166	32.7%
Voluntarily unemployed (homemaker or other reasons)	3	0.3%	501	46.2%
Involuntarily unemployed	48	4.5%	17	1.6%
Student	228	21.5%	195	18.0%
Retired	23	2.2%	17	1.5%
Drinking pattern (past 12 months)				
Drank any alcohol during past 12 months	593	70.6%	367	40.9%
Average number of drinking days (drinkers only)		56.57 days		17.49 days
Average number of drinks per occasion (drinkers only)		10.74 drinks		8.27 drinks
Average annual volume (drinkers only)		326.72 drinks		164.78 drinks
Drank five or more drinks on at least one occasion (drinkers only)		77.0%		40.2%

Results

As shown in Figure 1, more males than females reported being the victim of physical aggression by a partner in the past two years (p < .000).

FIGURE 1. Percent of respondents who reported having been a victim, by sex, Household Survey on Addictions, Mexico, 2005.

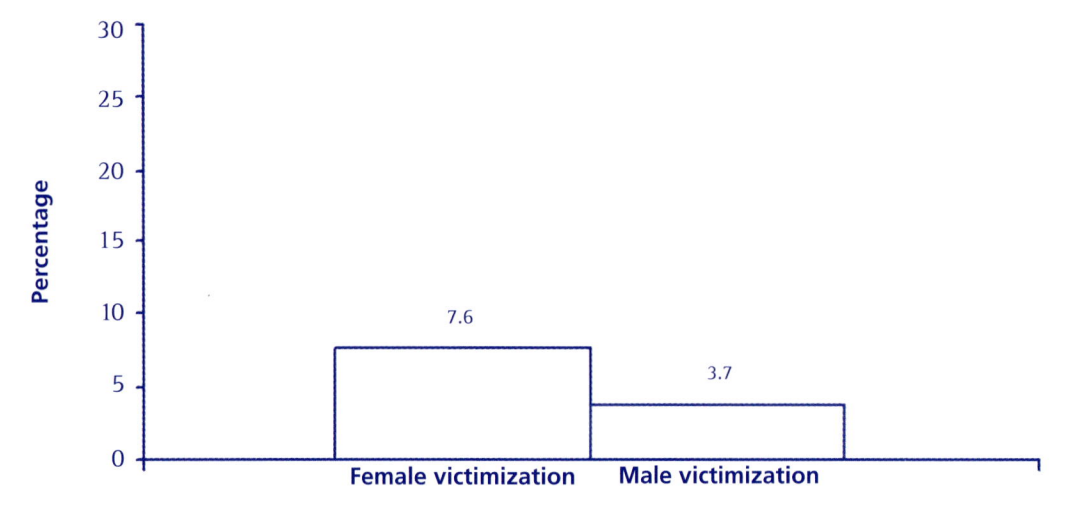

Female victimization: 7.6
Male victimization: 3.7

As shown in Figure 2, physical aggression by a partner was higher for the younger age groups than for the oldest age groups; however, these differences did not reach statistically significant levels. The mean age for male victims was 35.1 years, and for female victims it was 34.9 years.

FIGURE 2. Percent of respondents who reported having been a victim, by age group and sex, Household Survey on Addictions, Mexico, 2005.

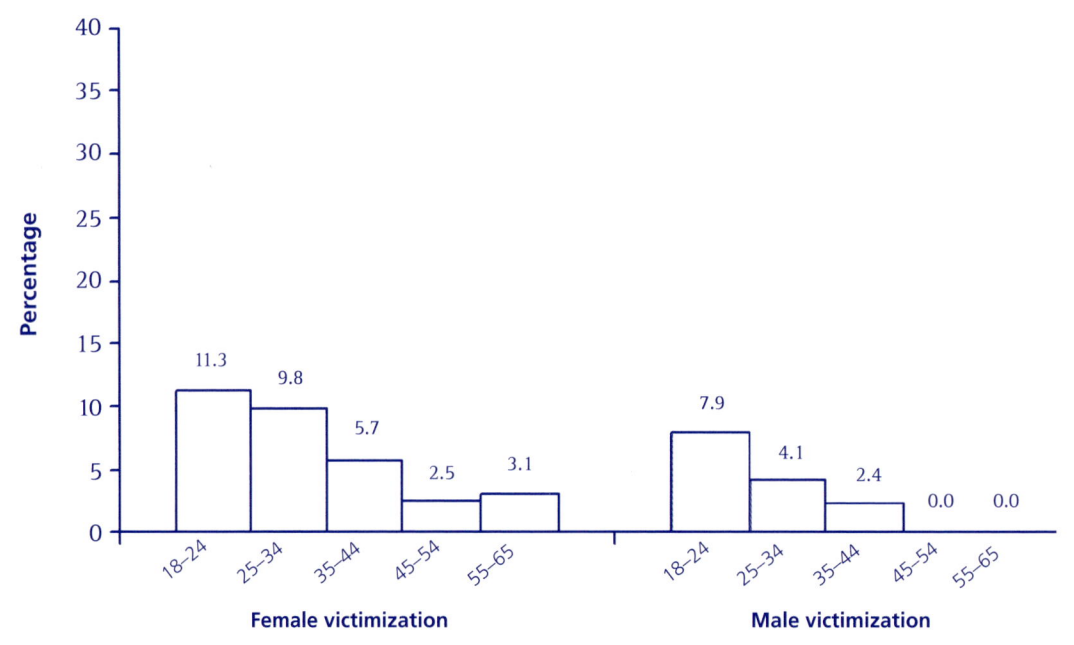

Female victimization:
- 18–24: 11.3
- 25–34: 9.8
- 35–44: 5.7
- 45–54: 2.5
- 55–65: 3.1

Male victimization:
- 18–24: 7.9
- 25–34: 4.1
- 35–44: 2.4
- 45–54: 0.0
- 55–65: 0.0

As shown in Figure 3, the percent reporting partner physical aggression varied by marital status. Cohabiting females, followed by divorced/separated females, were more likely to report aggression by their partner than were women in other marital status categories (p <. 000). For males, the highest rate of aggression by a partner was among divorced/separated and never-married respondents, but the rates among these two marital status groups were not significantly different statistically from never-married or married males.

FIGURE 3. Percent of respondents who reported having been a victim, by marital status and sex, Household Survey on Addictions, Mexico, 2005.

Female victimization
- Married: 6.8
- Cohabiting: 15.4
- Divorced/separated: 12.7
- Never married: 3.7

Male victimization
- Married: 1.1
- Cohabiting: 3.3
- Divorced/separated: 9.1
- Never married: 6.6

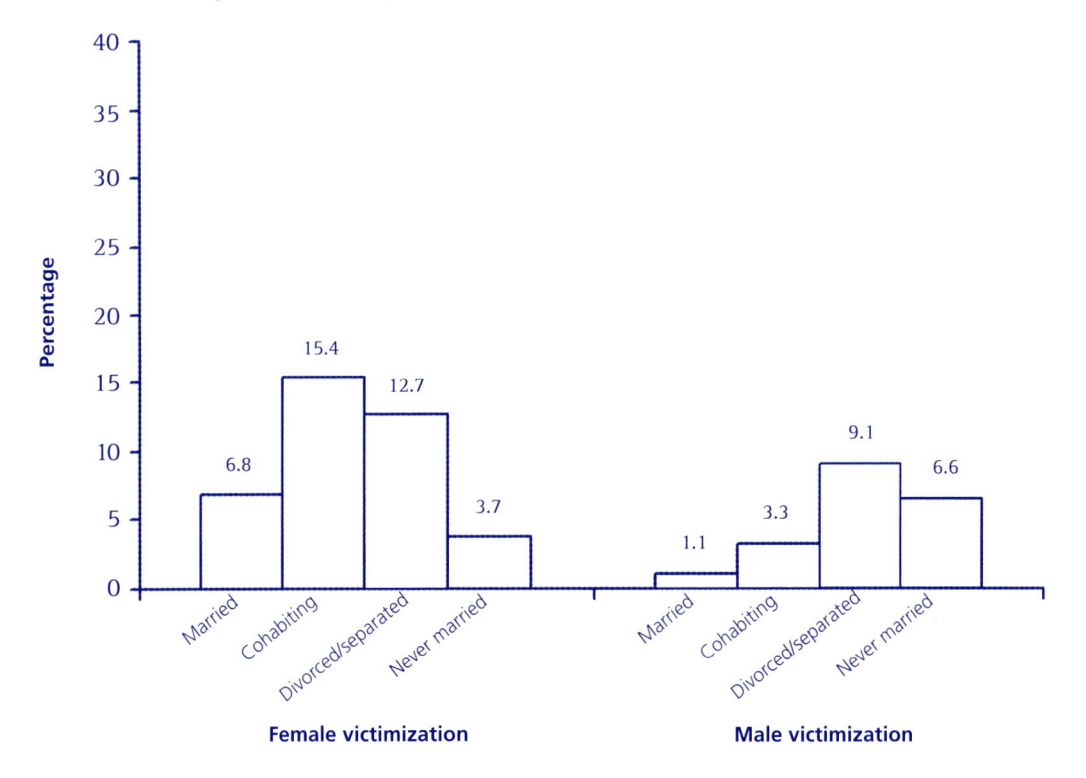

Figure 4 shows the frequency of each type of aggression, by sex. Female victims were more likely than male victims to report that they had been pushed (p < .001) or beaten up (p < .01). No other significant sex differences between types of aggressive acts were found.

Almost 20% (19.6%) of female victims sought medical attention and 19.2% filed a complaint, while no male victims reported doing either of these things.

FIGURE 4. Type of aggressive act against females and males as reported by victims, Household Survey on Addictions, Mexico, 2005.

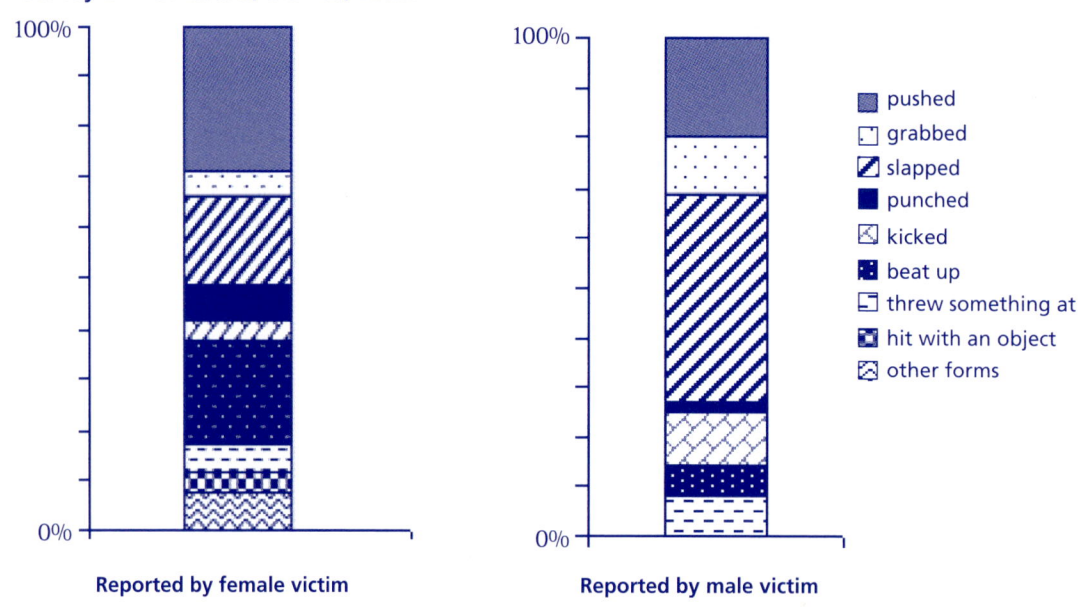

Reported by female victim

Reported by male victim

- pushed
- grabbed
- slapped
- punched
- kicked
- beat up
- threw something at
- hit with an object
- other forms

As shown in Figure 5, 12.9% of the male victims reported that both persons were drinking at the time the aggression occurred, 6.8% reported that only the male victim was drinking, 3.2 % that only the female aggressor was drinking, and 74.6% reported that neither partner had been drinking. Among female victims, 39.2% reported that only the male aggressor had been drinking, while 60% reported that no one had been drinking.

FIGURE 5. Percent of incidents in which no partner had been drinking, both partners had been drinking, only the male partner had been drinking, or only the female partner had been drinking, as reported by male and female victims, Household Survey on Addictions, Mexico, 2005.

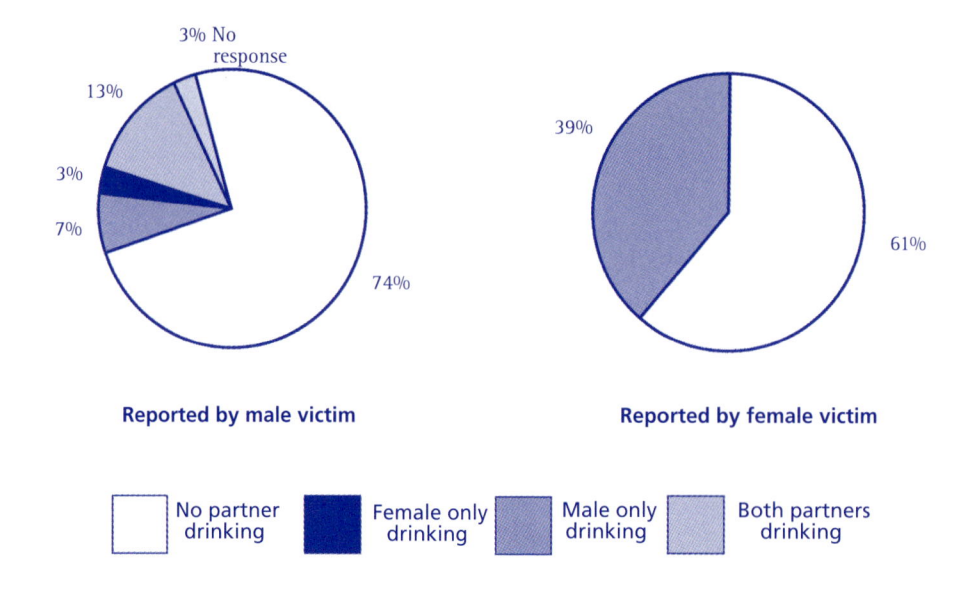

Reported by male victim: 74%, 13%, 7%, 3%, 3% No response

Reported by female victim: 61%, 39%

- No partner drinking
- Female only drinking
- Male only drinking
- Both partners drinking

The Relationship between Alcohol Consumption and Partner Aggression

Among male victims, 70.6% reported being current drinkers versus 29.4% who reported being abstainers (5.6% who were lifetime abstainers and 23.8% who defined themselves as being former drinkers). Among female victims, 40.9% reported being current drinkers versus 59.1% who reported being abstainers (28.2% who were lifetime abstainers and 30.9% who defined themselves as being former drinkers).

Respondents' Drinking Pattern and Partner Aggression

Figure 6 shows the percent of drinkers reporting partner physical aggression by whether the respondent had consumed five or more drinks on an occasion in the past year. Both male and female respondents who drank five or more drinks on at least one occasion in the past year were significantly more likely than those who had never consumed that many drinks to report partner aggression ($p < .001$).

FIGURE 6. Percent of respondents who reported victimization (aggression by a partner) by whether respondent had consumed five or more drinks on an occasion or had never consumed five drinks on an occasion, by sex, Household Survey on Addictions, Mexico, 2005.

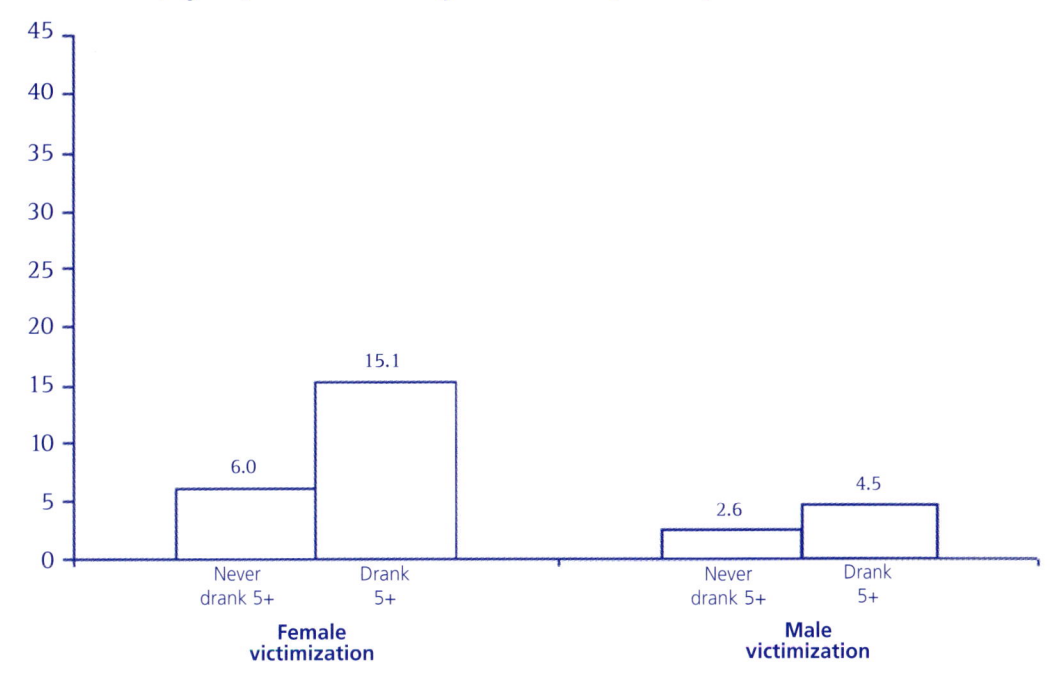

	Never drank 5+	Drank 5+
Female victimization	6.0	15.1
Male victimization	2.6	4.5

As shown in Figures 7, 8, and 9, female victims who reported aggression involving alcohol reported drinking more frequently, drinking more drinks per occasion, and having a greater annual consumption of alcohol, compared with females who reported aggression that did not involve alcohol and those who reported no aggression; these differences, however, were not statistically significant.

Male victims who reported aggression in which neither partner had been drinking reported drinking more frequently in the past year, compared with males who reported aggression with alcohol and males who reported no aggression, although this difference was not significant. Males who reported partner aggression involving alcohol reported more drinks per occasion and more annual consumption than did males who reported aggression that did not involve alcohol or no aggression, but again these differences were not statistically significant.

Because the sample of males who reported aggression by a partner in which one or both persons had been drinking was very small, logistic regression was conducted regressing any aggression by a partner (versus no aggression) on drinking variables and age. The only significant finding was for the number of drinks consumed on usual drinking occasions ($p < .042$) to be significantly greater for males who had experienced aggression by a partner compared to males who reported no aggression.

FIGURE 7. Mean number of drinking days in the year preceding the survey for respondents who had been victims in incidents involving alcohol, in incidents not involving alcohol, or who reported no victimization, by sex, Household Survey on Addictions, Mexico, 2005.

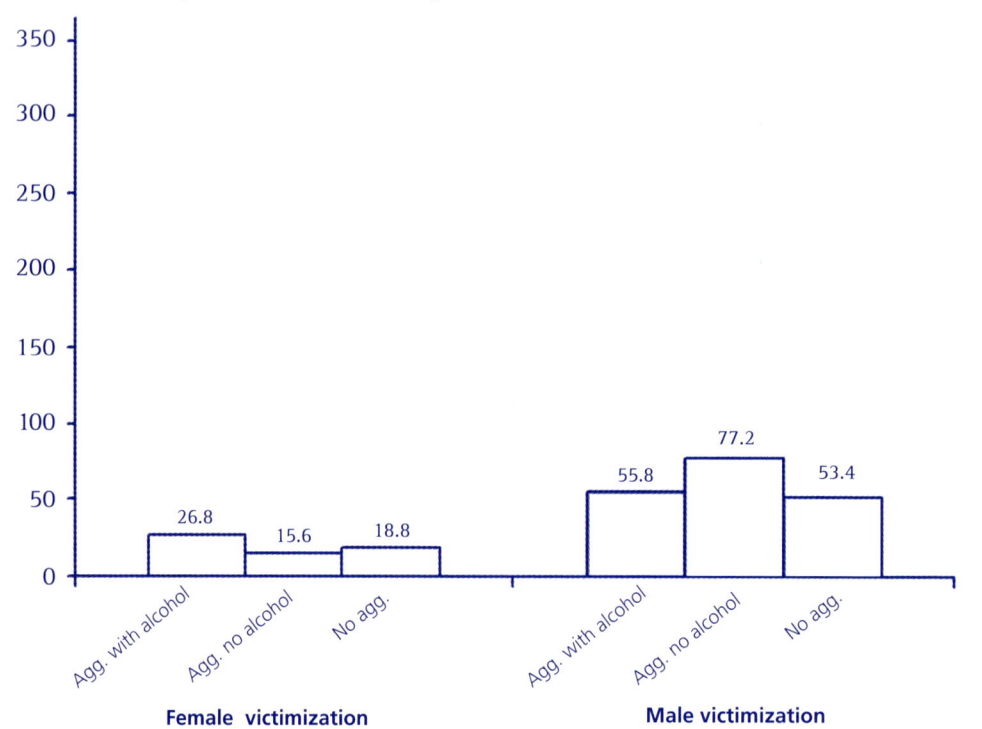

Female victimization
- Agg. with alcohol: 26.8
- Agg. no alcohol: 15.6
- No agg.: 18.8

Male victimization
- Agg. with alcohol: 55.8
- Agg. no alcohol: 77.2
- No agg.: 53.4

Mexico | 141

FIGURE 8. Mean number of drinks consumed on usual drinking occasions by respondents who had been victims in incidents involving alcohol, in incidents not involving alcohol, or who reported no victimization, by sex, Household Survey on Addictions, Mexico, 2005.

Female victimization:
- Agg. with alcohol: 2.9
- Agg. no alcohol: 2.0
- No agg.: 2.6

Male victimization:
- Agg. with alcohol: 8.6
- Agg. no alcohol: 6.6
- No agg.: 6.4

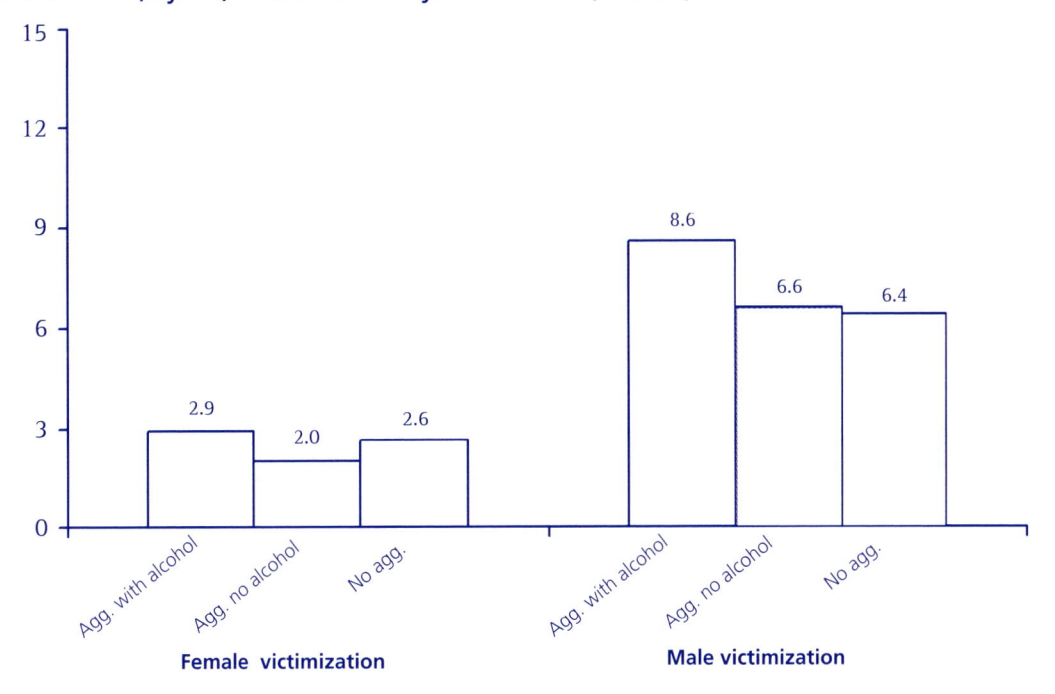

FIGURE 9. Overall mean number of drinks consumed annually by respondents who had been victims in incidents involving alcohol, in incidents not involving alcohol, or who reported no victimization, by sex, Household Survey on Addictions, Mexico, 2005.

Female victimization:
- Agg. with alcohol: 124.0
- Agg. no alcohol: 73.2
- No agg.: 72.9

Male victimization:
- Agg. with alcohol: 949.0
- Agg. no alcohol: 741.0
- No agg.: 72.9

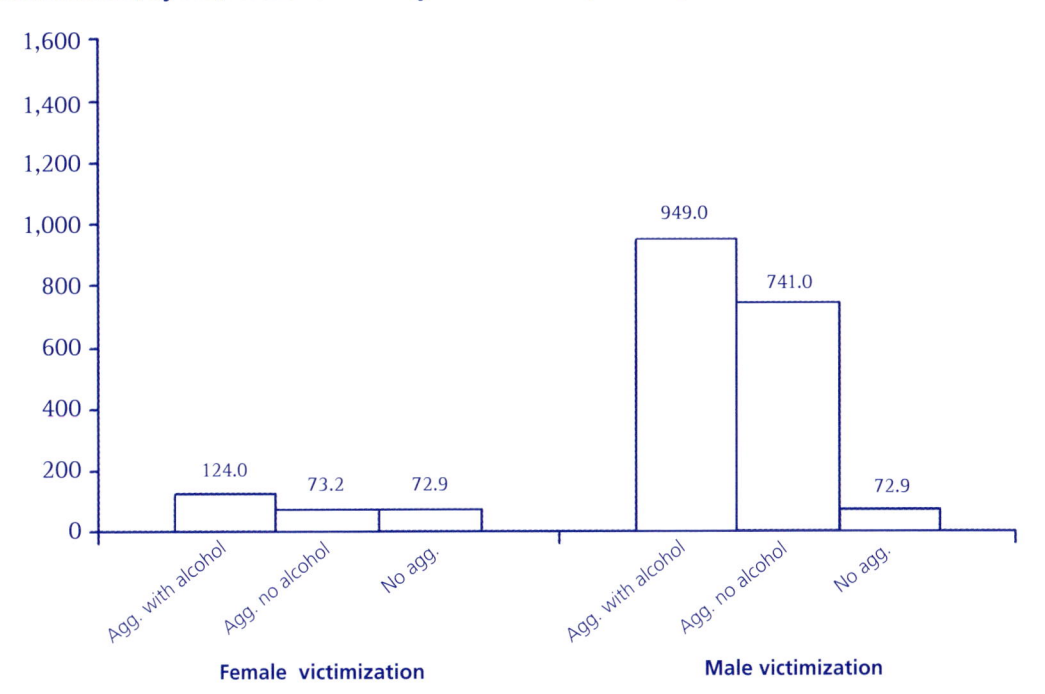

Discussion

The rates of partner aggression obtained in this study are somewhat lower than rates found in previous surveys. One reason for the lower rate might be that the results covered only four cities, rather than being national in scope. Another reason is that the survey asked only about physical aggression and did not include questions about sexual assault or other forms of abuse. In terms of aggression type, the type of aggressive acts reported by females were similar to those obtained in the ENDIREH 2003, with the highest rates being recorded for being pushed and being beaten up.

One of the most important strengths of this study is that it includes the prevalence of aggressive acts experienced by males, an issue that had not been addressed by most previous research in Mexico, perhaps because gender studies of masculinity have not achieved the importance that women's studies have. This study confirms that females are more likely than males to be the victims of partner aggression, especially more severe types of partner aggression such as being beaten up. Prevalence is especially high for younger females.

In relation to marital status, it is clear that females living in common-law relationships and divorced males and females are more likely to report partner aggression than are persons from other marital status groups. This pattern with regard to marital status is similar to results from national surveys on violence against women. The question that arises is what might be the reasons for this phenomenon: Legal status? Intolerance to women's autonomy? Traditionalism?

Another strength of the present study is the measurement of usual drinking pattern, which was investigated not in a single question (i.e., presence or absence) as in most other studies, but in a standardized set of questions and international measures that allow comparison with previous National Surveys on Addictions. The results of the latest (2005) study point to a higher risk of victimization among those who drink higher quantities per occasion, suggesting that future interventions need to particularly target heavier drinkers.

Female victims reported that if anyone was drinking during the aggressive incident, it was the male. In relation to female drinking patterns, those experiencing aggression when the male partner had been drinking compared to females who reported no aggression tended to be heavier drinkers themselves. This relationship was not, however, statistically significant. The fact that no female victims reported drinking at the time of the incident of physical aggression deserves further investigation. Other studies have shown that women in Mexico tend to hide their own consumption.

One limitation of this study is that the male and female aggressors' pattern of consumption was not investigated and it was not possible to compare drinking patterns between male/females aggressors and male/female victims.

A further limitation is that the survey asked only about acts of physical aggression and did not include other forms of partner abuse more involved with violence against women. According to Krahé, Bieneck, and Möller (2005), several critics have argued that the picture of gender symmetry with regard to "men's and women's equal involvement in intimate partner violence portrayed . . . " by similar questions, ". . . is largely due to the fact that decontextualized instances of violence are recorded that fail to distinguish motivationally distinct forms of intimate partner violence in which men and women are differentially involved." However, by including information on male victimization, the present study reveals various ways in which partner aggression is similar and how it is different for men and women and points to directions for future research.

The relationship between partner aggression and drinking pattern suggests a need to raise awareness among policymakers regarding the need for further study of the relationship between alcohol and violence, both as part of population-based studies and as part of research in clinical settings. Despite efforts made in Mexico to provide treatment to victims of violence, it is important to point out that a portion of these victims may also have alcohol abuse or alcohol dependence problems that deserve to be treated at the same time. This points to the need for universities, particularly as regards the medical and law professions, to provide adequate training in gender equity as a way to raise awareness regarding partner violence and to encourage the adoption of interventions that address issues of alcohol consumption and violence as interrelated problems.

Acknowledgments

The authors wish to thank the National Council against Addictions (Consejo Nacional contra las Adicciones, or CONADIC) for its financial support, as well as CONADIC's equivalents in Baja California, Chihuahua, Monterrey, and Quéretaro, and the National Institute of Psychiatry (INP).

References

Agoff C, Rajsbaum A, Herrera C (2006). Perspectivas de las mujeres maltratadas sobre la violencia de pareja en México. Salud Pública de México. 48 Suplemento (2):307–314.

Angelucci M. (2007). Love on the Rocks: Alcohol Abuse and Domestic Violence in Rural Mexico. Discussion paper No. 2706. March. University of Arizona and The Institute for the Study of Labor (IZA)

Baker Ch, Norris F, Diaz D, Perilla J, Murphy A, Hill E (2005). Violence and PTSD in Mexico. Gender and Regional Differences. Soc Psychiatry Psychiatr Epidemiol 40:519–528.

Castro R, Peek-Asa C, Ruiz A (2003). Violence against women in Mexico: a study of abuse before and during pregnancy. American Journal of Public Health 93(7): 1110–1116.

Cuevas S, Blanco J, Juárez C, Palma O, Valdez-Santiago R. (2006). Violencia y embarazo en usuarias del sector salud en estados de alta marginación en México. Salud Pública de México. 48 Suplemento (2):239–249.

Freyermuth G (2004). La violencia de género como factor de riesgo en la maternidad. In: Torres Falcón M: Violencia contra las mujeres en contextos urbanos y rurales. Ed. El Colegio de México, Programa Interdisciplinario de Estudios de la Mujer, 447p.

Krahé B, Bieneck S, Möller I (2005). Understanding gender and intimate partner violence from an international perspective. Sex roles 52(11/12):807–827.

Mexico, Código Penal para el Distrito Federal (2006). Ley de Asistencia y Prevención a la violencia familiar. Ed. Sista. México.

Mexico, ENA. (1998). Encuesta Nacional de Adicciones. Instituto Mexicano de Psiquiatría. Secretaría de Salud.

Mexico, ENA. (2002). Encuesta Nacional de Adicciones, Instituto Nacional de Estadística, Geografía e Informática. México.

Mexico, ENDIREH, INEGI. (2004). Encuesta Nacional sobre la dinámica de las relaciones en los hogares, 2003. Instituto Nacional de Estadística, Geografía e Informática. México.

Mexico, ENDIREH, INEGI. (2007). Encuesta Nacional sobre la dinámica de las relaciones en los hogares, 2006. Instituto Nacional de Estadística, Geografía e Informática. *http:www.inegi.gob.mx/contenidos/español/sistemas/endire/2006/panorama_gra.pps .México.* Visited on August, 2007.

Mexico, Ley General de Acceso de las Mujeres a una Vida Libre de Violencia y tipificación del feminicidio como delito de lesa humanidad. (2006). H. Congreso de la Unión de Diputados, LIX Legislatura. México.

Natera G, Juárez García F, Tiburcio M. (2004). Validez factorial de una escala de violencia hacia la pareja en una muestra nacional mexicana. Salud Mental. 27(2), April, 31-38.

Natera G, Tiburcio M, Villatoro J. (1997). Marital violence and its relationship to excessive drinking in Mexico. Contemporary Drug Problems 24, Winter: 787-804.

Olaiz G, Rojas R, Valdez R, Franco A, Palma O. (2006). Prevalencia de diferentes tipos de violencia en usuarias del sector salud en México. Salud Pública de México 48(2), suplemento 2: 232-238.

Ramírez-Rodríguez JC. (2006). La violencia de varones contra sus parejas heterosexuales: realidades y desafíos. Un recuento de la producción mexicana. Salud Pública de México. 48 Suplemento (2):315-327.

Ramos L, Borges G, Cherpitel C, Medina-Mora ME, Mondragón L. (2002). Violencia doméstica, un problema oculto en el sistema de salud. El caso de los servicios de urgencias. Revista de Salud Fronteriza/Journal of Border Health. VII(1), January-June: 42-55.

Rivera-Rivera L, Allen B, Rodríguez-Ortega G, Chávez-Ayala R, Lazcano-Ponce E. (2006). Violencia durante el noviazgo, depresión y conductas de riesgo en estudiantes femeninas (12-24 años) Salud Pública de México. 48 Suplemento (2):288-296.

Rivera-Rivera L, Lazcano-Ponce E, Salmerón-Castro J, Salazar-Martínez E, Castro R, Hernández-Avila M. (2004). Prevalence and determinants of male partner violence against Mexican women_ a population-based study. Salud Pública de México 46(2), March-April, 113-121.

Valdez-Santiago R. (2004a). Del silencio privado a las agendas públicas: el devenir de la lucha contra la violencia doméstica en México. In: Torres Falcón M: Violencia contra las mujeres en contextos urbanos y rurales. Ed. El Colegio de México, Programa Interdisciplinario de Estudios de la Mujer,417-447.

Valdez-Santiago R. (2004b). Respuesta médica ante la violencia que sufren las mujeres embarazadas. In: Torres Falcón M: Violencia contra las mujeres en contextos urbanos y rurales. Ed. El Colegio de México, Programa Interdisciplinario de Estudios de la Mujer, 447p.

UNHAPPY HOURS:

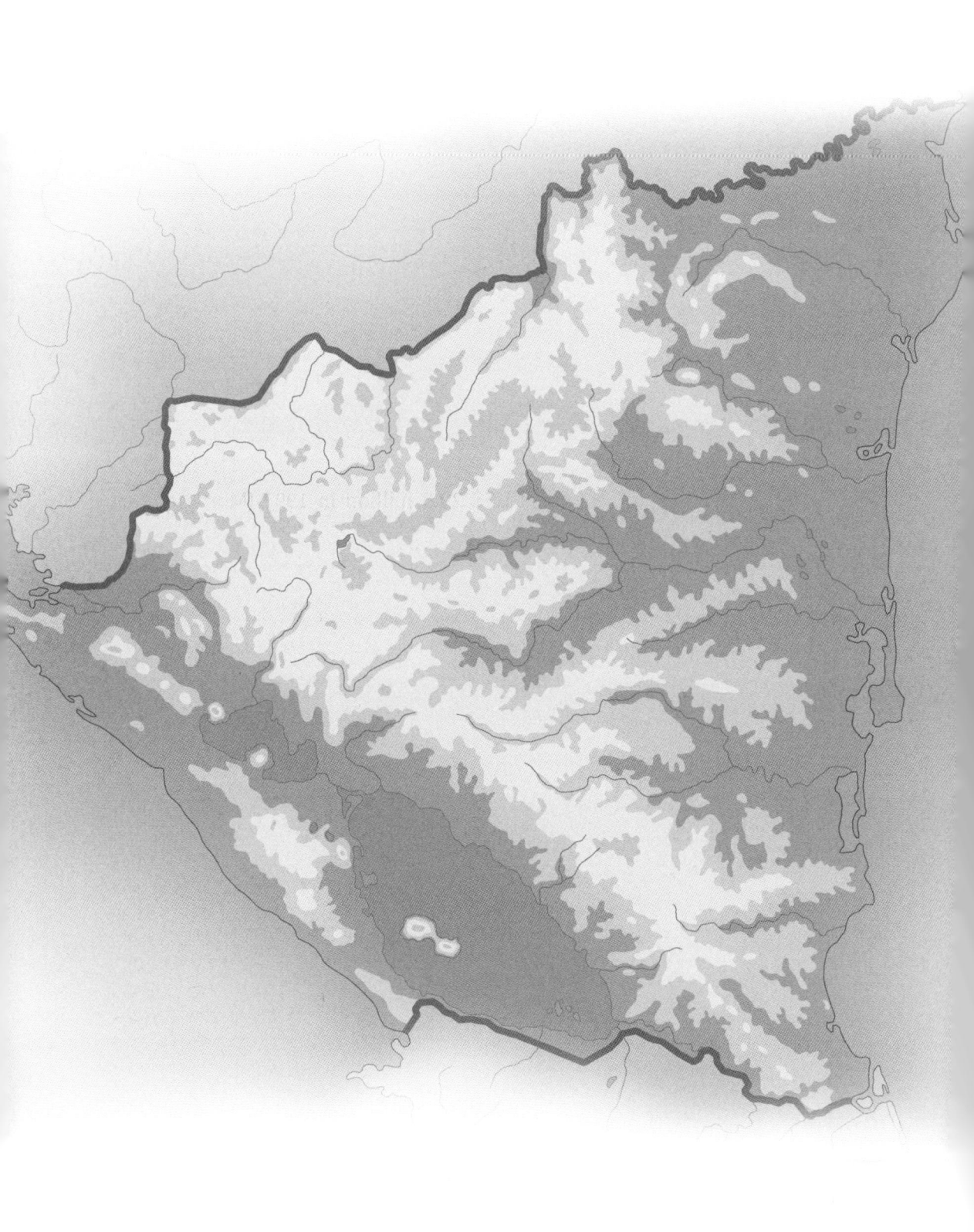

Nicaragua: Alcohol and Partner Physical Aggression in Bluefields, Estelí, Juigalpa, León, and Rivas
—*José Trinidad Caldera Aburto, Sharon Bernards, and Myriam Munné*

Introduction

Partner violence against women in Nicaragua leads to serious health problems, including more inpatient treatment and surgery than that seen among non-abused women, mortality from injuries, sexually transmitted diseases, depression, and low birthweight babies (Ellsberg, Caldera, et al, 1999; Morrisson and Orlando, 1999; Valladares, Ellsberg, et al 2002). The economic costs of domestic violence against women in Nicaragua (including lost earnings, lower educational levels in children, and increases in medical treatment costs) was estimated to exceed US$ 29.5 million in 1997 (Morrisson and Orlando, 1999; Watts and Zimmerman, 2002a; 2002b). Husbands' use of violence against their wives is a widely accepted practice, and many women have traditionally viewed violence as an expected part of their lives (Ellsberg, et al, 1997). In a sample in León, among ever-married women who had experienced physical aggression by their partners at least once in their lifetime, almost all reported that they had experienced an incident within the home (71% reported an incident in the bedroom); 22% reported that they had experienced an incident of partner violence outside the home, with most of these incidents occurring on the street (Ellsberg, et al, 2000).

In Nicaragua, violence against women has been acknowledged as a public health problem since the 1980s. Women's involvement in the country's revolutionary struggle led to women's greater participation in government and fostered the development of women's non-governmental organizations (NGOs). At this writing, more than 150 women's groups are part of the national Network of Women Against Violence (Ellsberg et al, 2001; Ellsberg et al, 1997). Nicaragua's Network of Women against Violence lobbied the country's National Assembly to improve laws designed to protect women suffering violence and to increase penalties for offenders, especially sexual abusers. The Penal Code was reformed in 1992 (Law 150) and again in 1996 (Law 230) to allow women to seek protection (for example, by prohibiting the offending spouse from entering the woman's residence or workplace, requiring that he or she receive counseling, and confiscating weapons). In addition, the law recognized psychological injuries as well as physical ones, and considered aggression by a family member as an aggravating circumstance that warranted a sentence of up to six years in jail (Ellsberg et al, 1997)

In 1993, the first shelter for battered women opened its doors in Estelí, followed some years later by a shelter opening in Managua; by 1997, there were women's health centers in nearly every major Nicaraguan city (Ellsberg et al, 1997). In 1994, Women and Children's Police Stations ("comisarías") began to be developed; by 2007, there were 25 in operation. Comisarías include teams of social workers, psychologists and investigators (Policía Nacional de Nicaragua; Wessel and Campbell, 1997). In 1993, among women in León who had ever been married and who reported physical aggression by a partner during their lifetime, 80% did not seek help, citing shame, fear of reprisal, and deeming it unnecessary as the most common reasons (Ellsberg, Pena, et al, 2000). Between 2005 and 2006, the number of cases reported to the comisarías increased 51% , although only 32.7% of the cases went on to the judicial system; instead, the majority of cases were settled by extrajudicial agreement (Policía Nacional de Nicaragua).

Existing Knowledge of Rates of Partner Aggression in Nicaragua

The first scientific study about violence against women in Nicaragua was conducted in 1995 by Mary Ellsberg (Ellsberg, Herrera, et al, 1999). It found that the percentage of women in León who suffered physical aggression by a former or current partner some time in their lives was 40% (8% among dating women and 52% among ever-married women). Among ever-married women, 27% reported physical violence by a former or current partner in the year before the survey. The most common types of aggressive acts reported in the past year were incidents of pushing (40%), punching and kicking them (27%), throwing an object at them (22%), slapping them (22%), and hitting them with an object (22%). In addition, 10% of the women reported having been beaten and 14% reported being threatened with a weapon or the use of a weapon (Ellsberg, Pena, et al., 2000). A 1997 study in Managua found the lifetime prevalence of partner physical abuse against ever-married women to be 69% and that of violence in the year preceding the study, 33% (Morrisson and Orlando, 1999). The 1998-1999 Demographic Health Survey (ENDESA), using a nationally representative sample of ever-married women found a lifetime prevalence of physical violence of 28% (25% in León and 28% in Managua), with 12% of women reporting minor and severe violence in the year before the survey (10.2% in León, 11.2% in Estelí, 9.2% in Rivas, 10.6% in and around Bluefields, and 14.0% in the area around Chontales Juigalpa) (Rosales et al, 1999). While ENDESA was nationally representative, possibly accounting for the lower rates, Ellsberg and colleagues (Ellsberg, Heise, et al, 2000) suggest that the lower rates might also have been the result of some of the women's reluctance to report aggression by their current partners because family members, including their husbands, were present during 35% of the interviews.

Involvement of Alcohol in Partner Aggression

In a study of physical aggression against ever-married women in León, 48% of the women reported that their husbands had used alcohol at the time of the incident (an additional 6% reported that the husband had been using another psychoactive substance) (Ellsberg, Pena, et al, 2000). In another study of pregnant women in León (Valladares et al, 2005), the husband's drunkenness was often reported by victims to be a precipitant for violence against them.

Methods
Survey and Sample

The survey was conducted from May to July 2005, using face-to-face interviews of adults older than 18 years of age in five Nicaraguan cities with populations of at least 60,000 that were representative of the country's geographic areas: Estelí in the north, Juigalpa in the east, Rivas in the south, León in the west, and Bluefields on the Atlantic coast. The survey excluded Managua residents because that city was much larger than the other cities in the sample and included areas considered dangerous for interviewers. All researchers wore white lab coats and carried university identification. Interviews were conducted in private (with the exception of three in which a partner was present and one in which a mother-in-law was present).

Table 1 shows the demographic characteristics of the survey sample. Of the 2,030 interviewees who participated in the survey, 614 were men (30.2% of the total) and 1,416 (69.8%), were women. The average age for male respondents was 36 years and for women it was 34 years; the distribution by age group was roughly the same for all cities. Most respondents were married (664, or 32.7%) or living together (564, or 27.8%). More than half of the women in the sample were not part of the labor force, compared to only 10% of men; conversely, most men in the sample were most likely to be employed (66.5%), while only 25.6% of women worked. Almost 57% of men and more than 90% of women reported that they had not drunk any alcohol in the year preceding the survey. Of those who did drink alcohol, the number of drinking days was low, although the number of drinks consumed per occasion was high. A large percentage of current drinkers had drunk five or more drinks on at least one occasion (93% of men drinkers and almost 63% of women drinkers). The percent of current drinkers in the five cities was lowest for men and women in Rivas (32.1% and 5.6% respectively) and highest in Bluefields (52% of men and 16.6% of women) (see Table 2).

TABLE 1. Age, marital status, employment status, and drinking pattern in the 12 months preceding the survey, for male and female respondents, GENACIS survey, Nicaragua, 2005.

	Men (N=614)		Women (N=1,416)	
Variable	Number	Percent or mean	Number	Percent or mean
Age		35.8 years		34.3 years
18–24 years	172	28.2	396	28.2
25–34 years	155	25.5	395	28.2
35–44 years	112	18.4	319	22.7
45–54 years	102	16.8	174	12.4
55–64 years	46	7.6	94	6.7
65 and older	22	3.6	25	1.8
Marital status				
Married	198	32.3	466	32.9
Cohabiting/Living with a partner	167	27.2	397	28.0
Divorced or separated	19	3.1	61	4.3
Never married	225	36.6	454	32.1
Widowed	5	0.8	38	2.7
Employment status				
In the labor force	408	66.5	361	25.6
Involuntarily unemployed	51	8.3	114	8.1
Not in the labor force	64	10.4	746	52.6
Student	74	12.1	181	12.8
Retired	17	2.8	14	1.0
Drinking pattern (past 12 months)				
Average number of drinking days (drinkers only)		44.3 days		31.3 days
Drank any alcohol during past 12 months	266	43.4%	149	10.5%
Average number of drinks per occasion (drinkers only)		12.3 drinks		7.0 drinks
Average annual volume (drinkers only)		685.6 drinks		345.2 drinks
Drank five or more drinks on one or more occasions (drinkers only)	247	(92.9%)	94	(63.1%)

TABLE 2. Number and percent of respondents who drank alcohol in the 12 months preceding the interview, by city and sex, GENACIS survey, Nicaragua, 2005.

	Men		Women	
	Number	Percent	Number	Percent
Bluefields	63	52.0	48	16.6
Estelí	50	40.9	20	7.1
Juigalpa	52	39.1	26	9.3
León	66	51.1	38	14.0
Rivas	35	32.1	17	5.6
Total	266	43.3	149	10.5

Measures That Differed from the Core Questions

Whether the respondent drank five or more drinks on a single occasion in the year preceding the survey was based on a graduated frequency measure as described in the chapter on methods of this publication. Respondents who indicated that they had a same-sex partner who also was involved in the aggression were excluded from these analyses (20 men and 18 women for victimization; 20 men and 17 women for aggression).

Results

As shown in Figure 1, the percent of men and women who reported physical aggression by a partner or physical aggression toward a partner in the past two years was approximately 6%. Of those who reported being involved in partner physical aggression, 26.5% of men and 34.8% of women were victims only, 26.5% of men and 39.1% of women were aggressors only, and 46.9% of men and 26.1% of women had been both victims and aggressors.

The percent of men who reported aggression by a partner ranged from 2.9% in Rivas to 10.2% in León; among women victims, rates of aggression ranged from 3.7% in Juigalpa to 10.8% in León (see Table 3). Among male aggressors, the lowest rate (2.5%) was reported in Estelí and the highest, in León (9.4%). A similar pattern was found among female aggressors (2.6% in Estelí vs. 13.7% in León). Overall, the highest rate of partner aggression was found in León.

Figure 1. Percent of respondents who reported having been a victim or aggressor, by sex, GENACIS survey, Nicaragua, 2005.

[Bar chart showing:
- Female victimization: 6.0
- Female aggression: 6.4
- Male victimization: 6.1
- Male aggression: 6.1]

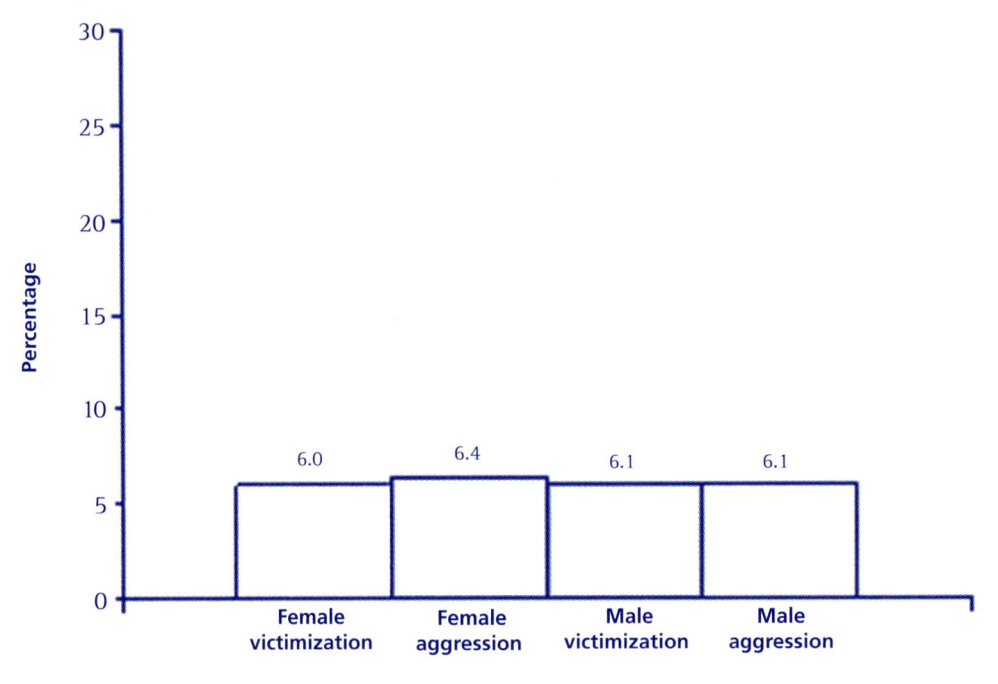

TABLE 3. Number and percent of respondents who reported physical aggression by a partner or aggression toward a partner, by city and sex, GENACIS survey, Nicaragua, 2005.

| | Aggression from partner |||| Aggression towards partner ||||
| | Men || Women || Men || Women ||
City	No.	%	No.	%	No.	%	No.	%
Bluefields	5	4.2	15	5.2	10	8.3	20	7.0
Estelí	5	4.2	16	5.8	3	2.5	7	2.6
Juigalpa	10	8.1	10	3.7	6	4.8	10	3.7
León	13	10.2	29	10.8	12	9.4	37	13.7
Rivas	3	2.9	14	4.7	5	4.8	16	5.3
Total	36	6.1	84	6.0	36	6.1	90	6.4

The average age of female victims was 29.2 years; of female aggressors, 29.8 years; and for both male victims and aggressors, 29.3 years. In general, aggression by and towards a partner decreased with age for both sexes, except that men 18–24 years old were less likely than men aged 25–34 years old to report being the victim of partner aggression (see Figure 2).

Among female and male victims and aggressors, the rate of partner physical aggression was higher for those who were cohabiting with their current partner, compared to other marital status groups (see Figure 3). However, this difference was significant (p<.01) only for cohabiting compared to never married female victims and female aggressors. Results should be treated with caution given the low numbers of respondents reporting partner aggression within some marital status groups.

FIGURE 2. Percent of respondents who reported having been a victim or aggressor, by age group and sex, GENACIS survey, Nicaragua, 2005.

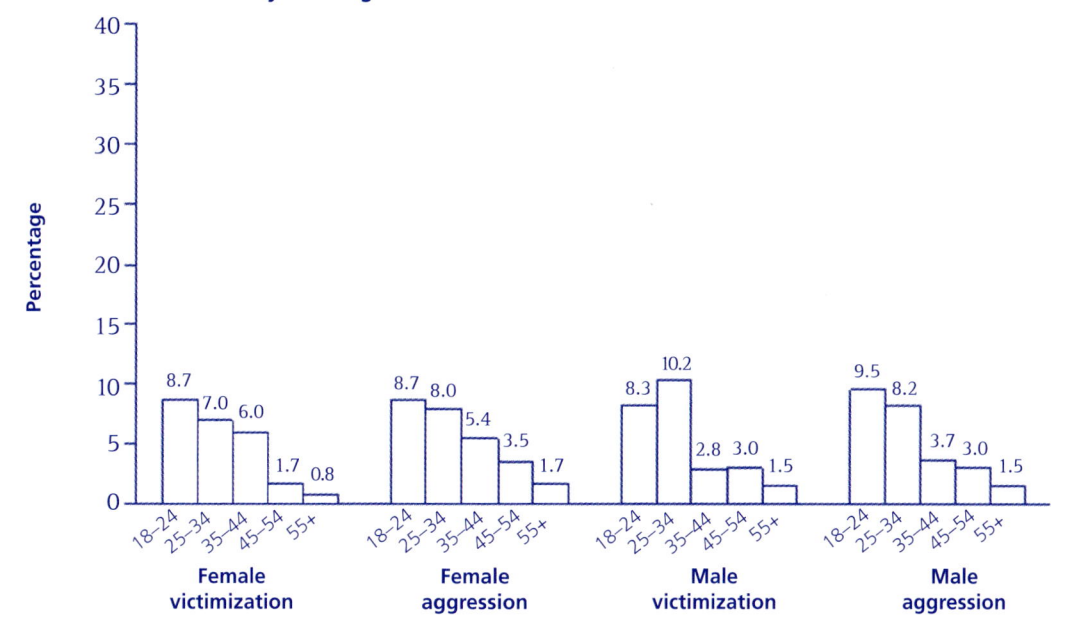

Figure 3. Percent of respondents who reported having been a victm or aggressor, by marital status and sex, Nicaragua, 2005.

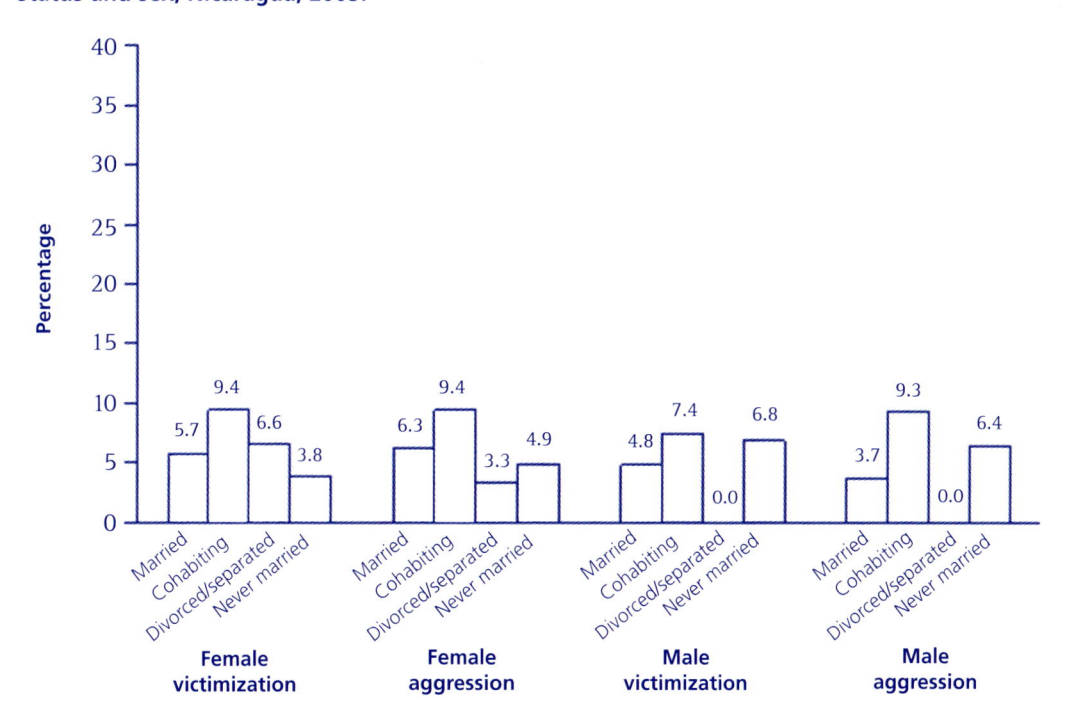

Figure 4 shows that female aggressors were more likely than their male counterparts to have slapped their partner, as reported by male and female victims and aggressors (significant only for male victims versus female victims at p<.01). Male victims reported being pushed more than female aggressors reported pushing (p<.01). Other differences between men and women victims and aggressors were not statistically significant. Acts coded as "other" include hitting, pulling hair, and biting.

FIGURE 4. Type of aggressive act against females as reported by female victims and male aggressors, and against males as reported by male victims and female aggressors, GENACIS survey, Nicaragua, 2005.

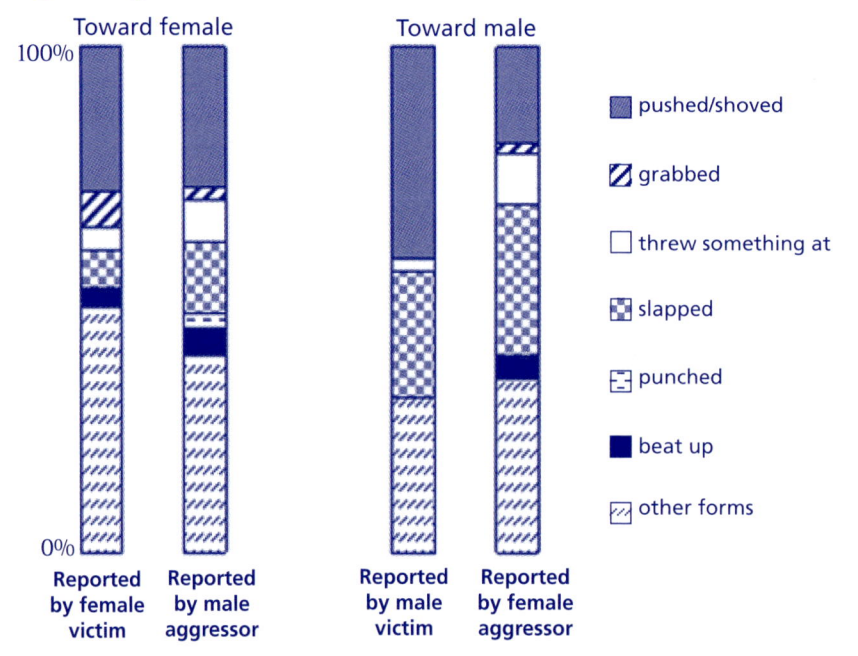

As shown in Figure 5, female victims rated the aggression as more severe and themselves as more afraid, upset, and angry than did female aggressors or male victims and aggressors; male victims gave the lowest ratings for the measures. For all four measures, female victims gave higher ratings than did male victims (severity and anger p<.01 and fear and upset p<.001, after controlling for age) and higher ratings than male aggressors (significant for fear p<.01, and upset and anger p<.05). Female aggressors rated themselves as more angry than did male victims (p<.05). Ratings by male aggressors were not statistically different from those of female aggressors. In addition to higher severity ratings, a significantly larger percentage of female than male victims reported seeking medical attention immediately or the next day—20 out of 84 (23.8%) versus 3 out of 36 (8.3%), p <.05.

Figure 6 shows that approximately 36% of female victims and 33% of male aggressors, and 36% of male victims and 30% of female aggressors reported alcohol consumption at the time of aggression. The male partner was the only drinker in most of the incidents involving alcohol. The following significant differences were found, although they should be considered with caution due to low numbers: more female victims than male victims reported that only the aggressive partner was drinking (p<.01); more male victims than female victims reported that only the respondent (i.e., the victim) was drinking (p=.001); more female aggressors than male aggressors reported that only the partner was drinking (p=.001); more male aggressors than female aggressors reported they were the only ones drinking (p<.001). Differences between female victims and male aggressors and between male victims and female aggressors were not statistically significant (i.e. p<.01).

FIGURE 5. Mean ratings of severity of aggression, fear, upset, and anger by male and female victims and aggressors, GENACIS survey, Nicaragua, 2005.

Severity
- Female victim: 5.4
- Female aggressor: 3.7
- Male victim: 3.5
- Male aggressor: 4.3

Fear
- Female victim: 6.2
- Female aggressor: 3.9
- Male victim: 3.5
- Male aggressor: 4.1

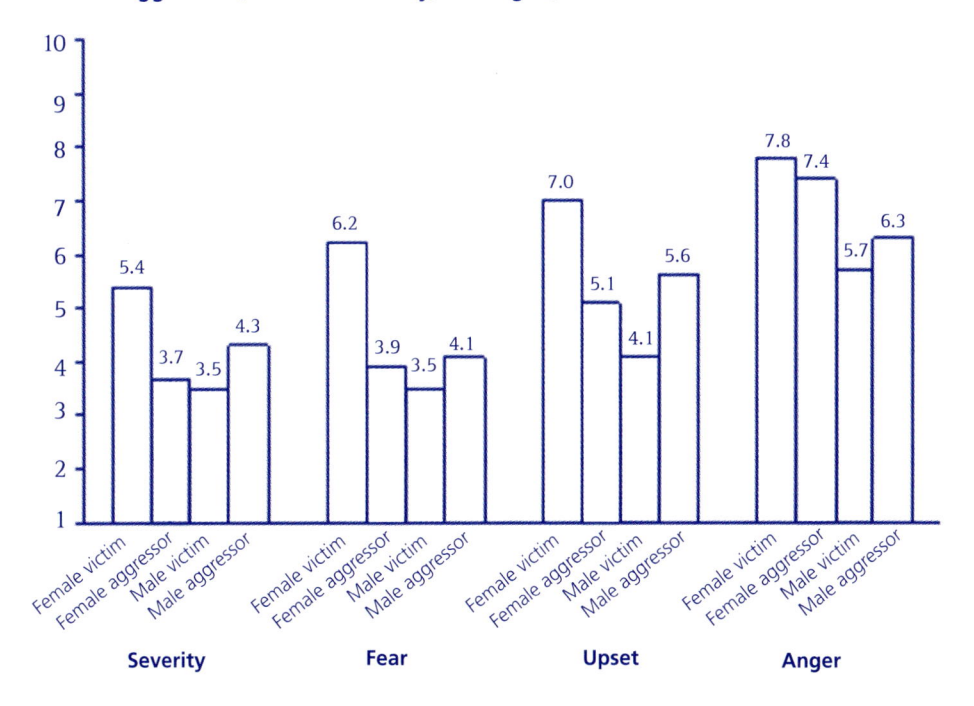

Upset
- Female victim: 7.0
- Female aggressor: 5.1
- Male victim: 4.1
- Male aggressor: 5.6

Anger
- Female victim: 7.8
- Female aggressor: 7.4
- Male victim: 5.7
- Male aggressor: 6.3

FIGURE 6. Percent of incidents in which no partner had been drinking, both partners had been drinking, only the male partner had been drinking, or only the female partner only had been drinking, as reported by male and female victims and aggressors, GENACIS survey, Nicaragua, 2005.

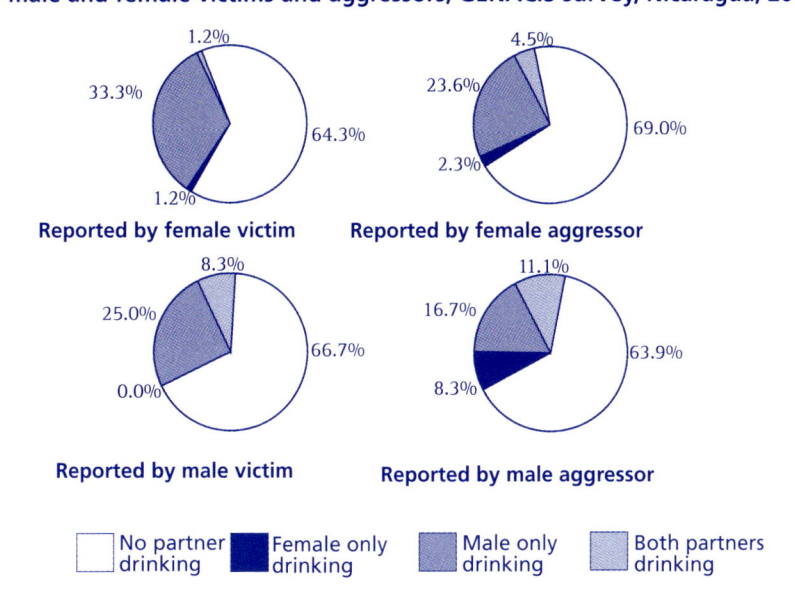

Reported by female victim: 33.3%, 1.2%, 64.3%, 1.2%

Reported by female aggressor: 23.6%, 4.5%, 69.0%, 2.3%

Reported by male victim: 25.0%, 8.3%, 66.7%, 0.0%

Reported by male aggressor: 16.7%, 11.1%, 63.9%, 8.3%

Legend: No partner drinking | Female only drinking | Male only drinking | Both partners drinking

After controlling for age, ratings of severity were higher for incidents involving alcohol, compared to incidents not involving alcohol, for female victims (6.6 versus 4.8, p<.05) and female aggressors (5.2 versus 3.1, p=.001). It was not possible to do a statistical comparison of severity ratings for males because of low numbers.

Relationship between Alcohol Consumption and Partner Aggression

Respondents who drank alcohol in the year preceding the survey were more likely than those who had not drunk alcohol to report being both victims and aggressors of partner physical aggression. In particular, 10.4% of men who drank compared to 2.7% of male abstainers, and 9.5% of women who drank versus 5.6% of female abstainers reported being victims. The percent of men who reported being aggressive toward a partner was 10.7% among drinkers and 2.4% among abstainers, and the percent of women aggressors was 7.4% among drinkers and 6.3% among abstainers. After controlling for age, these differences were statistically significant only for male victims (p=.001) and male aggressors (p<.001). These results should be treated with caution due to low numbers of male abstainers and female drinkers.

Respondents' Drinking Pattern and Partner Aggression

The following analyses of the relationship between partner physical aggression and respondents' drinking pattern could only be conducted for men, because the number of women who reported having drunk in the year preceding the survey was too low. However, these results should be treated with caution even for men. The number of men who never drank as many as five drinks on a single occasion was too low to allow a comparison to be made between them and those who did drink that much.

The mean number of drinking days (Figure 7) and the total number of drinks per year (Figure 9) were higher for male victims than for those reporting no partner aggression, and the mean number of drinks per occasion (Figure 8) was higher for male victims and aggressors compared to those reporting no partner physical aggression. After controlling for age, however, there were no statistically significant differences.

Discussion

The GENACIS survey results found lower rates of partner aggression than those found in earlier research on partner physical aggression against women, except that the ENDESA study found a similar rate as that found in León (Rosales et al, 1999). These differences might be related to survey methods, such as the focus of the questionnaire and the sex of the interviewers. Previous surveys that focused on violence against women only questioned women and interviews were conducted by female interviewers. The GENACIS survey, on the other hand, focused primarily on alcohol consumption and problems and included both men and women respondents and interviewers. Whereas respondents in the GENACIS survey may have been more reluctant to report aggression by and toward a partner, the privacy problems in the ENDESA study (Rosales et al, 1998; Ellsberg, Heise, et al, 2000) were minimized in the present study.

Nicaragua

FIGURE 7. Mean number of drinking days in the year preceding the survey for male respondents by whether the respondent had been a victim of partner aggression and whether the respondent had been aggressive toward a partner, GENACIS survey, Nicaragua, 2005.

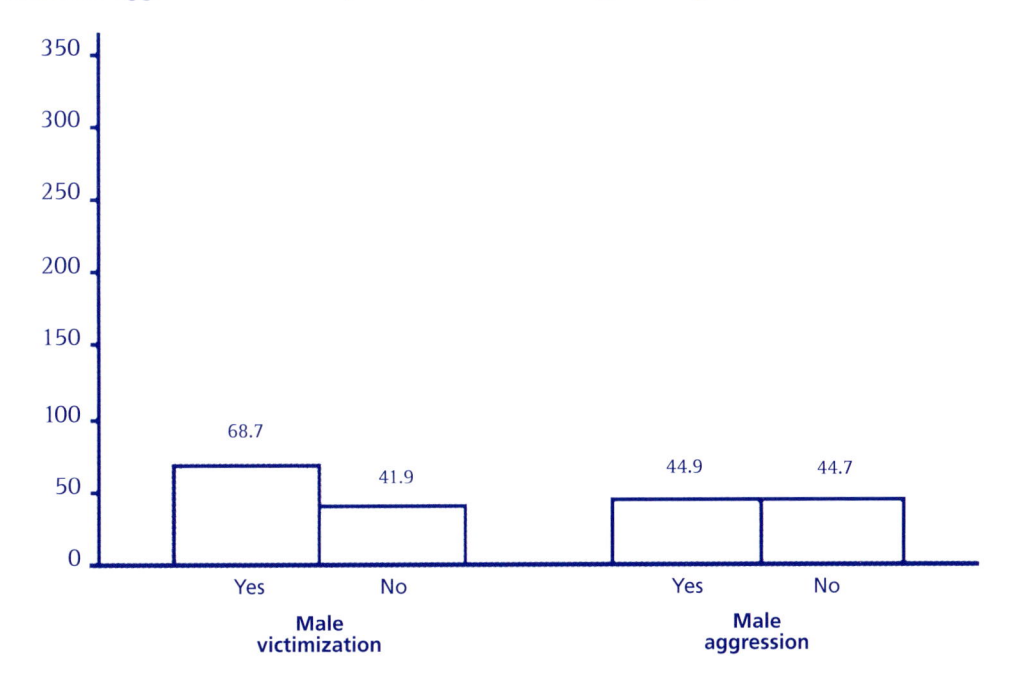

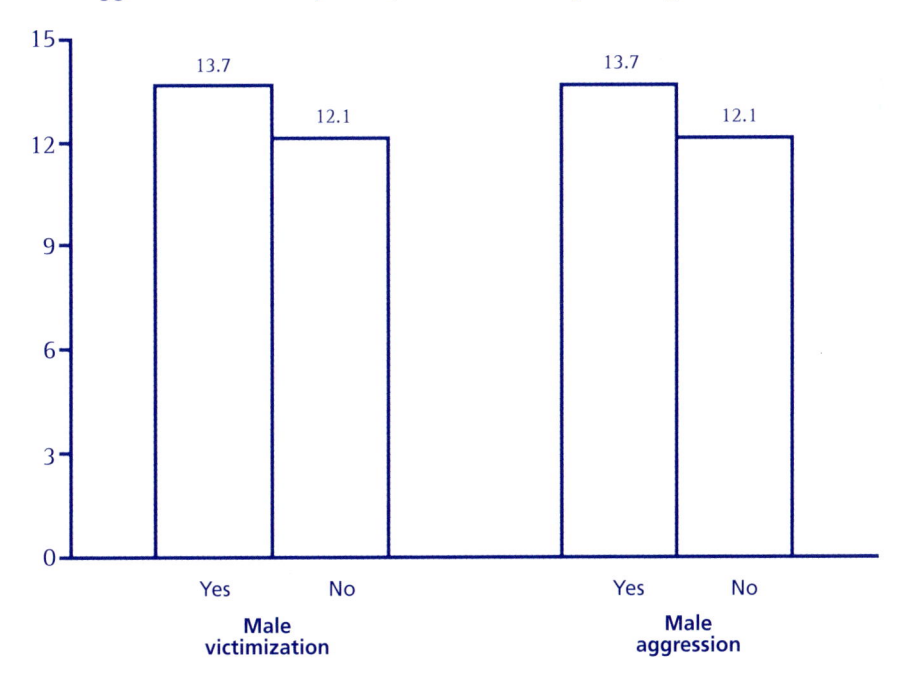

Male victimization		Male aggression	
Yes	No	Yes	No
68.7	41.9	44.9	44.7

FIGURE 8. Mean number of drinks consumed on usual drinking occasions by male respondents by whether the respondent had been a victim of partner aggression and whether the respondent had been aggressive toward a partner, GENACIS survey, Nicaragua, 2005.

Male victimization		Male aggression	
Yes	No	Yes	No
13.7	12.1	13.7	12.1

FIGURE 9. Total number of drinks consumed annually by male respondents by whether the respondent had been a victim of partner aggression and whether the respondent had been aggressive toward a partner, GENACIS survey, Nicaragua, 2005.

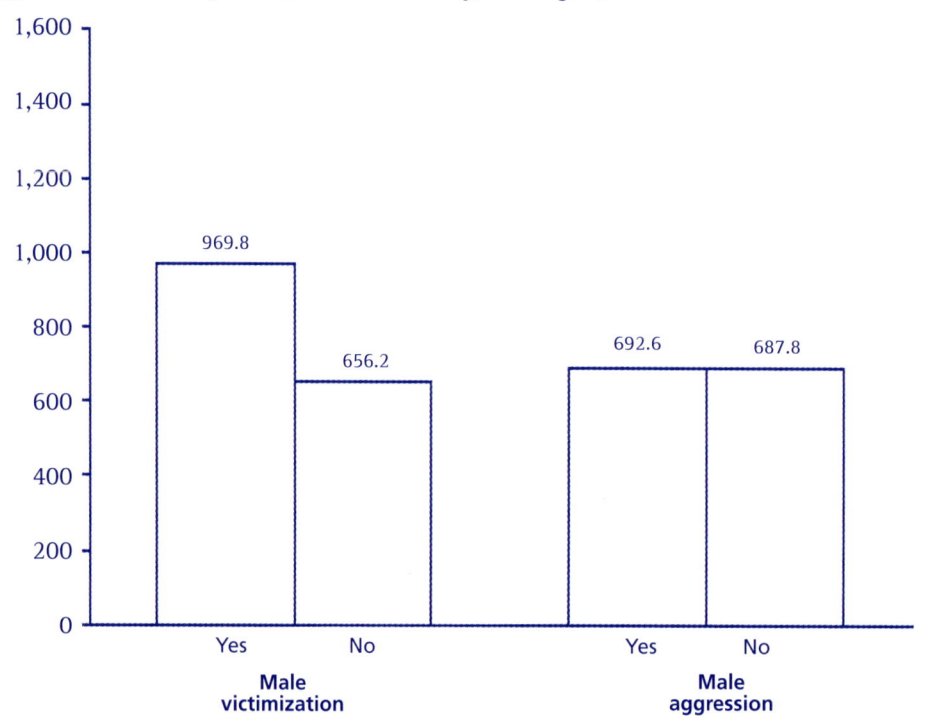

Male victimization: Yes 969.8, No 656.2
Male aggression: Yes 692.6, No 687.8

Results from the GENACIS survey are consistent with previous findings, showing that partner aggression is most common among young adults and generally decreases with age. It should be noted in this regard, however, that previous studies included respondents aged 15 years old and older, while the present study was limited to respondents 18 years old and older. This difference might also partly account for the lower rates of aggression found in the GENACIS survey study, because the highest rate of aggression in the ENDESA survey was reported by 15–19-year-olds.

Partner physical aggression for male and female victims and aggressors was higher among cohabiting respondents than in any other marital status groups (although these results should be interpreted with caution, given the small number of cases). In Nicaragua, cohabiting partners must live together for 10 years before they can be legally recognized as having the same rights and obligations as married partners; thus, those who choose cohabiting relationships, compared to those in formal marriages, might be more willing to take risks overall. This result also might be confounded with age, in that cohabiting is more common among younger than among older adults.

The GENACIS survey study also differed from previous research in that it also included physical aggression against men . While the percentages of men and women reporting physical victimization and aggression toward a partner were similar, some differences did emerge. More men (46.9%) than women (26.1%) reported that they had been both a victim and an aggressor (although not necessarily in the same incident), while more women than men reported being only a victim or only an aggressor. The findings also indicated different forms and severity of aggression for men and women. For example, slapping was more likely to be done by women than by men; however, aggression by male partners was more severe than aggression by female partners. Female victims rated the severity of the aggression and their feelings of fear, anger, and upset higher than did male victims and male aggressors. In addition, female victims were more likely than male victims to seek medical attention after the incident. Thus, there were important differences, despite the similarities in the percent of men and women reporting physical aggression by a partner.

The GENACIS project was the first known study in Nicaragua to explore the association between partner aggression and alcohol consumption for both sexes. Regardless of the victim's sex and whether the aggression was reported by the victim or the aggressor, more than 30% of incidents involved alcohol consumption, usually by the male partner. It should be noted that this finding might have resulted by chance, because a larger percentage of men drank alcohol and drank more frequently than women and, thus, were more likely to be drinking at any time, including during aggressive incidents. A comparison of drinkers versus nondrinkers, however, indicated that men and women who drink are more likely than those who do not drink to be both victims and aggressors. There was also some evidence to suggest that men who drank more drinks per occasion were more likely than men who drank fewer to report being victims or aggressors, although this difference was not statistically significant. It was not possible to determine the causal relationship between alcohol and partner aggression using these data. (For example, while alcohol consumption might lead to or aggravate the level of aggression between partners, it also is possible that being involved in partner aggression results in heavier drinking, particularly as a coping mechanism for victims). The finding that female victims and aggressors rated the severity of the aggression higher in incidents in which alcohol was involved than in incidents in which neither of the partners had been drinking suggests a possible increased risk of more severe aggression after alcohol consumption. While partner aggression involves other factors besides alcohol consumption (in the current study, alcohol consumption did not take place in the majority of incidents), previous findings and findings in the current study point to the need for further research in Nicaragua to examine the context within which alcohol consumption and aggression within intimate relationships occur and how alcohol might serve to precipitate or escalate that aggression. It is particularly important to further examine the social and physical contexts in which partner aggression occurs among younger adults to develop prevention, treatment, and assistance strategies for victims that are appropriate for this age group.

The GENACIS survey is the only survey in Nicaragua that collected data from both men and women about their victimization and aggression involving an intimate partner. The survey also collected information on drinking during the physical aggression incidents and about usual drinking patterns. Analyses of the relationship between a respondent's drinking and experiences with partner aggression were limited to males, because of a high abstention rate among females in the sample. Although the results of the GENACIS survey should be treated with caution because the reported cases of partner aggression were low, these results do suggest that it would be valuable to conduct further research using a large representative sample of the Nicaraguan population to examine gender differences in how partner aggression is experienced and the role that alcohol plays.

Acknowledgements
We are grateful to the interviewer team, the field supervisor, the Pan American Health Organization (PAHO), and GENACIS for support for this project.

References
Ellsberg M, Caldera T, Herrera A, Winkvist A, Kullgren G. (1999). Domestic violence and emotional distress among Nicaraguan women: Results from a population-based study. *Am Psychological Association, 54*, 30-36.

Ellsberg M, Heise L, Penna R, Agurto S, Winkvist A. (2000). Researching violence against women: Methodological considerations from three Nicaraguan studies. Umea University, SE-901 85 Umea, Sweden.

Ellsberg M, Herrera A, Liljestrand J, Winkvist A. (1999). Wife abuse among women of childbearing age in Nicaragua. *Am J of Public Health, 89*: 241-4

Ellsberg M, Liljestrand J, Winkvist A. (1997).The Nicaraguan Network of Women Against Violence: Using research as action for change. *Reproductive Health Matters*, No. 10.

Ellsberg M, Peña R, Herrera A, Liljestrand J, Winkvist A. (2000). Candies in hell: women's experiences of violence in Nicaragua. *Soc Sci & Med, 51*, 1595-1610.

Ellsberg M, Winkvist A, Peña R, Stenlund H. (2001). Women's strategic responses to violence in Nicaragua. J. Epidemiol. *Community Health, 55*, 547-555.

Morrisson A, Orlando M.(1999). Social and economic costs of domestic violence: Chile and Nicaragua. In Morrison A. and Biehl M. (eds.) *Too Close to Home: Domestic Violence in the Americas.* Washington, D.C.: Inter-American Development Bank, p.51-80.

Policia Nacional de Nicaragua. *www.policia.gob.ni/expospn.pdf*

Rosales J, Loaiza E, Primante D, Barberena A, Blandon L, Ellsberg M. (1999). Encuesta Nicaraguense de Demografia y Salud, 1998. Managua, Nicaragua: Instituto Nacional De Estadisticas y Censos, INEC and Macro International, Inc.

Valladares E, Ellsberg M, Pena R, Hogberg U, Persson L. (2002). Physical partner abuse during pregnancy: a risk factor for low birth weight in Nicaragua. *Obstet Gynecol. 100*, 700-705.

Valladares E, Pena R, Åke L. and Högberg U. (2005). Violence against pregnant women. Prevalence and characteristics: A population based study in Nicaragua. *Bjog, 112*, 1243-1248.

Watts C, Zimmerman C. (2002a). Violence against Women: Effects on Reproductive Health. *Out Look* 20(1), page 2

Watts C, Zimmerman C. (2002b). Violence against women: Global scope and magnitude. *Lancet, 359*, 1232-1237.

Wessel L, Campbell J. (1997). Providing sanctuary for battered women: Nicaragua's casas de la mujer. *Issues Ment Health Nurs, 18*, 455-476.

UNHAPPY HOURS:

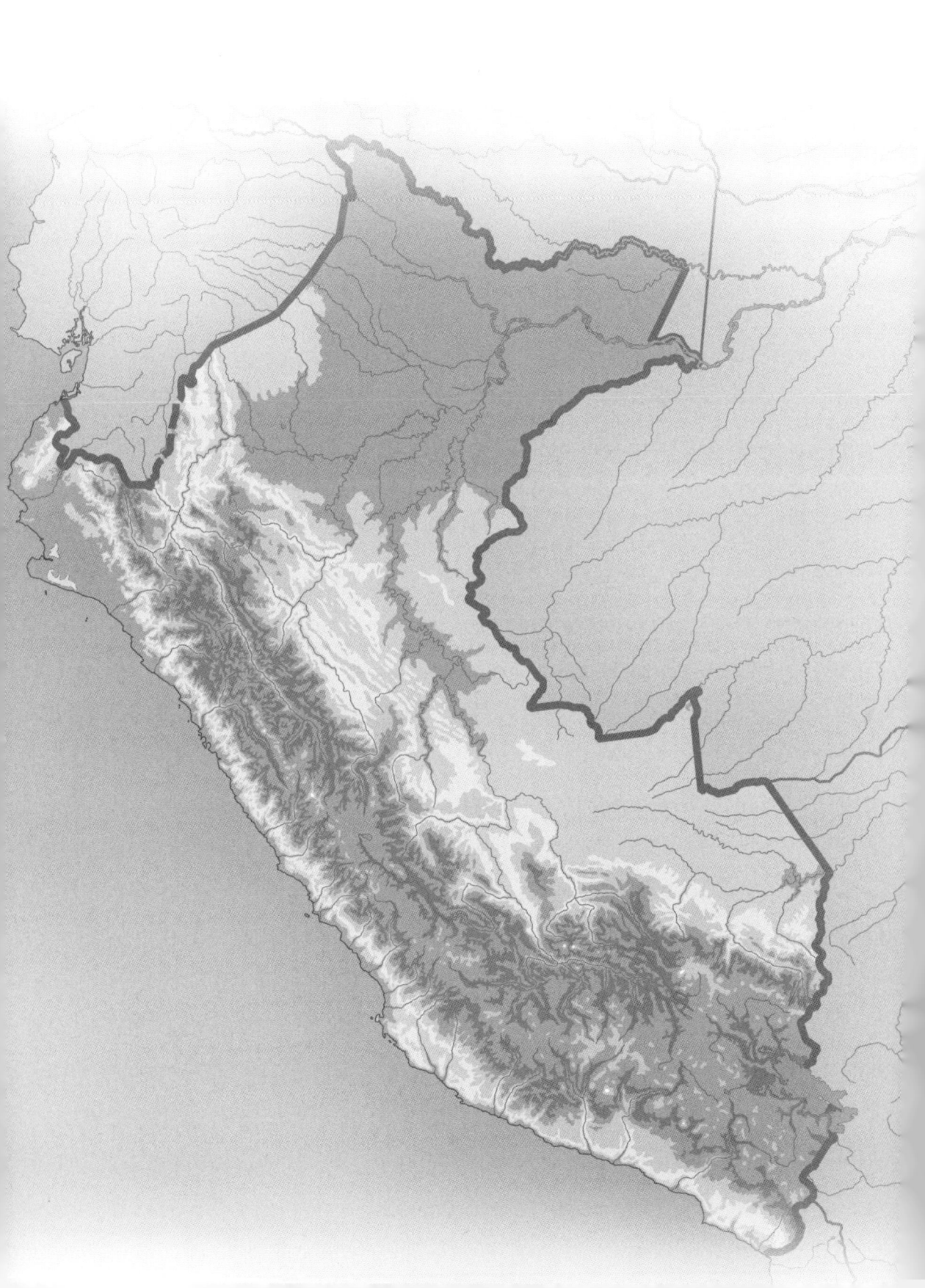

Peru: Alcohol and Partner Physical Aggression in Lima and Ayacucho—*Marina Piazza*

Introduction

Partner aggression is a significant public health problem that has received increasing attention in Peru during the last 15 years. The issue's heightened profile is reflected in the growing number of publications focusing on it, the development of preventive and therapeutic services to address it, and the adoption of policy and legal norms that incorporate a gender, human rights-based, and public health perspective. Nevertheless, partner aggression is still considered to be an accepted practice, media attention is insufficient, and the various approaches to intervention remain fragmented. In addition, most research has focused on violence against women, with a gap in knowledge about female-to-male violence.

Peru's Ministry of Women and Social Development (known by its Spanish acronym of MIMDES) has a National Program against Sexual and Family Violence that has the mandate to design and implement policies and activities for the prevention, treatment, and support to persons involved in sexual and domestic violence. MIMDES has developed a network of 43 Women's Emergency Centers. Nongovernment organizations have also been very active in developing services for victims and in fostering prevention efforts and research. Other services for victims of domestic violence who are seeking help include police stations, the Ombudsman's Office, health services, the National Department of Justice, and the Institute of Forensic Medicine. Two national laws—# 26260 and # 28236—provide protection to victims of family violence. In addition, Peru is a signatory nation to the Inter-American Convention on the Prevention, Punishment, and Eradication of Violence against Women (also known as the Convention of Belem do Pará) and the Convention on the Elimination of all Forms of Discrimination against Women (known as CEDAW).

Despite these efforts, the acceptance of partner aggression still persists, captured in an expression popular throughout the Peruvian Andes—"the more I love you, the more I beat you"—although the level of acceptance varies across different cultural environments. As another example, alcohol use is treated as an extenuating circumstance in the legal evaluation of the damage caused by the aggression of a person under the influence of psychoactive substances at the moment of the aggression. By contrast, it is an aggravating factor for a driver in a traffic collision who has a blood alcohol concentration above 0.5 g/100ml.

Regional differences were shown in the Peru data from a 2002 World Health Organization (WHO) multisite study of sexual and physical violence against women, with 60.9% of women in the Andean region of Cuzco and 48.4% of women in the capital city of Lima reporting lifetime physical violence (Güesmez, Palomino, and Ramos, 2002).

Past-year physical violence was also more prevalent in Cuzco (24.7%) than in Lima (16.9%). Within the region of Cuzco, physical violence was reported to a greater extent in urban (28.2%) versus rural areas (23.7%).

The 2004 National Demographic and Health Survey examined the most recent experience of physical violence among women who had been married or had lived with a partner at least once in their lifetime (Perú, Instituto Nacional de Estadística e Informática 2004). Types of physical aggression included being hit, attempted strangulation, being set on fire, being threatened with a weapon, or being forced against one's will into a sexual act. About 42% of women reported having been the victims of violence at least once during their most recent relationship. This rate was found to be greater among divorced, separated, or widowed females (63%) than among those living with a partner/spouse (37%). Rates were higher among those who had completed high school (45%), as compared to those who had attended or completed elementary school, or those with an education above the secondary level. When comparing by geographical regions, the highest rates were observed in the highlands (47%) and jungle areas (46%), with lower rates being recorded for the rest of the coast (38%) and in Lima (37%). The types of aggression most frequently reported were being shaken or pushed by one's partner (35%) and having been slapped or having the arm twisted (29%). About 10% reported having been forced into a sexual act against one's will, and 15% reported having experienced physical violence during the past year. Females in younger age groups reported higher rates of recent physical violence than their counterparts in the older groups.

Besides these population-based estimates, relevant statistics from service providers are also available. For example, the Institute of Forensic Medicine reported 92,655 clinical forensic exams for injuries due to domestic violence in 2005. During that same year, the National Police of Peru registered 76,255 reports of domestic violence. The victims were approximately 90% females and 10% males. Two-thirds (66%) of these reports concerned physical violence. Of the female victims, approximately 40% described themselves as housewives, 20% as vendors, and 15% did technical work. In terms of the relationship of the aggressor to the female victim, 40% of reported aggressors were partners, 31% were spouses, 16% were other family members, 8% were former partners, and 5% were former spouses.

Pattern of Alcohol Consumption and Relationship to Partner Aggression

A survey on drug use conducted in 2002 reported a lifetime alcohol use prevalence rate of 94.0% and a past-year prevalence rate of 75.2% for a national representative sample of residents aged 12–64 who resided in cities with populations of more than 20,000 (Perú, Comisión Nacional para el Desarrollo y Vida sin Drogas, 2002). This study also measured the disapproval level of alcohol use. Approximately three of every four subjects interviewed stated that they did not approve of alcohol use. The disapproval level was greater among respondents who had not used alcohol during the last month (83.3%) than among those who reported use during the last month (68.4%).

Another national epidemiological study in 2003 reported similar rates for alcohol use (Castro de la Mata and Zavaleta Martínez-Vargas, 2003). Among males, 21.3% reported drinking 1–2 times during the past year, 20.0% 3–6 times, and 9.6 % 7–11 times; 22.6%

reported drinking at least once per month, 9.2% at least once a week, and 0.2% daily; 7.6% reported not having consumed alcohol during the last year, and 9.4% reported never having consumed alcohol in their lifetime. Among females, 24.9% reported drinking 1–2 times during the past year, 20.5% 3–6 times, and 6.0% 7–11 times; 16.6% reported drinking at least once a month, 2.7% at least once a week, and 0.5% daily; 14.3% reported not having consumed alcohol in the last year, and 14.5% not having consumed alcohol in their lifetime.

There are very limited data on alcohol involvement in partner aggression. A WHO study of partner aggression toward women indicated that being under the influence of alcohol was the main situation that would give rise to partner aggression (Güesmez, Palomino, and Ramos, 2002). This reason was mentioned more by women in Cuzco (63.5%) than women in Lima (29.5%). Other reported situations related to physical violence were jealousy (Lima 29.9%, Cuzco 28.2%), economic difficulties (Lima 19.1%, Cuzco 11.5%), that the female victim disobeyed her partner (Lima 16.9%, Cuzco 15.3%), problems with the woman's or her partner's family (Cuzco 17.1%, Lima 12.3%), and problems with work (Lima 12.3%, Cuzco 7.2%).

Logistic regression models based on a sample of 15,991 females from the 2000 Demographic and Health Survey conducted in Peru (Flake, 2005) revealed that a partner's alcohol consumption was a significant family-level risk marker for a woman's abuse. Individual-level predictors for women reporting partner abuse included low educational attainment, early marriage or cohabitation, and a family background marked by violence. At the community level, living in a noncoastal area and having an urban residence increased the likelihood of abuse when other factors were controlled.

Data on partner aggression collected at police stations and compiled in National Police Reports indicate that about 26% of the aggressors were under the influence of alcohol. In addition, 8% of aggressors reported being motivated by problems with alcohol; other reported reasons for aggression included intimate relationship issues (43%), family issues (21%), and economic reasons (12%) (Perú, Policia Nacional del Perú, 2005).

Research Objectives
The purpose of this chapter is to assess the relationship between drinking pattern and risk of partner physical aggression among adults in the general population and to examine the role of alcohol consumption at the time of partner aggression. Additionally, the chapter aims to determine if the association between drinking level and partner aggression varied between two cities located in different regions: Lima, with a population of 8.8 million, representing 30% of the total Peruvian population and located in the coastal area, and Ayacucho, with a population about 70,000 and located in the central highlands.

Methods
The study used data from personal face-to-face interviews conducted with a multistage probability sample survey of residents aged 18–64 of Lima (n = 1,110) and Ayacucho (n = 421). The sampling frame used data and boundary maps from the 1996 Population Count, including *conglomerados*, or basic areas similar to U.S. census

tracts, which are the smallest geographically defined units for which data on population are available. The first sampling stage involved sampling census tracts, each with a total of approximately 40 households distributed over one or several blocks. A second stage involved sampling households, and, finally, persons within each household. For Lima, the sample was drawn from 144 census tracts, and in Ayacucho it was drawn from 50 census tracts.

The Gender, Alcohol, and Culture: An International Study (GENACIS) questionnaire was adapted taking into account special local language expressions and rephrasing some questions to enhance clarity. In order to facilitate the understanding of the response options, a set of cards was created. The table of equivalencies of beverages' alcoholic content was adapted using the Peruvian Technical Norms for Alcoholic Beverages (Perú, Instituto de Derechos del Consumidor y Propiedad Intelectual, 2003), and an inventory specifying the alcoholic content of local beverages was developed for use in this study. The study was approved by the Institutional Review Board of the Universidad Peruana Cayetano Heredia.

Interviewer training took place in Lima in July 2005 and in Ayacucho in September 2005. Interviewers were psychologists, anthropologists, sociologists, and social workers. Training issues included privacy, confidentiality, and interviewing techniques. A pilot study was conducted consisting of 30 interviews in each of the two cities that provided input for necessary adjustments to be made to the questionnaire. Following completion of the interviews, respondents were offered information about community resources for alcohol and drug treatment.

General characteristics of male and female participants in the survey are shown in Table 1. This table also presents drinking patterns. In general, approximately 8 of every 10 males and 6 of every 10 females reported having drunk alcohol during the last year. Rates for Ayacucho were higher than those for Lima. Among those who reported alcohol use during the last year, the frequency of use (measured by the average number of drinking days) was higher for males than females. This was true for Lima (males 23.3, females 12) and Ayacucho (males 12.1, females 7.5). In terms of the amount of alcohol consumed per occasion (measured by number of drinks per occasion), on average in Lima males drank almost twice as much (7.0 drinks) as females (3.7 drinks). This pattern was similar for Ayacucho (males 6.9, females 4.3 drinks). The annual volume of alcohol consumption was greater for males than females. Gender differences were greater in Lima (males 229.8 drinks, females 59.3 drinks) than in Ayacucho (males 141.1 drinks, females 54.6 drinks). Males reported higher rates than females of drinking five or more drinks on one or more occasions. This drinking pattern was more prevalent in Ayacucho (males 90.5%, females 76.4%) than in Lima (74.0% males, 46.7% females).

Overall drinking patterns by gender revealed more male than female alcohol use as assessed by different alcohol use measures, including percent of users during the last year, frequency of use, amount of drinks per occasion, annual volume of alcohol consumption, and drinking five or more drinks per occasion. Male and female drinkers in Lima drank more frequently than did drinkers in Ayacucho and had a higher annual volume of use (males). In contrast, drinkers in Ayacucho were more likely than drinkers from Lima to report drinking five or more drinks on one or more occasions during the past year.

TABLE 1. Age, marital status, employment status, and drinking pattern in the 12 months preceding the survey, for male and female respondents, GENACIS survey, Lima and Ayacucho, Peru, 2005.

	Lima				Ayacucho			
	Male (N=376)		Female (N=734)		Male (N=140)		Female N=281	
	Number	Percent or mean	Number	Percent or mean	Number	Percent or mean	Number	Percent or mean
Age		37.1 years		37.5 years		31.0 years		32.5 years
18 to 24 years	79	21.0%	139	18.9%	51	36.5%	73	26.0%
25 to 34 years	109	29.0%	185	25.2%	41	29.3%	94	33.5%
35 to 44 years	79	21.0%	185	25.2%	34	24.3%	80	28.5%
45 to 54 years	49	13.0%	145	19.8%	9	6.4%	20	7.1%
55 years and older	60	16.0%	80	10.9%	5	3.6%	14	5.0%
Marital status								
Married	119	31.7%	260	35.2%	39	27.9%	87	31.0%
Cohabiting/Living with partner	85	22.6%	192	26.2%	47	33.6%	64	22.8%
Divorced or separated	10	2.6%	60	8.2%	2	1.4%	40	14.2%
Never married	162	43.1%	200	27.3%	51	36.4%	82	29.2%
Widowed	0	0	22	3.0%	1	0.7%	8	2.9%
Employment status								
Working for pay (includes temporarily not working due to illness, pregnancy)	299	79.5%	268	36.5%	99	70.7%	135	48.2%
Voluntarily not working (includes homemaker, not working by choice)	6	1.6	377	51.4%	4	2.9%	88	31.4%
Involuntarily unemployed	13	3.5%	8	1.1%	2	1.4%	3	1.1%
Student	42	11.2%	66	9.0%	34	24.3%	53	18.9%
Retired	16	4.3%	15	2.0%	1	0.7%	1	0.4%
Drinking pattern (past 12 months)								
Drank any alcohol during past 12 months	307	81.7%	441	60.1%	118	84.3%	179	63.9%
Average number of drinking days (drinkers only)		23.3 days		12.0 days		12.1 days		7.5 days
Average number of drinks per occasion (drinkers only)		7.0 drinks		3.7 drinks		6.9 drinks		4.3 drinks
Average annual volume (drinkers only)		229.8 drinks		59.3 drinks		141.1 drinks		54.6 drinks
Drank five or more drinks on one or more occasions (drinkers only)	223	74.0%	190	46.7%	105	90.5%	136	76.4%

Results
Rates of Physical Aggression

Rates of male-to-female and female-to-male physical aggression as reported by aggressors and victims were estimated. Results are presented for each city separately, with those for Lima appearing in Figures 1a–10a and those for Ayacucho being shown in Figures 1b–10b. In addition, comparisons were made between the two cities.

The percent of males and females reporting physical aggression by a partner (the victim) and physical aggression toward a partner (the aggressor) are shown in Figures 1a and 1b. In Lima, a larger percentage of females than males reported being the victim of aggression by a partner. In this city, females also reported being aggressive toward a partner in a greater proportion than males, but these differences were not significant (Figure 1a). In Ayacucho (Figure 1b), more females (19.8%) than males (10.0%) reported being the victim of partner aggression ($p < .05$). Within each of the two cities, no other pair-wise differences between the percent of males and females victims and aggressors were found to be significant. Significant differences between cities were found for female victims (Lima 8.4%, Ayacucho 19.8%, $p < .001$) and male aggressors (Lima 6.5%, Ayacucho 12.9%, $p < .05$).

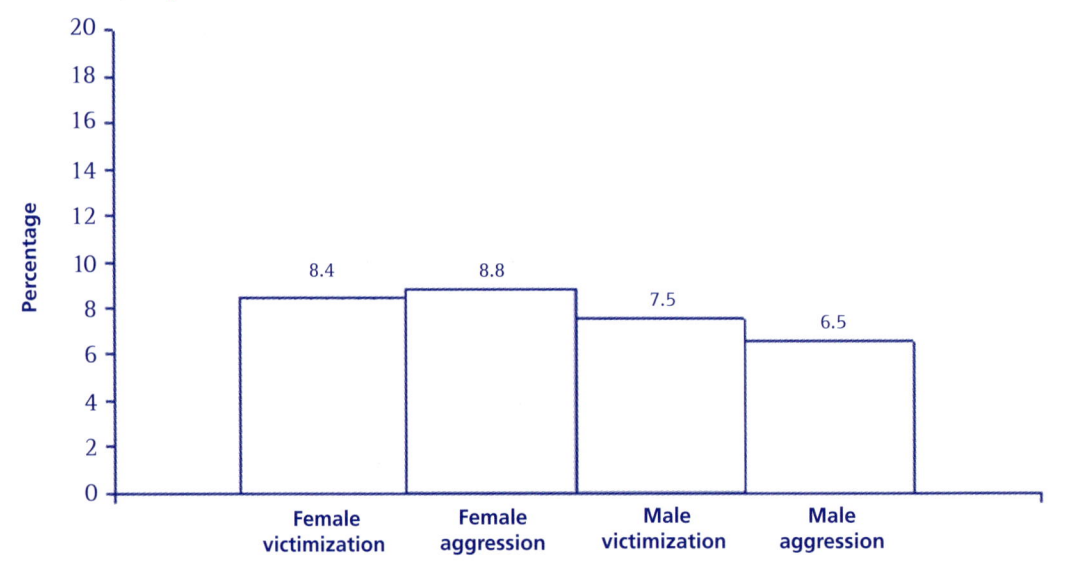

FIGURE 1a. Percent of Lima respondents who reported having been a victim or aggressor, by sex, GENACIS survey, Peru, 2005.

Category	Percentage
Female victimization	8.4
Female aggression	8.8
Male victimization	7.5
Male aggression	6.5

FIGURE 1b. Percent of Ayacucho respondents who reported having been a victim or aggressor, by sex, GENACIS survey, Peru, 2005.

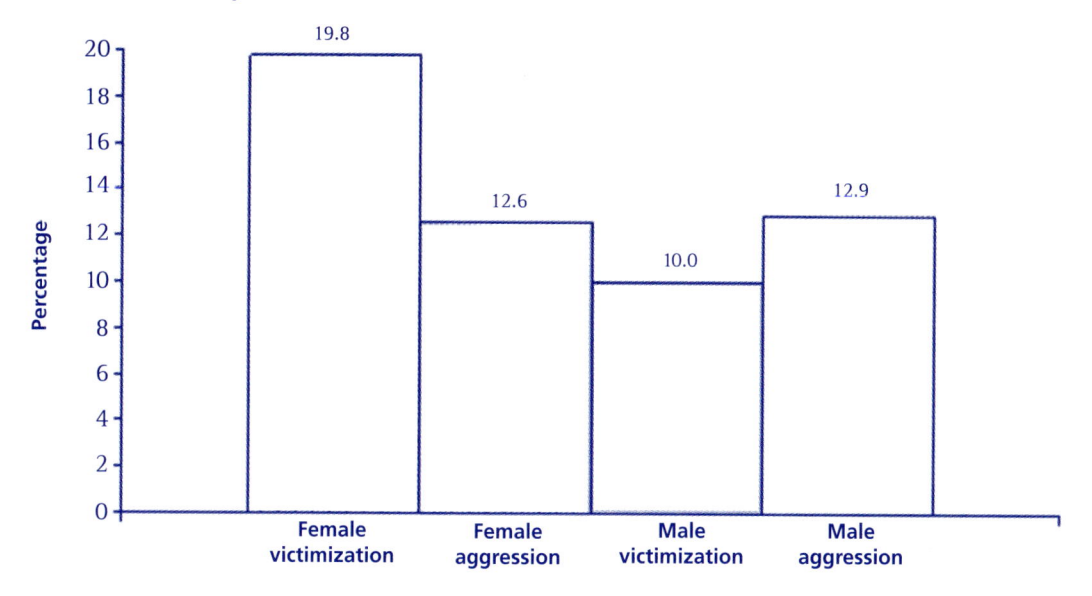

In terms of the extent that persons reported both victimization and aggression, among females in Lima who reported any partner aggression, 35.4% reported being only a victim, 38.4% reported being only an aggressor, and 26.3% reported being both a victim and an aggressor. Among males in Lima, 36.8% reported being only a victim, 26.3% reported being only an aggressor, and 36.8% reported being both a victim and an aggressor. In contrast, in Ayacucho, females were more likely to report being only a victim, while males were more likely to report being only an aggressor (females: 50.0% victim only, 21.4% aggressor only, 28.6% both victim and aggressor; males: 25.0% victim only, 41.7% aggressor only, 33.3% both victim and aggressor).

Rates of Physical Aggression by Age

As shown in Figures 2a and 2b, reports of partner physical aggression tended to decline with age. This pattern was observed for victims and aggressors of both sexes and in both cities.

FIGURE 2a. Percent of Lima respondents who reported having been a victim or aggressor, by age group and sex, GENACIS survey, Peru, 2005.

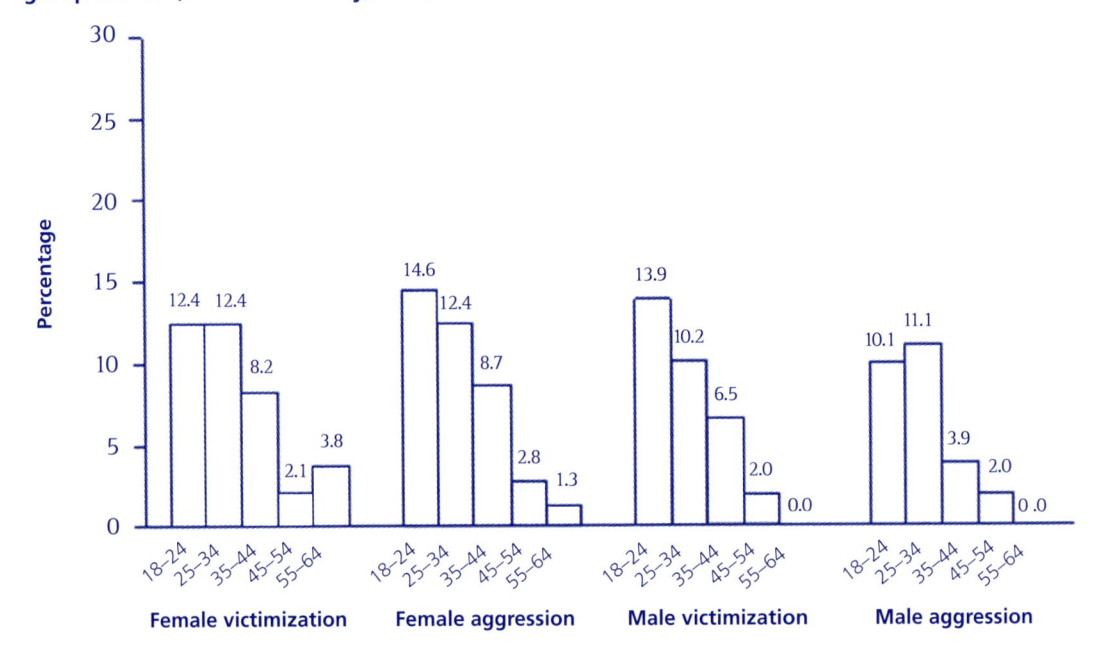

Female victimization (18–24 to 55–64): 12.4, 12.4, 8.2, 2.1, 3.8
Female aggression: 14.6, 12.4, 8.7, 2.8, 1.3
Male victimization: 13.9, 10.2, 6.5, 2.0, 0.0
Male aggression: 10.1, 11.1, 3.9, 2.0, 0.0

FIGURE 2b. Percent of Ayacucho respondents who reported having been a victim or aggressor, by age group and sex, GENACIS survey, Peru, 2005.

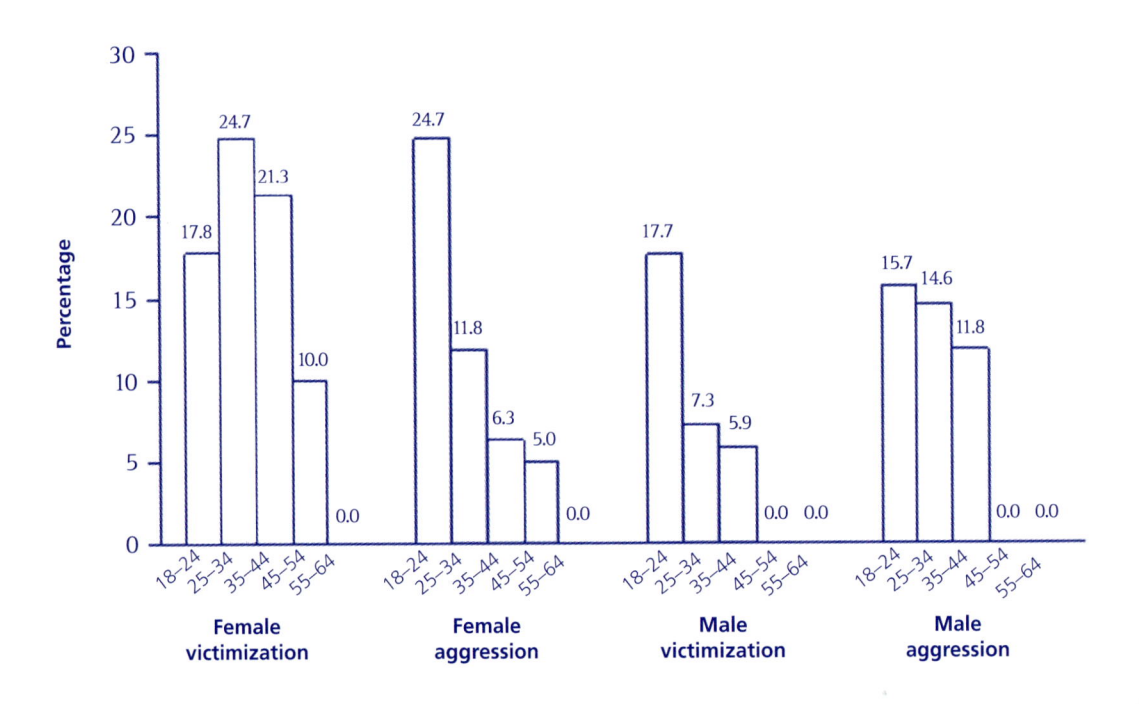

Female victimization (18–24 to 55–64): 17.8, 24.7, 21.3, 10.0, 0.0
Female aggression: 24.7, 11.8, 6.3, 5.0, 0.0
Male victimization: 17.7, 7.3, 5.9, 0.0, 0.0
Male aggression: 15.7, 14.6, 11.8, 0.0, 0.0

Rates of Physical Aggression by Marital Status

Figures 3a and 3b show rates of partner physical aggression as reported by female and male victims and aggressors, by marital status. The numbers of males who were divorced or separated in both cities were too small to be included in these analyses. Among female victims and male aggressors in both cities, and female aggressors in Lima, the rate of partner aggression was higher for those who cohabited with a partner during the past year than for other marital status groups. These results were significant for both Lima and Ayacucho when comparing female victims who cohabited with those who had never married ($p < .01$). Among female aggressors in Lima, those who cohabited reported significantly more partner aggression than married females ($p < .001$).

Never-married men in both cities reported a higher rate of aggression by a partner than did men in other marital status groups. The same pattern was observed among female aggressors in Ayacucho, significant when compared to married female aggressors ($p < .01$). In contrast, never-married women in both cities were least likely to report victimization, significant for never-married compared to married ($p < .01$) and cohabiting ($p < .001$) in Ayacucho, and never-married compared to cohabiting ($p < .01$) in Lima. Male aggressors and male victims in both cities, and female aggressors in Lima, were least likely to be married compared to all other marital statuses. No other pair-wise comparisons were statistically different. These results should be interpreted with caution, however, due to low numbers, particularly for males in Ayacucho.

FIGURE 3a. Percent of Lima respondents who reported having been a victim or aggressor,[a] by marital status and sex, GENACIS survey, Peru, 2005.

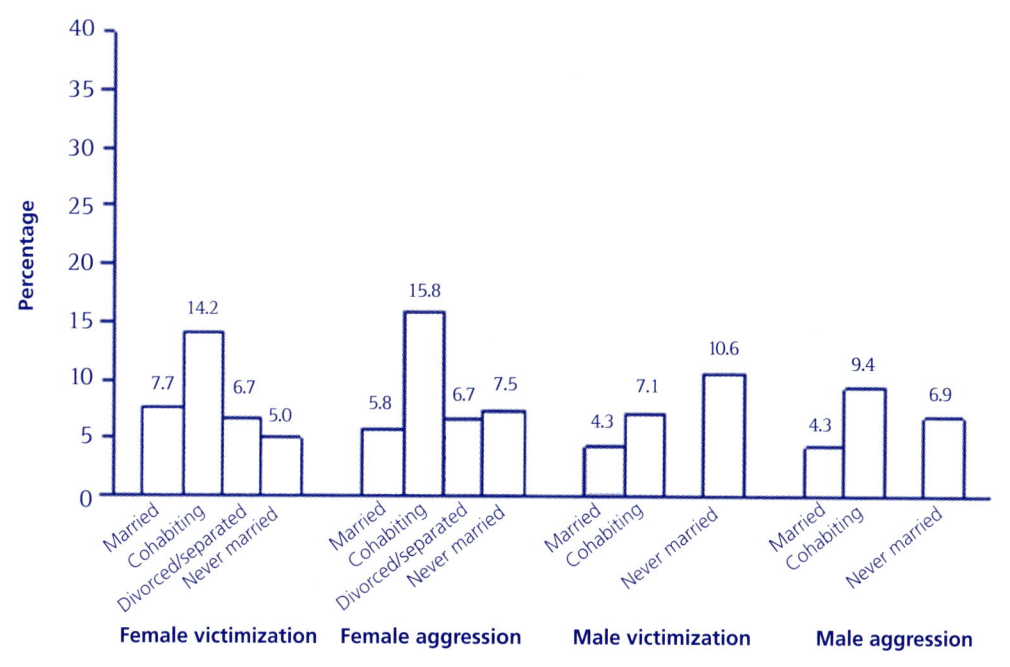

Category	Married	Cohabiting	Divorced/separated	Never married
Female victimization	7.7	14.2	6.7	5.0
Female aggression	5.8	15.8	6.7	7.5
Male victimization	4.3	7.1	—	10.6
Male aggression	4.3	9.4	—	6.9

[a]Excludes widowed respondents and divorced/separated males due to low number of cases.

FIGURE 3b. Percent of Ayacucho respondents who reported having been a victim or aggressor,[a] by marital status and sex, GENACIS survey, Peru, 2005.

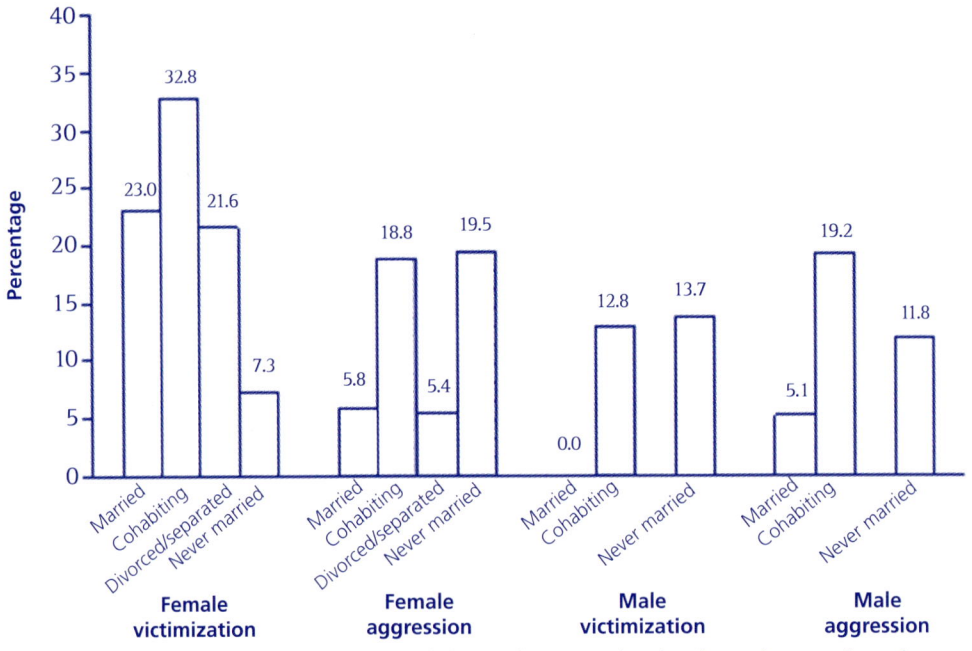

Female victimization: Married 23.0, Cohabiting 32.8, Divorced/separated 21.6, Never married 7.3
Female aggression: Married 5.8, Cohabiting 18.8, Divorced/separated 5.4, Never married 19.5
Male victimization: Married 12.8, Cohabiting 0.0, Never married 13.7
Male aggression: Married 5.1, Cohabiting 19.2, Never married 11.8

[a]Excludes widowed respondents and divorced/separated males due to low number of cases.

Types of Aggression

In Lima, the most frequent form of aggression was slapping, reported by approximately 40% of respondents (Figure 4a). More severe types of aggression, such as punching and beating up, were more likely to be used against female than against male partners. This pattern was reported by both female victims and male aggressors. Nevertheless, these differences did not meet the criterion of $p < .01$ for significance and should be treated with caution due to the small numbers of cases.

The data for Ayacucho presented in Figures 4b–10b came from female respondents only, due to the small number of males who reported being victims and aggressors. As seen in Figure 4b, slapping was the most common form of aggression reported by victims and aggressors. Female victims in Ayacucho reported being punched or beaten up more often than female aggressors reported using these acts. However, these differences did not meet the criterion for significance.

Peru | 173

FIGURE 4a. Type of aggressive act against females as reported by female victims and male aggressors, and against males as reported by male victims and female aggressors, GENACIS survey, Lima, Peru, 2005.

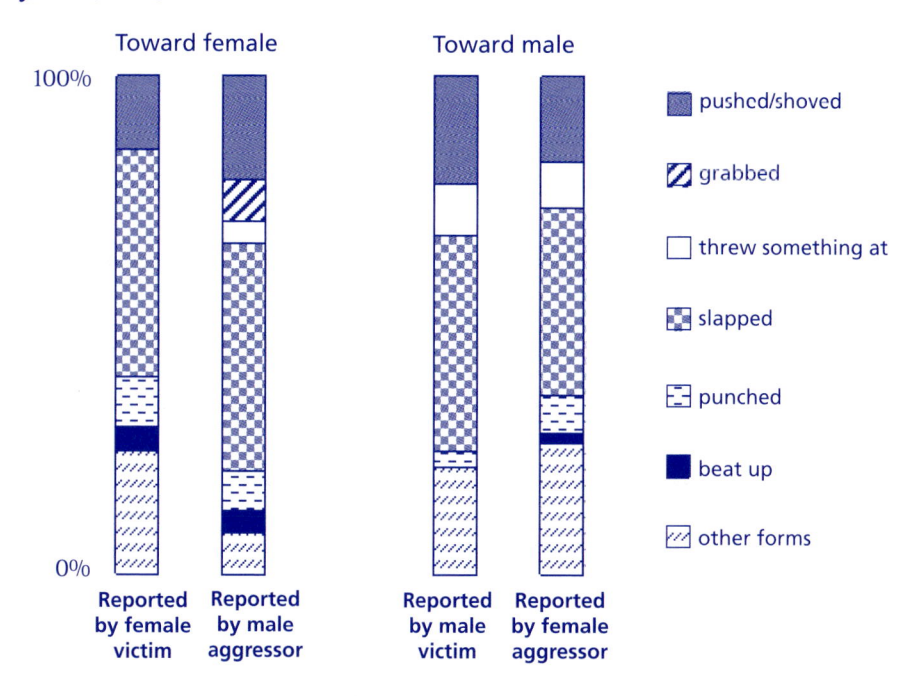

FIGURE 4b. Type of aggressive act against females as reported by female victims and against males as reported by female aggressors, GENACIS survey, Ayacucho, Peru, 2005.

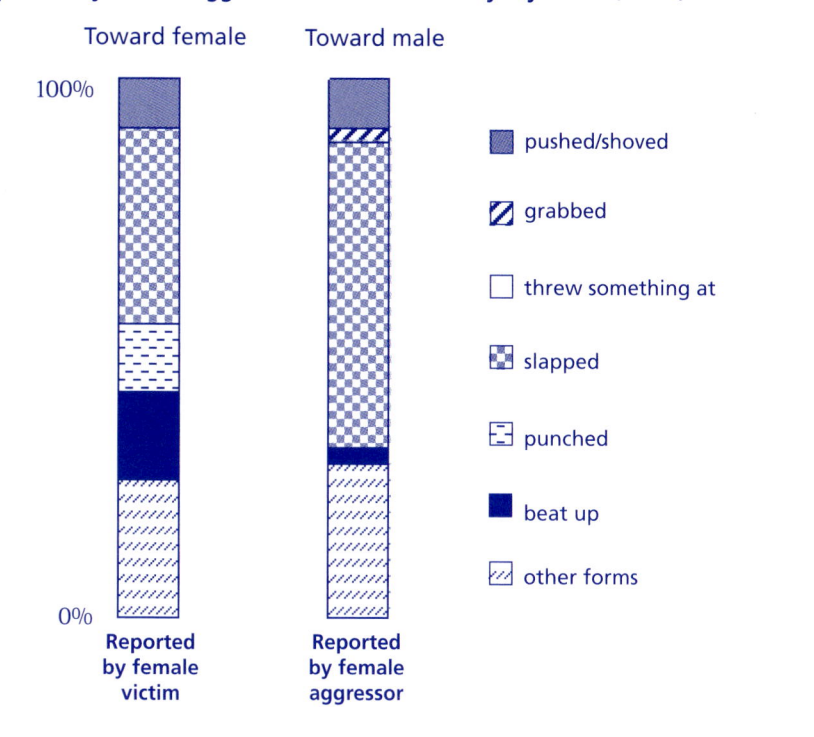

Severity of Aggression

Average ratings of the level of severity of the aggressive act and the emotional impact, as measured by how scared, upset, and angry the respondent felt at the time of the aggression, revealed that in Lima, female victims gave higher ratings than male victims on all four measures, (significant after controlling for age: $p < .001$ for fear, upset, and anger), as shown in Figure 5a. Female victim ratings were also higher than those of male aggressors (significant after controlling for age: $p = <.001$ for upset, $p < .01$ for anger). Ratings by male aggressors and male victims were not significantly different from those of female aggressors. In addition, in Lima, more female (23.0%) than male victims (3.6%) reported seeking medical attention at the time of the aggression or the next day ($p < .05$).

FIGURE 5a. Mean ratings of severity of aggression, fear, upset, and anger by male and female victims and aggressors, GENACIS survey, Lima, Peru, 2005.

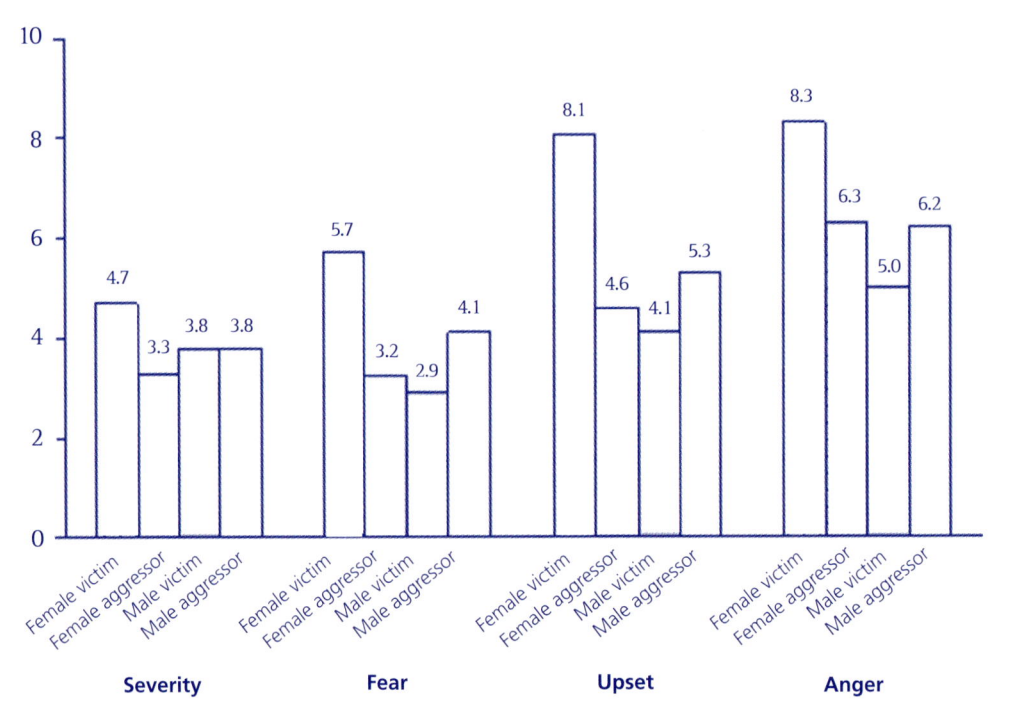

As shown in Figure 5b, female victims in Ayacucho rated all four dimensions of aggression higher than did female aggressors; however, none of these differences was significant after controlling for age. Approximately 13% of female victims in Ayacucho sought medical attention. There were no significant differences between Lima and Ayacucho in terms of women's ratings of severity of aggression. Analyses of differences on these ratings by sex could not be done for the Ayacucho sample due to the small number of males in the sample.

FIGURE 5b. Mean ratings of severity of aggression, fear, upset and anger by female victims and aggressors, GENACIS survey, Ayacucho, Peru, 2005.

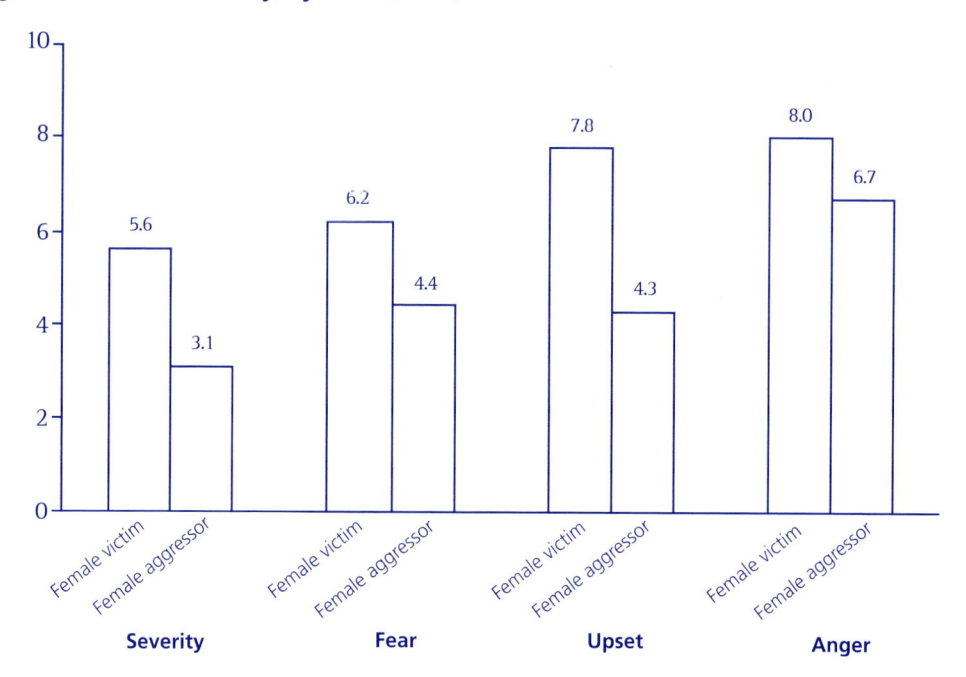

Category	Female victim	Female aggressor
Severity	5.6	3.1
Fear	6.2	4.4
Upset	7.8	4.3
Anger	8.0	6.7

As shown in Figure 6a, in Lima, female victims were more likely than the other groups of respondents to report that one or both partners were drinking during the incident. Comparing reports of victims by sex, more female victims reported the male partner was drinking than male victims reported the female partner was drinking ($p = .001$). More male victims than female victims reported being the only drinker ($p < .01$). Similarly, more male aggressors than female aggressors reported being the only drinker ($p < .01$).

A similar pattern was found in Ayacucho, where approximately 44% of females reported that one or both partners were drinking during the incident (Figure 6b). Similarly, in Ayacucho, males were more likely to be the sole drinker in the incident as reported by female victims and female aggressors. Comparing reports by female victims and aggressors from Lima and Ayacucho identified no significant differences in the proportion who reported alcohol involvement in the aggressive incident.

Severity ratings were compared for situations in which the aggression involved alcohol and those in which it did not. Analyses controlled for the possible confounding effect of age. In Ayacucho, severity ratings by female victims were significantly higher for incidents that involved alcohol (6.5) than for incidents in which no one was drinking (4.9) ($p < .05$). In Lima, the ratings of female victims were not significantly different in aggressive situations involving alcohol (4.8) and those not involving alcohol (4.6). It was not possible to examine severity ratings by alcohol involvement for female aggressors, male victims, or male aggressors due to low numbers.

FIGURE 6a. Percent of incidents in which no partner was drinking, both partners were drinking, only the male was drinking, or only the female was drinking, as reported by male and female victims and aggressors, GENACIS survey, Lima, Peru, 2005.

Reported by female victim: 3.3%, 38%, 0.0%, 59.0%

Reported by female aggressor: 6.4%, 19.1%, 1.6%, 72.9%

Reported by male aggressor: 4.2%, 20.8%, 0.0%, 75.0%

Reported by male victim: 3.6%, 17.9%, 3.6%, 74.9%

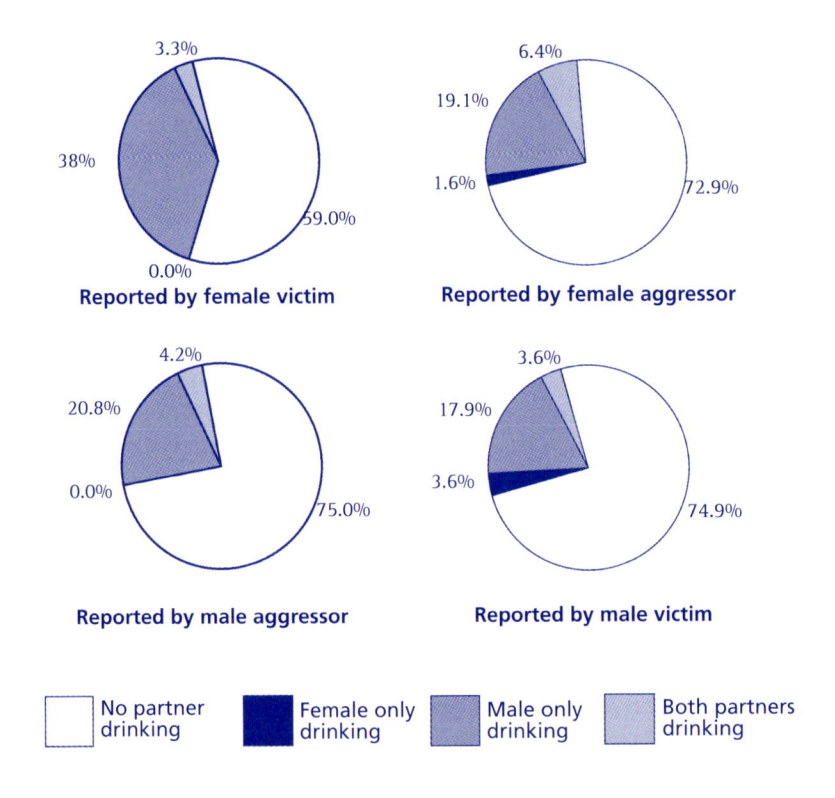

Legend: No partner drinking | Female only drinking | Male only drinking | Both partners drinking

FIGURE 6b. Percent of incidents in which no partner was drinking, both partners were drinking, only the male was drinking, or only the female was drinking, as reported by female victims and aggressors, GENACIS survey, Ayacucho, Peru, 2005.

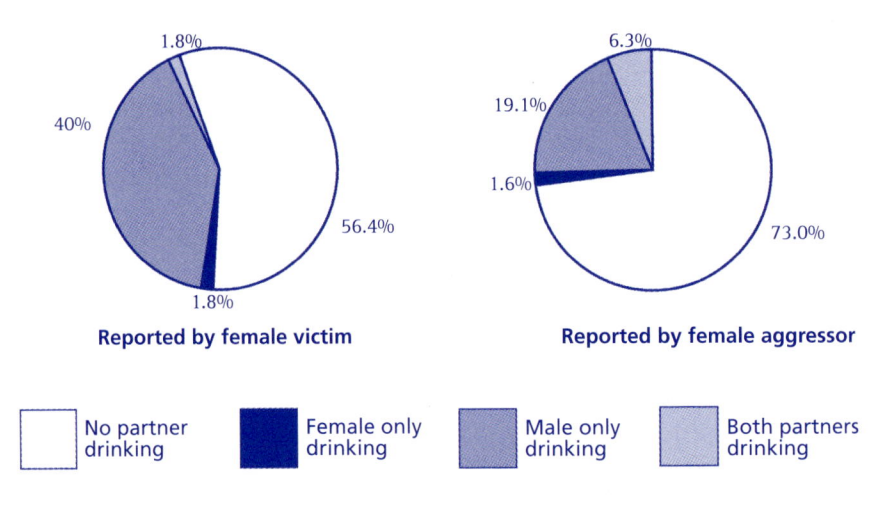

Reported by female victim: 1.8%, 40%, 1.8%, 56.4%

Reported by female aggressor: 6.3%, 19.1%, 1.6%, 73.0%

Legend: No partner drinking | Female only drinking | Male only drinking | Both partners drinking

The Relationship between Alcohol Consumption and Partner Aggression

In Lima, the percent of victims and aggressors was higher among those who drank alcohol in the past year compared to those who abstained. Among female drinkers, 10.3% reported being the victim of partner aggression and 10.7% reported aggression toward a partner compared to 5.5% and 5.8%, respectively, for female abstainers. Among male drinkers in Lima, 8.3% reported being the victim of partner aggression and 7.6% reported aggression toward a partner versus 4.4% and 1.5%, respectively, for male abstainers. Female drinkers in Ayacucho also reported higher rates than female abstainers of victimization by a partner (22.6% versus 14.9%) and aggression toward a partner (13.4% versus 10.9%). Logistic regression of partner physical aggression (yes/no) on whether respondent drank in the past year (yes/no) controlling for age resulted in odds ratios that were greater than 1, but were significant only for female victims and female aggressors in Lima ($p < .05$).

Respondents' Drinking Pattern and Partner Aggression

Among respondents who consumed alcohol in the past year, the percent of those reporting aggression by a partner and toward a partner was higher for respondents who drank five or more drinks on at least one occasion in the past year than for those who did not drink this amount. This pattern was similar for both cities (Figures 7a and 7b). However, this difference was significant only for female victims in Ayacucho after controlling for age ($p < .05$).

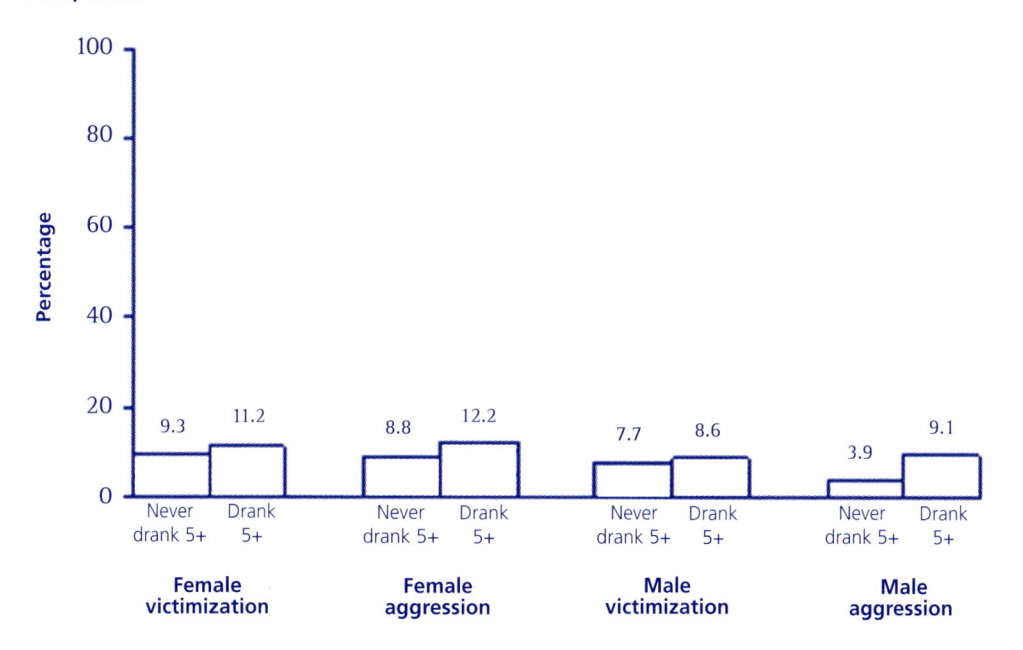

FIGURE 7a. Percent of respondents who reported victimization (aggression by a partner) and aggression (aggression toward a partner) by whether the respondent had consumed five or more drinks on an occasion or never consumed five drinks on an occasion, by sex, GENACIS survey, Lima, Peru, 2005.

	Never drank 5+	Drank 5+
Female victimization	9.3	11.2
Female aggression	8.8	12.2
Male victimization	7.7	8.6
Male aggression	3.9	9.1

FIGURE 7b. Percent of female respondents reporting victimization (aggression by a partner) and aggression (aggression toward a partner) by whether the respondent had consumed five or more drinks on an occasion or never consumed five drinks on an occasion, GENACIS survey, Ayacucho, Peru, 2005.

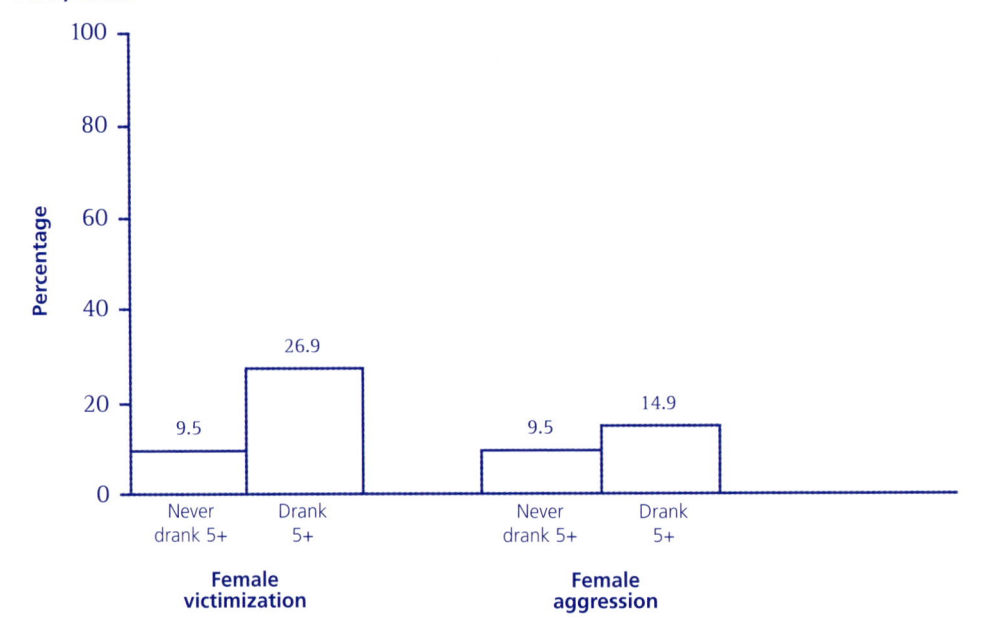

The mean number of days in the year preceding the survey on which respondents consumed any alcohol was compared for victims and aggressors versus those who reported no partner aggression. In Lima, there were no significant differences in frequency of drinking between respondents who reported being victims of partner aggression or aggressive toward a partner compared to respondents of the same sex who reported no aggression (Figure 8a). In Ayacucho, the number of drinking days was higher for female aggressors compared to females who reported no aggression toward a partner ($p < .05$). Female victims did not differ significantly from females who reported no victimization (Figure 8b).

The number of drinks consumed on usual drinking occasions is shown in Figures 9a and 9b. In Lima, the number was higher for female victims ($p < .05$) and female aggressors ($p < .01$) than for females who reported no aggression (no significant differences for males). In Ayacucho, no significant differences were found between females who reported partner aggression and those who did not. Figures 10a and 10b show the total number of drinks during the past year for respondents who reported partner aggression compared to those who did not. No significant differences were found.

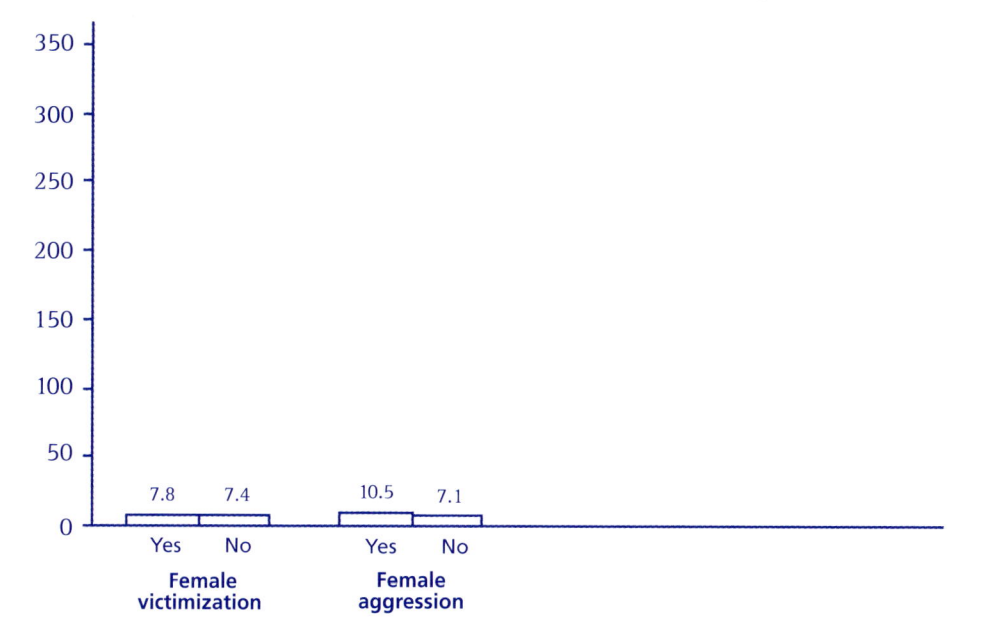

FIGURE 8a. Mean number of drinking days in the year preceding the survey by whether the respondent had been a victim of partner aggression and whether the respondent had been aggressive toward a partner, by sex, GENACIS survey, Lima, Peru, 2005.

	Female victimization		Female aggression		Male victimization		Male aggression	
	Yes	No	Yes	No	Yes	No	Yes	No
	10.4	12.2	10.2	12.3	17.5	23.5	27.1	22.7

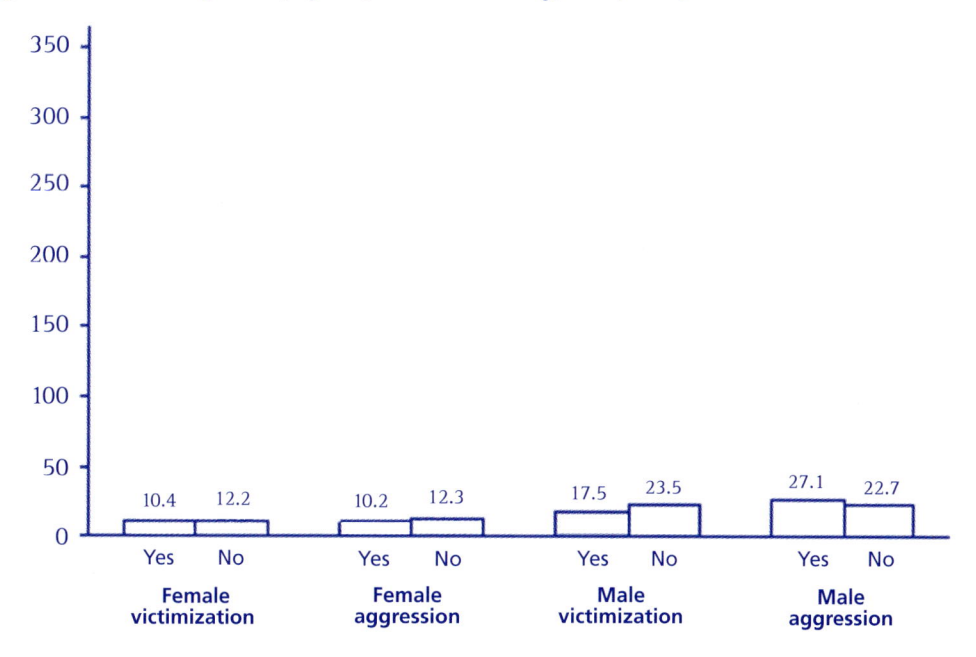

FIGURE 8b. Mean number of drinking days in the year preceding the survey for female respondents by whether the respondent had been a victim of partner aggression and whether the respondent had been aggressive toward a partner, GENACIS survey, Ayacucho, Peru, 2005.

	Female victimization		Female aggression	
	Yes	No	Yes	No
	7.8	7.4	10.5	7.1

FIGURE 9a. Mean number of drinks consumed on usual drinking occasions by whether the respondent had been a victim of partner aggression and whether the respondent had been aggressive toward a partner, by sex, GENACIS survey, Lima, Peru, 2005.

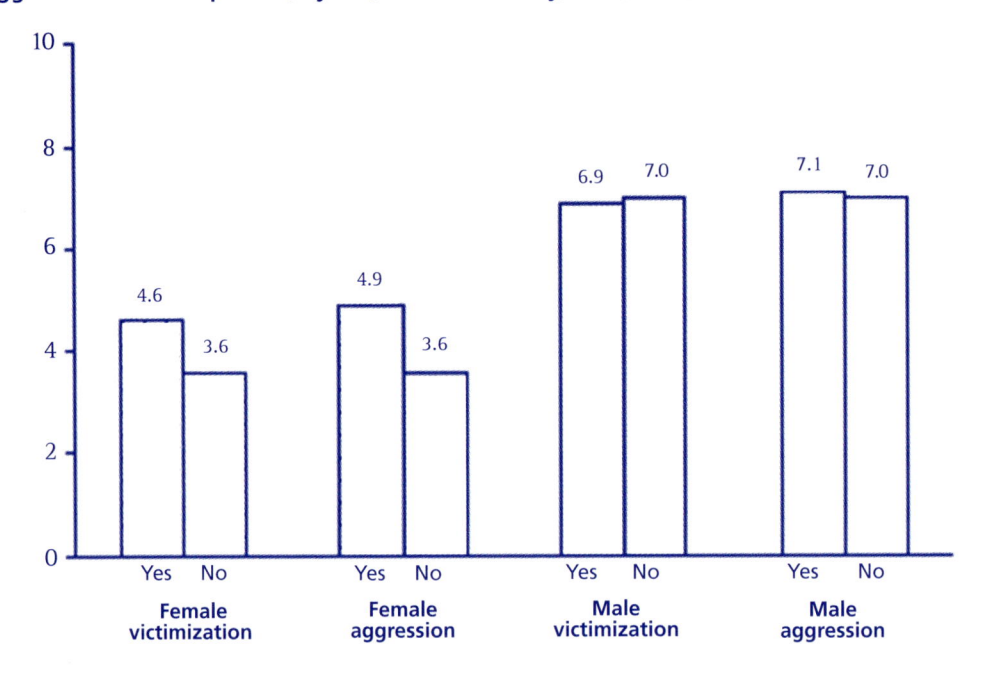

	Yes	No
Female victimization	4.6	3.6
Female aggression	4.9	3.6
Male victimization	6.9	7.0
Male aggression	7.1	7.0

FIGURE 9b. Mean number of drinks consumed on usual drinking occasions by female respondents, by whether the respondent had been a victim of partner aggression and whether the respondent had been aggressive toward a partner, GENACIS survey, Ayacucho, Peru, 2005.

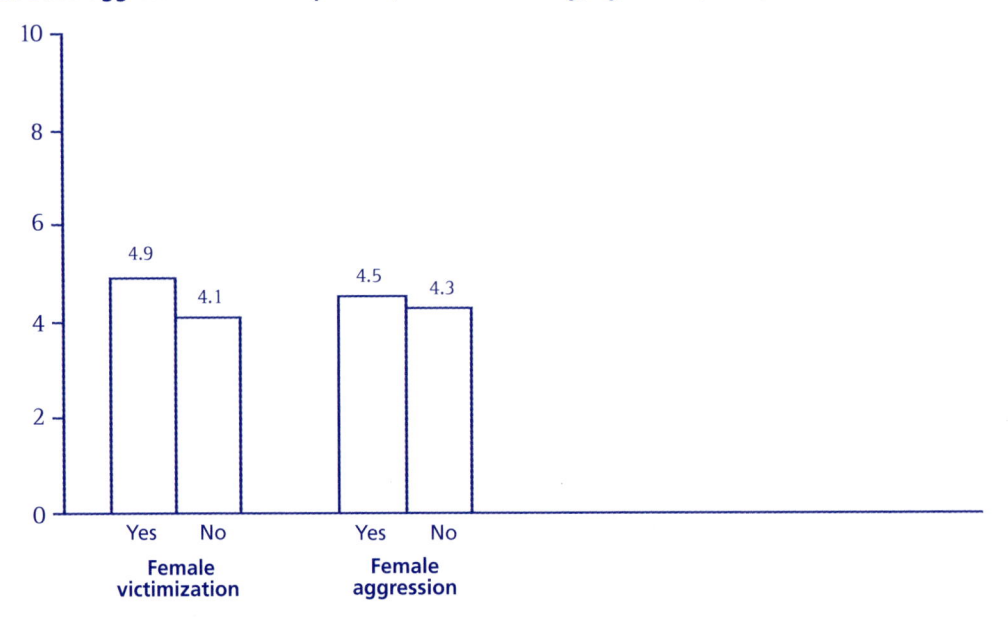

	Yes	No
Female victimization	4.9	4.1
Female aggression	4.5	4.3

Peru | **181**

FIGURE 10a. Overall mean number of drinks consumed annually by whether the respondent had been a victim of partner aggression and whether the respondent had been aggressive toward a partner, by sex, GENACIS survey, Lima, Peru, 2005.

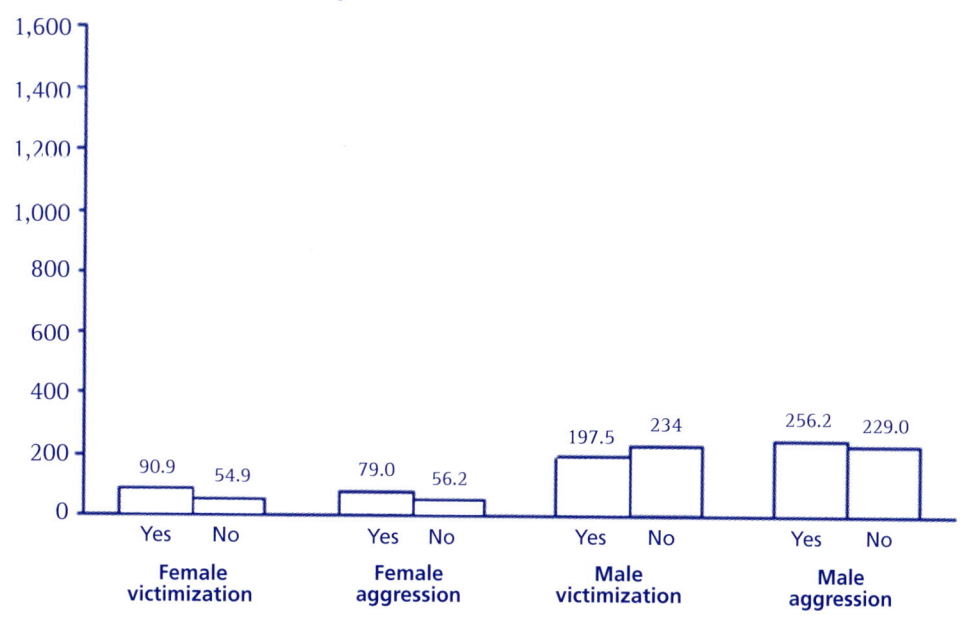

	Yes	No
Female victimization	90.9	54.9
Female aggression	79.0	56.2
Male victimization	197.5	234
Male aggression	256.2	229.0

FIGURE 10b. Overall mean number of drinks consumed annually by female respondents by whether the respondent had been a victim of partner aggression and whether the respondent had been aggressive toward a partner, GENACIS survey, Ayacucho, Peru, 2005.

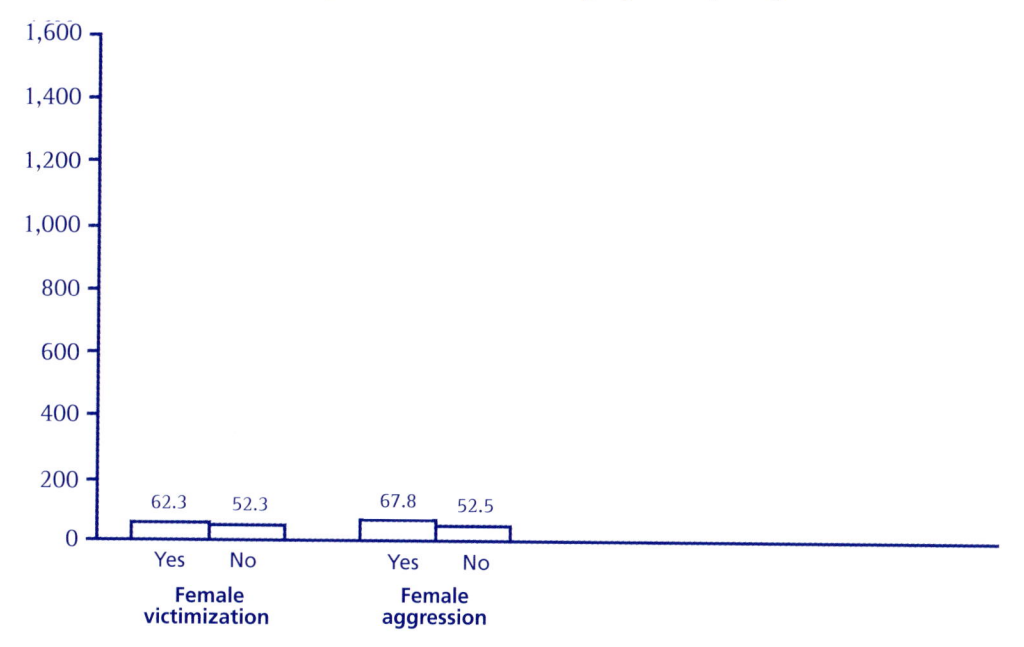

	Yes	No
Female victimization	62.3	52.3
Female aggression	67.8	52.5

Discussion

This study represents an important contribution to knowledge about partner physical aggression in Peru by including physical violence toward both women and men. Another important contribution of this investigation is that it analyzes partner aggression both from the perspective of the victim and from the perspective of the aggressor. The research described in this chapter also addresses the relationship between alcohol consumption and partner aggression. Additionally, this study compares partner aggression and alcohol consumption patterns in two very different cultural contexts, that of the national capital of Lima and the Andean city of Ayacucho.

The study's findings show that partner physical aggression is an important problem for both men and women in Peru. However, this study found higher rates of physical aggression toward females than toward males. This represents important knowledge given the lack of comparable information regarding partner violence by sex in Peru. When comparing results for Ayacucho and Lima, the rates of physical aggression toward females are consistent with previous studies that found higher rates in cities located in the Andean region, as compared to Lima. Significant male–female differences by city were also found, with the rate of partner aggression being twice as high for female victims as for male victims in Ayacucho, but with similar rates for males and females being found in Lima.

Physical aggression was higher among the younger population and tended to decline with age. Similar results were found in the 2004 National Health and Demgraphics Study, which revealed a greater frequency of physical violence toward younger females. In terms of marital status, the percent of males and females who reported being victims, and the percent of males who reported being aggressors, was higher for those who had cohabited with a partner in the past year than for those who were divorced or never married. While married males were least likely to report being the victim or aggressor in partner aggression, the rate of victimization by a partner was lower for never–married than for married females. Marital status results differ from the 2004 National Demographic and Health Survey, which found higher rates of aggression toward divorced, separated, or widowed females than toward females living with a partner or spouse. These differences may be explained by the fact that the latter survey explored the most recent experience of physical violence only for females who had been married or living with a partner; combining these two groups would likely have resulted in a lower rate of partner aggression, given the low rate found among married individuals in the current study. Findings in this study suggest that never–married individuals are also at risk of partner aggression, particularly male victims, and should therefore also be included in surveys of partner aggression.

The current study identified slapping as the most frequent type of aggression in both cities. This behavior was reported by 40% or more of respondents. More severe types of aggression, such as punching and beating up, were more likely to be used against females than toward male partners. Although these differences were not statistically significant, they are consistent with findings from other countries presented in this book.

In terms of seeking medical attention in relation to the aggression, significantly more female victims than male victims reported doing this in Lima. Female victims also rated the severity of the incident significantly higher than did male victims, and the emotional impact of the aggression, in terms of fear, upset, and anger, was greater for female victims than for male victims and male aggressors.

The study findings are also interesting with regard to differences by sex in the two settings. Rates of physical aggression toward females are consistent with previous studies that found higher rates in cities located in the Andean region, as compared to Lima. The distribution of the victim–aggressor categories among males and females differed in the two cities as well. Women in Ayacucho were more likely than their counterparts in Lima to report being only the victim and less likely to report being only the aggressor, while men in Ayacucho were less likely than their counterparts in Lima to report being only the victim and more likely to report being only the aggressor. One possible explanation for the regional differences is greater gender-role traditionalism in the Andean region than in Lima, with the traditional value of men's domination of women making male-to-female violence more acceptable (see Archer 2006). In addition, women tend to have less education in Ayacucho than in Lima. Low educational attainment was found to be a risk factor for experiencing partner aggression for women in a previous survey in Peru (Flake, 2005).

As described in the Results section, examination of drinking patterns revealed higher rates, higher frequency of use, greater amount of alcohol used per occasion, and greater annual volume of alcohol consumption for males than for females. The results for frequency of drinking are similar to those from other studies in Peru. For example, frequency of drinking during the past year was similar to that in the Castro de la Mata and Zavaleta Martínez-Vargas study (2003). In that study, among those who drank at least once during the last year, 67.3% reported drinking less than once a month, 24.8% once a month, 7.4% once a week, and 0.5% reported daily use. In the current study, more drinkers in Ayacucho than in Lima reported consuming five or more drinks on an occasion, while there was a greater reported frequency and higher annual volume of use among male drinkers in Lima compared to Ayacucho.

Partner aggression was related to the pattern of drinking five or more drinks on at least one occasion during the past year. This result was found consistently for males and females in both cities. Female respondents from Lima who reported partner aggression also consumed more drinks per occasion that did female respondents who reported no aggression. Also, female respondents from Ayacucho who reported aggression toward a partner drank more frequently in the past year than did respondents who reported no aggression. Comparisons for men were limited by the small numbers who reported partner aggression, but overall the results suggest a link between drinking pattern and partner aggression. However, these results should be interpreted with caution, given the small sample sizes for some of the analyses.

In general, gender differences in drinking patterns seemed to be greater in Lima than in Ayacucho. However, a pattern was evident in both Lima and Ayacucho in terms of the association between alcohol consumption and partner aggression: in both cities, male alcohol consumption was more related to male physical aggression toward females than to female aggression towards males (as reported by victims and aggressors of both sexes). Alcohol involvement was also related to the severity of the aggression for female victims in Ayacucho.

Acknowledgments

The author would like to acknowledge the contributions made by Sharon Wilsnack, Sharon Bernards, and Kathyrn Graham during the preparation of this chapter and at the same time express her gratitude to Inés Bustamante and Duncan Pedersen for their contributions to the GENACIS study in Peru.

References

Archer J. Cross-Cultural Differences in Physical Aggression Between Partners: A Social-Role Analysis. *Personality and Social Psychology Review*, Vol. 10, No. 2, 133-153 (2006).

Castro de la Mata R, Zavaleta Martínez-Vargas A. Epidemiología de drogas en la población urbana peruana 2003. Encuesta de hogares. Lima: CEDRO. Monografía de investigación 23, 2003.

Flake D. Individual, Family, and Community Risk Markers for Domestic Violence in Peru. *Violence Against Women*, Vol. 11, No. 3, 353-373 (2005).

Güesmez AN. Palomino, M. Ramos. Violencia sexual y física contra las mujeres en el Perú. Estudio Multicéntrico sobre la violencia de pareja y la salud de las mujeres. Lima: Flora Tristán, Universidad Peruana Cayetano Heredia (UPCH), Organización Mundial de la Salud (OMS), 2002.

Peru, Comisión Nacional para el Desarrollo y Vida sin Drogas (DEVIDA). II Encuesta Nacional sobre Prevención y Consumo de Drogas 2002. Informe Ejecutivo proyecto RLA/AD/PER/99/D77. Lima: Mix Negociaciones, 2003.

Peru, ENDESA Continua. PERÚ Encuesta Demográfica y de Salud Familiar. Informe Principal Instituto Nacional de Estadística e Informática (INEI), Dirección Nacional de Censos y Encuestas Dirección Técnica de Demografía e Indicadores Sociales, 2004.

Peru, Instituto de Derechos del Consumidor y Propiedad Intelectual, 2003.

Peru, Policia Nacional del Perú. Anuario Estadístico Policial, 2005.

UNHAPPY HOURS:

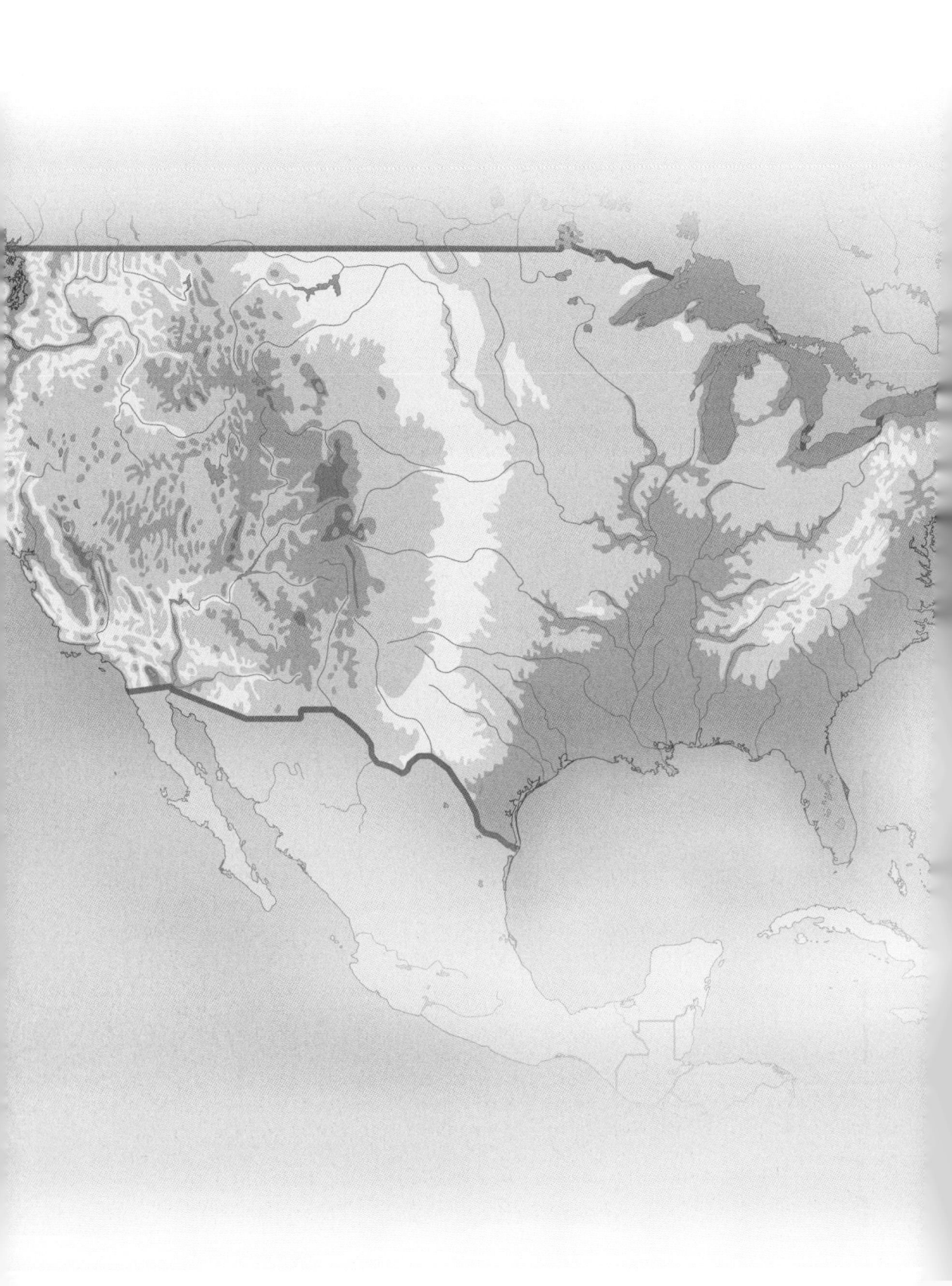

United States: Alcohol and Partner Physical Aggression—Findings from a National Sample of Women

—Sharon C. Wilsnack, Richard W. Wilsnack, and Arlinda F. Kristjanson

Introduction

Intimate partner violence in the United States is widely recognized as a major social problem, although estimates of the problem's magnitude vary. Estimates of women's lifetime exposure to intimate partner violence range from 25% to 54%, depending on the population sampled, criteria for intimate partner violence, and methods of data collection (Thompson and Kingree, 2006). In general population surveys conducted by Straus and Kaufman Kantor (Straus, 1995), the annual prevalence of minor assaults by husbands against wives (and by wives against husbands) rose from about 8% in 1985 to about 9% in 1992, but the prevalence of severe assaults by husbands (but not by wives) declined, from 3% to 2%. In the 1992–1994 National Survey of Families and Households, 18% of coresident couples reported physical violence between the partners in the past 12 months (Fox and Benson, 2006). Similarly, a 1995 national survey of couples found that violence had occurred in 18% of couples in the preceding 12 months (Schafer, Caetano, and Clark, 1998). The 1995–1996 National Violence against Women Survey found that 1.5% of all women and 0.9% of all men had been physically assaulted by a partner in the past 12 months (Tjaden and Thoennes, 2000a). According to the United States Department of Justice's Bureau of Justice Statistics (2000), the number of intimate partner violence incidents has declined over the past decade, but still remains very large: 1.1 million incidents in 1993; 876,000 incidents in 1998; and 693,000 incidents in 2001 (Rennison, 2003).

Women who have been victims of intimate partner violence have worse physical and mental health than non-victims (Plichta, 2004; Dutton, Green, Kaltman, Roesch, Zeffiro, and Krause, 2006), including three to five times greater likelihood of depression, suicidal tendencies, and substance abuse (Golding, 1999), although most of the evidence for these effects is cross-sectional. Estimates provided by the U.S. National Center for Injury Prevention and Control of the direct medical consequences of intimate partner violence for women in 2003 included more than 807,000 overnight hospital stays, more than 971,000 outpatient visits to physicians, more than 1,000,000 physical therapy visits, and total health care costs of US$ 4 billion (United States, 2003).

Research in the United States has predominantly focused on men assaulting women, but several recent general population surveys have found that women reported similar or slightly higher rates of aggression and violence toward their partners than men did (Straus, 1995, 2006; Archer, 2000; Anderson, 2002; Caetano, McGrath, Ramisetty-Mikler, and Field, 2005; Richardson, 2005; Williams and Frieze, 2005). As previously noted, an exception is the 1995-1996 National Violence against Women Survey, which found higher rates of physical assault by male than by female partners (Tjaden and Thoennes, 2000b).

Gender differences in violence may be smaller in general population samples than in institutional samples (e.g., in clinics or shelters), and men may be more likely than women to engage in intimate partner violence that involves sexual abuse or stalking, or that leads to involvement of the criminal justice system (Saunders, 2002; see also Muehlenhard and Kimes, 1999). A consistent pattern in the United States, however, is that intimate partner violence severe enough to cause injury is more likely to be carried out by men against women (Cascardi, Langhinrichsen, and Vivian, 1992; Straus, 1995; Archer, 2000; Tjaden and Thoennes, 2000b). In 2002, in U.S. homicides resulting from intimate partner violence, 76% of the victims were women (Fox and Zawitz, 2004).

Alcohol Involvement in Partner Aggression

According to data from the U.S. National Health and Nutrition Examination Surveys for the period 1999-2002 (Fryar, Hirsch, Porter, Kottiri, Brody, and Louis, 2007), 24.5% of men aged 20 or older and 35.6% of women aged 20 or older were lifetime abstainers or former drinkers. In terms of heavy drinking, among men, 10.4% typically drank more than 14 drinks in a week (13.8% of drinkers), while among women, only 6.3% drank more than seven drinks in a week (9.8% of drinkers). Heavy episodic drinking (five or more drinks in a day) was relatively common among drinkers. A majority of male drinkers, particularly young adults (51.4% overall, 74.1% of male drinkers in their 20s), had engaged in heavy episodic drinking at least once in the past year, and a large minority of women had done this as well (23.4% of drinkers, and 40.5% of drinkers in their 20s).

A substantial proportion of incidents of intimate partner violence in the United States involves alcohol. Studies of persons convicted of a violent crime against an intimate partner have found that about one-half of the offenders had been drinking prior to the crime (Slade, Daniel, and Heisler, 1991; Greenfield et al., 1998). General population surveys of intimate partner violence, however, have found lower rates of alcohol involvement. For example, the 1995-1996 National Violence against Women Survey found that 33.6% of partners and 6.9% of victims had been using alcohol at the time of the assault (Thompson and Kingree, 2006[1]). The link between drinking and intimate partner violence also has been found in recent research on men in treatment for alcohol abuse, which found that intimate partner violence is more likely to occur on drinking occasions or days (Fals-Stewart, 2003; Murphy, Winters, O'Farrell, Fals-Stewart, and Murphy, 2005). In addition, several studies of both treatment and nontreatment populations have found that alcohol use by the male partner at the time of intimate partner violence is related to greater severity of male violence toward female partners (Kyriacou et al., 1999; Testa, Quigley, and Leonard, 2003; Fals-Stewart, Leonard, and Birchler, 2005) or greater risk of injury (Thompson and Kingree, 2006[1]).

---

[1] These studies of *associations between intimate partner violence and drinking* are based on large general population samples and thus are most useful for comparison with the findings of the Gender, Alcohol, and Culture: An International Study (GENACIS) project. Other studies cited are based on clinical samples (Gerber, Ganz, Lichter, Williams, and McCloskey, 2005; Weinsheimer, Schermer, Malcoe, Balduf, and Bloomfield, 2005; Stuart, Meehan, Moore, Morean, Hellmuth, and Folansbee, 2006), case-control samples (Hotaling and Sugarman, 1986; Lipsky, Caetano, Field, and Larkin, 2005), or samples of U.S. Army personnel (Pan, Neidig, and O'Leary, 1994; Bell, Harford, McCarroll, and Senier, 2004; Bell, Harford, Fuchs, McCarroll, and Schwartz, 2006), or are meta-analyses (Stith, Rosen, Middleton, Busch, Lundeberg, and Carlton, 2000). All cited studies of intimate partner violence prevalence are based on representative general population samples.

With regard to the relationship between intimate partner violence and drinking patterns of the victims and aggressors, research in the United States has consistently found that male violence toward female partners is more prevalent among men who drink heavily (e.g., Hotaling and Sugarman, 1986; O'Leary and Schumacher, 2003;[1] Bell, Harford, McCarroll, and Senier, 2004; Caetano, McGrath, Ramisetty-Mikler, and Field, 2005;1) and/or have problems related to their drinking (e.g., Chen and White, 2004;[1] Schafer, Caetano, and Cunradi, 2004;[1] Stith, Smith, Penn, Ward, and Tritt, 2004; Bell, Harford, Fuchs, McCarroll, and Schwartz, 2006). A smaller number of studies have found consistently that male drinking or problem drinking is positively associated with the severity of men's violence toward their partners, either as a general association between violence and typical drinking pattern (e.g., Cunradi, Caetano, and Schafer, 2002;[1] Pan, Neidig, and O'Leary, 1994) or as a specific association with drinking at the time of the violent incident (e.g., Brecklin 2002).

Most U.S. research on alcohol and intimate partner violence has focused on men's drinking, and less is known about how women's drinking pattern may be associated with intimate partner violence. Some studies have found that women's violence toward male partners is to some extent associated with women's drinking (Kaufman Kantor and Asdigian, 1997a;[1] Caetano, McGrath, Ramisetty-Mikler, and Field, 2005;[1] Martino, Collins, and Ellickson, 2005[1]) and problem drinking (Chen and White, 2004;[1] Caetano, McGrath, Ramisetty-Mikler, and Field, 2005;[1] Stuart, Meehan, Moore, Morean, Hellmuth, and Folansbee, 2006). It is more uncertain whether women's drinking or problem drinking is associated with assaults by their male partners. Several studies have found such an association (e.g., Cunradi, Caetano, and Schafer, 2002;[1] Gerber, Gantz, Lichter, Williams, and McCloskey, 2005; Weinsheimer, Schermer, Malcoe, Balduf, and Bloomfield, 2005), but there is only scarce time-ordered evidence that women's drinking precedes assaults by male partners (Chen and White, 2004;[1] Caetano, McGrath, Ramisetty-Mikler, and Field, 20051) or increases after such assaults (Kilpatrick, Acierno, Resnick, Saunders, and Best, 1997;[1] Martino, Collins, and Ellickson, 20051). The uncertainty is increased by studies that have not found a relationship between women's drinking and violence by a male partner (Kaufman Kantor and Asdigian, 1997b;[1] Kilpatrick, Acierno, Resnick, Saunders, and Best, 1997;[1] Testa, Livingston, and Leonard, 2003;[1] Lipsky, Caetano, Field, and Larkin, 2005).

Interventions in Intimate Partner Violence

Attempts to prevent intimate partner violence in the United States did not become common or widespread until the 1970s. These efforts have been directed mainly at men who abuse women and have relied primarily on the criminal justice system. By 1980, 47 U.S. states had passed laws that allowed police to make arrests without warrants for intimate partner violence and to enforce protection orders that prohibited offenders from contacting victims, using physical abuse or the threat of physical abuse, or damaging the victim's property (Zorza, 1992; Fagan, 1996; Danis, 2003). The conventional assumption of such law enforcement was that intimate partner violence can be deterred by sufficiently certain, swift, and severe punishment.

However, such law enforcement has not worked as intended. Arrests for intimate partner violence often have not led to prosecution, partly because of lack of support from prosecutors and partly because many victims have been reluctant to press charges (Rebovich, 1998) for fear of retribution by their partners, economic hardships (such as loss of child support), and an unsympathetic legal environment (Buzawa and Buzawa, 1992; Goodman, Bennett, and Dutton, 1999). To address these problems, states and communities in the United States have adopted policies that make arrests for intimate partner violence mandatory and do not permit charges to be dropped after they have been made. Despite these efforts, only a fraction of episodes of intimate partner violence lead to police intervention, according to the U.S. Department of Justice (1998). Furthermore, courts have been reluctant to put violent male partners in jail or prison, preferring instead to order such men to participate in treatment programs outside the criminal justice system (Hanna, 1998; Stuart, Temple, and Moore, 2007).

Treatment programs for men involved in intimate partner violence are relatively short-term (6-32 weeks) meetings for groups of men; individual, couples, or family therapy for intimate partner violence is not regarded as appropriate in most states (Tolman and Edleson, 1995; Austin and Dankwort, 1999; Babcock, Green, and Robie, 2004). Programs are usually guided by some combination of two philosophies: (1) a feminist approach that seeks to change men's beliefs that they have a right to control and dominate their partners, and (2) a cognitive-behavioral or social learning approach that emphasizes learning behavioral alternatives to violence (through skills training and anger management techniques) and learning to reevaluate the effects of violent behavior (Tolman and Edleson, 1995; Babcock, Green, and Robie, 2004).

Effects of treatment programs and law enforcement are usually evaluated by how much reduction of recidivism (recurrence of intimate partner violence) occurs (Tolman and Edleson, 1995). Such evaluations are flawed in several ways: subsequent arrests are incomplete measures of intimate partner violence; efforts to obtain better data from victim reports are limited by loss of contact with victims for follow-ups (Babcock, Green, and Robie, 2004); and apparent benefits of treatment programs may be exaggerated by higher dropout rates among the men most likely to become violent again (younger, less educated, more likely to be unemployed, and with higher rates of conflict with their partners) (Aldarando and Sugarman, 1996; Saunders, 1996). It would be helpful to know about other outcomes (including frequency and severity of subsequent violence, psychological as well as physical abuse and threats, and the welfare of children in the household), but such data are rarely, if ever, available (Tolman and Edleson, 1995; Sartin, Hansen, and Huss, 2006).

The best available data on outcomes of interventions are not encouraging. Arrests of violent male partners, without other mandated interventions, are unlikely to benefit women or may have mixed results, because some women will be victims of retaliatory violence as well as paying the social costs of involvement with the police and courts (Tolman and Edleson, 1995; Danis, 2003). In general, policies making arrests mandatory and preventing charges against male partners from being dropped have not been any more successful (Schmidt and Sherman, 1998; Zorza 1998). Protection orders are sought primarily by women who have already been injured by intimate partner violence, and a majority of violent partners violate protection orders in some way within two years (Harrell and Smith, 1998).

The best hope of the criminal justice system in the United States has been mandated treatment. However, two recent meta-analyses of studies of men's treatment programs, examining both police reports and victim reports of recurrent violence, found that the benefits of treatment programs were quite small (Babcock, Green, and Robie, 2004) or possibly nonexistent (Feder and Wilson, 2005). The only way in which programs showed major benefits was that men who completed treatment were less likely than men who dropped out to engage in renewed violence, an effect that may reflect the characteristics of the men in the programs to a greater extent than the effects of the programs as such. One somewhat encouraging finding, however, is that an estimated one-third of men who engage in intimate partner violence cease their violence without judicial or treatment help (Rosenfeld 1992; Babcock, Green, and Robie, 2004).

In summary, intimate partner violence is a major social and health problem in the United States. Despite the large volume of research on this problem, the ways in which many factors cause or contribute to intimate partner violence remain unclear. Of particular relevance to this chapter are the limitations of research on associations between alcohol and intimate partner violence. In particular, research has often paid less attention to the female partner's drinking than to the male partner's drinking and often does not distinguish how intimate partner violence may be influenced by partners' long-term drinking patterns, as distinct from the effects of partners' drinking at the time the violence occurs. Data from a 2001 survey of a representative general population sample of women are presented here to address some of the unanswered questions about alcohol and intimate partner violence, and to allow comparisons with data from nine other countries in the Americas. Because the variables analyzed and reported in this book involve acts of *physical* aggression, and not other forms of violence or aggression toward a partner (e.g., verbal abuse, emotional abuse), we use the term "partner physical aggression" rather than "intimate partner violence" in the remainder of this chapter.

Methods
Sample
The U.S. sample consisted of 1,126 women from the 2001 survey of the National Study of Health and Life Experiences of Women (NSHLEW). The NSHLEW is a 20-year longitudinal study of drinking and problem drinking in women. The data were collected in 1981, 1986, 1991, 1996, and 2001 in personal interviews conducted with nationally representative samples of non-institutionalized English-speaking women aged 21 and older living in the contiguous 48 U.S. states (i.e., excluding Alaska and Hawaii); new subsamples of women aged 21–30 were added to the sample in 1991 and 2001. Women who consumed four or more drinks per week were over-sampled. Additional information about the NSHLEW design and methods can be found elsewhere (Wilsnack, Wilsnack, and Klassen, 1984; Wilsnack, Klassen, Schur, and Wilsnack, 1991; Wilsnack, Wilsnack, Kristjanson, Vogeltanz-Holm, and Windle, 2004; Wilsnack, Kristjanson, Wilsnack, and Crosby, 2006).

The 2001 sample included 483 women first interviewed in 1981 (aged 41 and older in 2001; 66.0% completion rate), 302 women first interviewed in 1991 (aged 31–40 in 2001; 75.3% completion rate), and 341 women aged 21–30 in 2001 (78.9% completion rate). Attrition analyses indicated that women lost to follow-up were older and less educated than women reinterviewed, but the two groups did not differ on baseline drinking behavior. Statistical weighting adjusted for the over-sampling of women who consumed four or more drinks per week, and for variations in nonresponse rates by sampling unit and by major demographic characteristics (age, education, marital status, and ethnicity). The weighted 2001 sample was demographically similar to women in the 2000 U.S. Census, with the exceptions that in the 2001 sample more women were classified as non-Hispanic white and fewer women reported less than a high school education.

The analyses reported here excluded 22 women who indicated that they were exclusively lesbian or that the partner physical aggression they reported involved a female partner. The 2001 weights for this heterosexual subsample were readjusted by a constant so that the total weighted n equaled the actual number of heterosexual respondents. Table 1 shows demographic characteristics and drinking patterns for the U.S. sample.

TABLE 1. Age, marital status, employment status, and drinking pattern in the 12 months preceding the survey, NSHLEW study, United States, 2001.

Variable	Weighted number[a]	Percent or mean
	1,103	
Age		47.7 years
21–24 years	82	7.5%
25–34 years	214	19.4%
35–44 years	240	21.7%
45–54 years	206	18.7%
55–64 years	141	12.8%
65 years and older	219	19.9%
Average age		
All women	1,103	47.7 years
Women reporting partner physical aggression	67	35.2 years
Marital status		
Married	641	58.1%
Cohabiting/Living with partner	72	6.5%
Divorced or separated	155	14.1%
Never married	123	11.2%
Widowed	112	10.1%
Employment status		
Working for pay	700	63.5%
Homemaker	148	13.4%
Voluntarily unemployed	33	3.0%
Involuntarily unemployed	40	3.7%
Student	15	1.3%
Retired	166	15.1%
Drinking pattern (past 12 months)		
Drank any alcohol during past 12 months	726	65.8%
Average number of drinking days (drinkers only)		45.7 days
Average number of drinks per occasion (drinkers only)		2.1[b] drinks
Average annual volume (drinkers only)		122.9[b] drinks
Drank six or more drinks on at least one occasion (drinkers only)	182[c]	21.7%

[a] Note that total numbers vary across variables due to missing data.
[b] Number of standard drinks. One drink = 12 grams of ethanol.
[c] Weights adjusted for drinkers only.

Interviews

Interviews were conducted by female interviewers from the National Opinion Research Center, University of Chicago. Seventy-two percent of the interviews were conducted face-to-face, in respondents' homes or other private settings; 28% were telephone interviews (generally due to distance or the respondent's preference for a telephone interview). Interviewers were selected for their interviewing skills and their personal comfort with questions about drinking behavior, sexual behavior, and other sensitive topics. The interviewers received extensive general and study-specific training. The 2001 survey used computer-assisted personal interviewing (CAPI); for potentially sensitive questions about sexual experience, respondents were offered the option of reading the questions on the laptop computer screen and entering their responses privately on the computer. The average interview length was approximately 90 minutes.

Measures that Differed from the Core Questions

The 2001 NSHLEW interview questionnaire included detailed questions about drinking patterns, drinking contexts, drinking-related problems, and a number of hypothetical antecedents and consequences of drinking behavior. The U.S. survey did not ask respondents about aggressive things they may have done to their male partners. Therefore, only the women respondents' self-reports of male-to-female partner aggression (i.e., aggression by their male partners) are reported in this chapter.

Partner Aggression Variables

The U.S. classification of event types differed slightly from the categorization used by the other countries in this book, in that the U.S. category *severe forms of aggression* was not an event category in analyses by the other countries. The events included in this category (e.g., broken bones, threatened with a weapon, shot at with a gun) were rated by the respondents as life-threatening aggression, and they rated themselves as being very upset and frightened at the time. These events could not be classified readily in any of the other event categories and so are treated as a separate category in the U.S. data.

Drinking Behavior

Annual volume was calculated in two ways. The first volume measure was generic annual volume, calculated by multiplying generic quantity by the number of drinking days in the past 12 months. The second measure used beverage-specific questions. Unlike the GENACIS 12-month beverage-specific questions, the U.S. questions asked about drinking different beverage types in the past 30 days. Thirty-day beverage-specific volume was calculated by multiplying usual quantity for beer, wine, and liquor in a drinking day by the number of days in which that beverage was consumed in the past month. The three 30-day beverage volumes were summed and the total was multiplied by 12 to approximate annual volume.

The U.S. measure of heavy episodic drinking (HED) differed slightly from the measure used by the other countries in this book. For comparability with previous waves of the NSHLEW, the U.S. HED question asked how often the respondent drank six or more drinks in a day. A dichotomous measure of HED (none vs. one or more days in the past 12 months) was used for the analyses reported here.

Results
Prevalence of Partner Aggression

Approximately 6% (6.1%) of the respondents (weighted n = 67; unweighted n = 86) reported experiencing some form of partner physical aggression in the preceding two years. As shown in Figure 1, the percent of women experiencing partner aggression decreased with age.

FIGURE 1. Percent of respondents who reported having been a victim of partner aggression, by age group, NSHLEW study, United States, 2001.

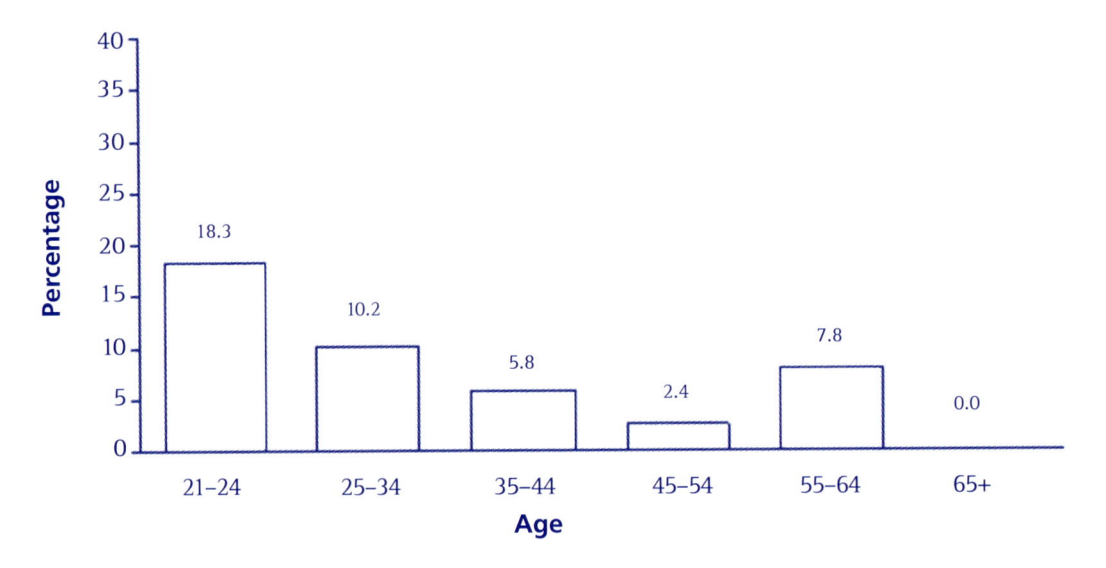

As shown in Figure 2, married and widowed women reported lower rates of partner aggression than women in other marital status groups. Widows may have experienced partner aggression in their lifetime, but did not report it having happened in the last two years; therefore they were excluded from the following pair-wise comparisons. Unmarried women who lived with a male partner ($p < .001$), divorced/separated women ($p < .001$), and women who had never been married ($p < .01$) were more likely to report partner aggression than were married women. There were no significant differences in the percent reporting partner aggression among cohabiting, divorced/separated, and never-married women (all p's $> .05$).

As shown in Figure 3, 43.7% of the women who experienced partner aggression reported that they were pushed or shoved in the most serious incident, 12.8% were grabbed, and 24.0% reported being slapped, punched, or hit, or having something thrown at them. Overall, 15.5% of the women reported more severe forms of aggression: 7.2% were beaten up (several aggressive acts combined; e.g., choked, slapped, and pushed;

FIGURE 2. Percent of respondents who reported having been a victim of physical aggression, by marital status, NSHLEW study, United States, 2001.

- Married: 3.9
- Cohabiting: 13.9
- Divorced/separated: 12.9
- Never Married: 9.8
- Widowed: 0.0

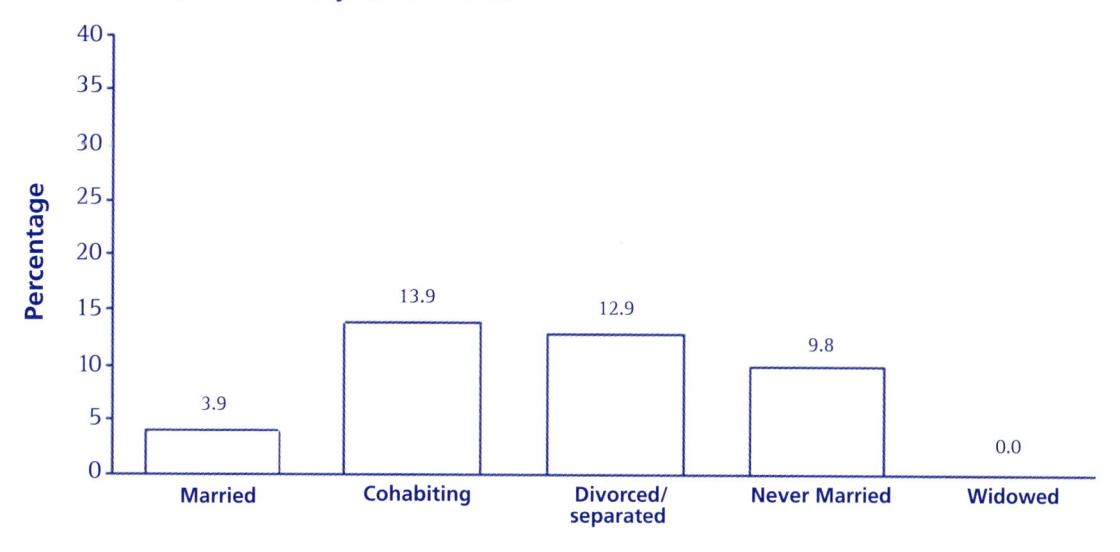

FIGURE 3. Type of aggressive act against females, as reported by female victims, NSHLEW study, United States, 2001.

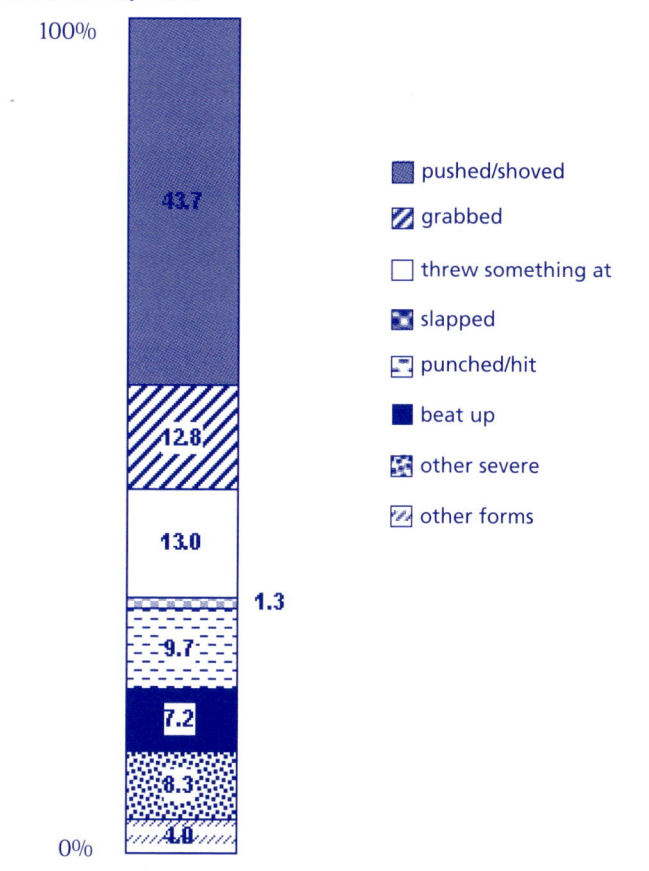

- pushed/shoved: 43.7
- grabbed: 12.8
- threw something at: 13.0
- slapped: 1.3
- punched/hit: 9.7
- beat up: 7.2
- other severe: 6.3
- other forms: 4.0

kicked and slugged), and 8.3% experienced other severe aggression, such as having bones broken, being threatened with a weapon, or being shot at with a gun. Four percent of the women reported other forms of aggression (e.g., "kicked," "torn shirt").

As shown in Figure 4, one or both partners had been drinking in 38.4% of the incidents. In 25.8% of incidents, it was only the male partner, in 11.8% both partners were drinking, and in one incident (0.8%) only the female respondent had been drinking.

FIGURE 4. Percent of incidents in which no partner had been drinking, both partners had been drinking, only the male partner had been drinking, or only the female partner had been drinking, as reported by female victims, NSHLEW study, United States, 2001.

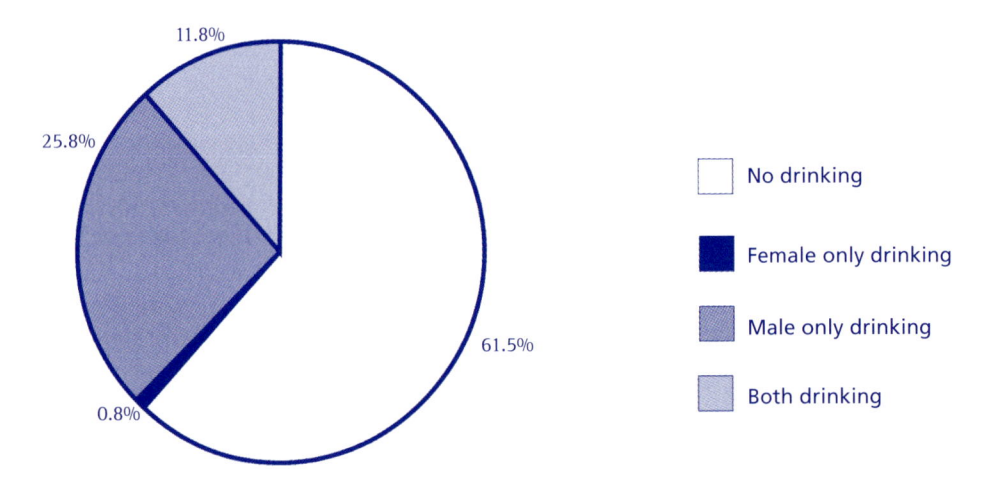

Respondents rated partner physical aggression on four descriptive scales: feelings of life-endangerment, being afraid, being upset, and being angry during the event. The mean ratings of the partner physical aggression events were 4.0, 5.6, 7.6, and 7.8, respectively. Aggressive events that involved drinking were rated as more life-threatening than events where drinking was not involved ($p < .001$). Ratings of being afraid, upset, or angry were also higher for events where drinking was involved, but the differences were not statistically significant (Figure 5).

The Relationship between Alcohol Consumption and Partner Aggression

Women who had consumed alcohol in the past 12 months were more likely than abstaining women to report partner physical aggression (8.3% vs. 1.9%, $p < .001$).

Respondents' Drinking Pattern and Partner Aggression

As shown in Figure 6, among women who drank in the past 12 months, women who reported one or more experiences of HED had higher rates of alcohol-related partner aggression (6.0%) than women drinkers who had not experienced HED (2.4%), although the difference was not statistically significant ($p = .168$). Drinking frequency, quantity, and volume for drinkers who reported alcohol-related aggression were consistently, but not significantly, higher than those of drinkers who experienced non-alcohol-related aggression or no partner aggression (Figures 7–9).

FIGURE 5. Mean ratings of endangerment, fear, upset, and anger by female victims, by whether alcohol was involved in aggression, NSHLEW study, United States, 2001.

	Endangerment	Fear	Upset	Anger
aggression with alcohol	5.5	5.7	8.2	8.4
aggression without alcohol	3.0	5.5	7.2	7.4

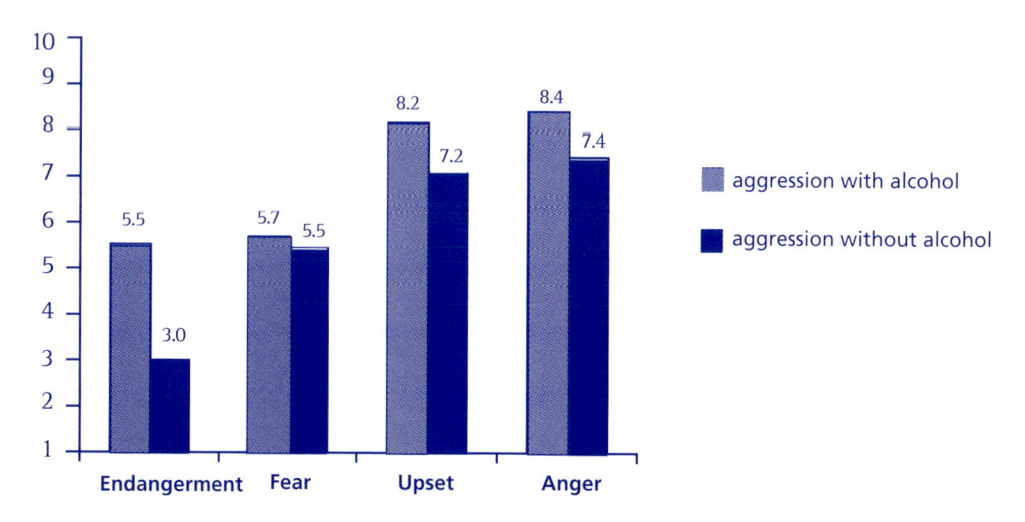

FIGURE 6. Percent of incidents in which one or both partners had been drinking or neither had been drinking by whether respondent had consumed six or more drinks on an occasion (drinkers only) or had never consumed six drinks on an occasion, NSHLEW study, United States, 2001.

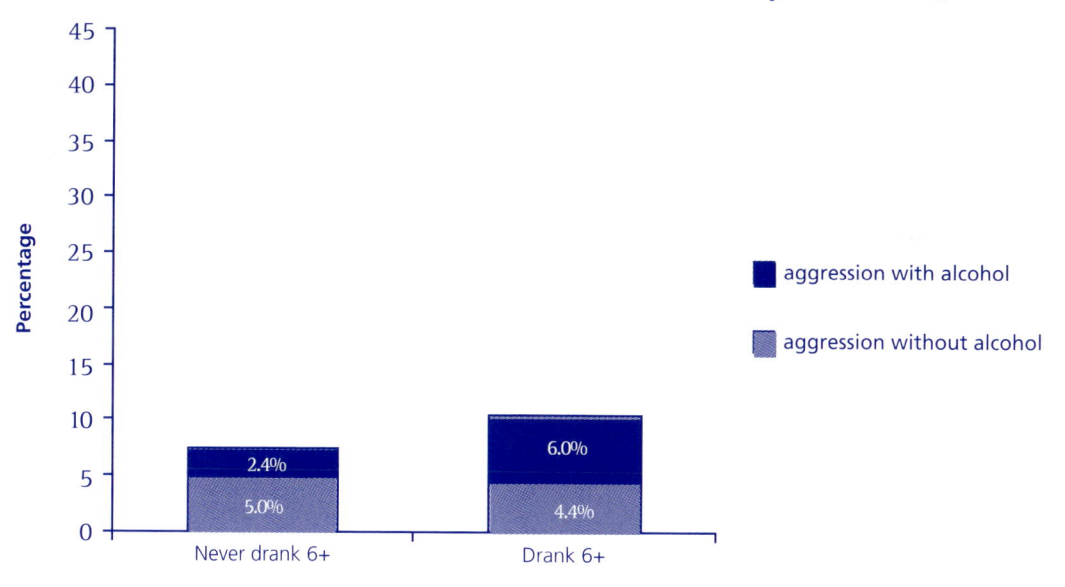

	Never drank 6+	Drank 6+
aggression with alcohol	2.4%	6.0%
aggression without alcohol	5.0%	4.4%

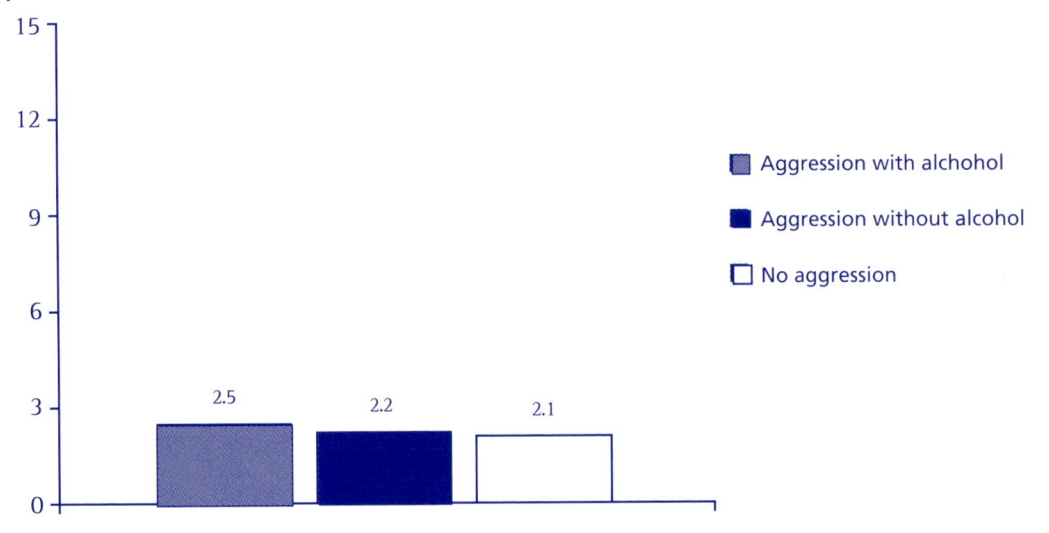

FIGURE 7. Mean number of drinking days in the year preceding the survey for female respondents who had been victims in incidents involving alcohol, in incidents not involving alcohol, or who reported no victimization, NSHLEW study, United States, 2001.

- Aggression with alchohol: 64.5
- Aggression without alcohol: 41.6
- No aggression: 45.4

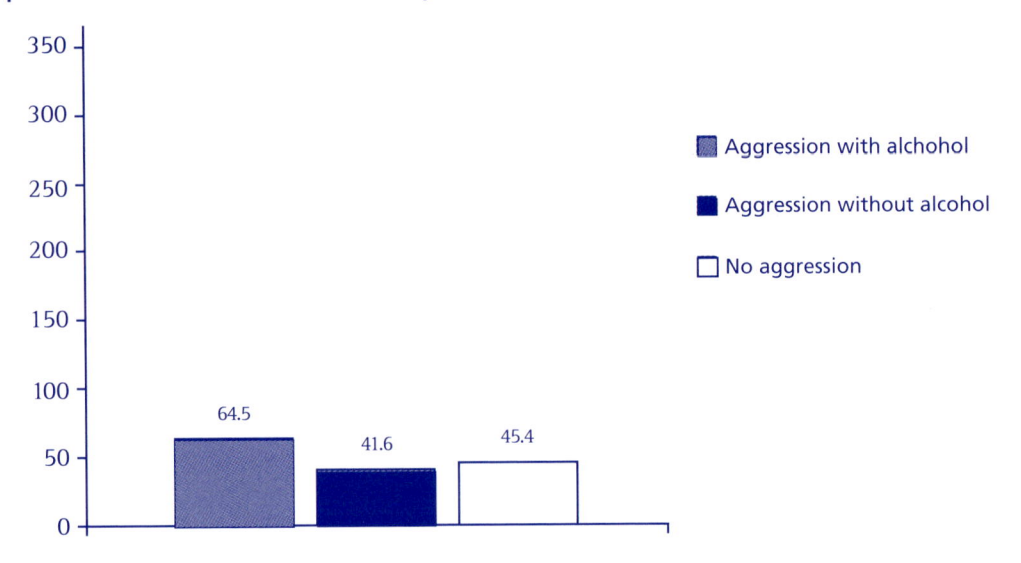

FIGURE 8. Mean number of drinks consumed on usual drinking occasions for female respondents who had been victims in incidents involving alcohol, in incidents not involving alcohol, or who reported no victimization, NSHLEW study, United States, 2001.

- Aggression with alchohol: 2.5
- Aggression without alcohol: 2.2
- No aggression: 2.1

FIGURE 9. Overall mean number of drinks consumed annually for female respondents who had been victims in incidents involving alcohol, in incidents not involving alcohol, or who reported no victimization, NSHLEW study, United States, 2001.

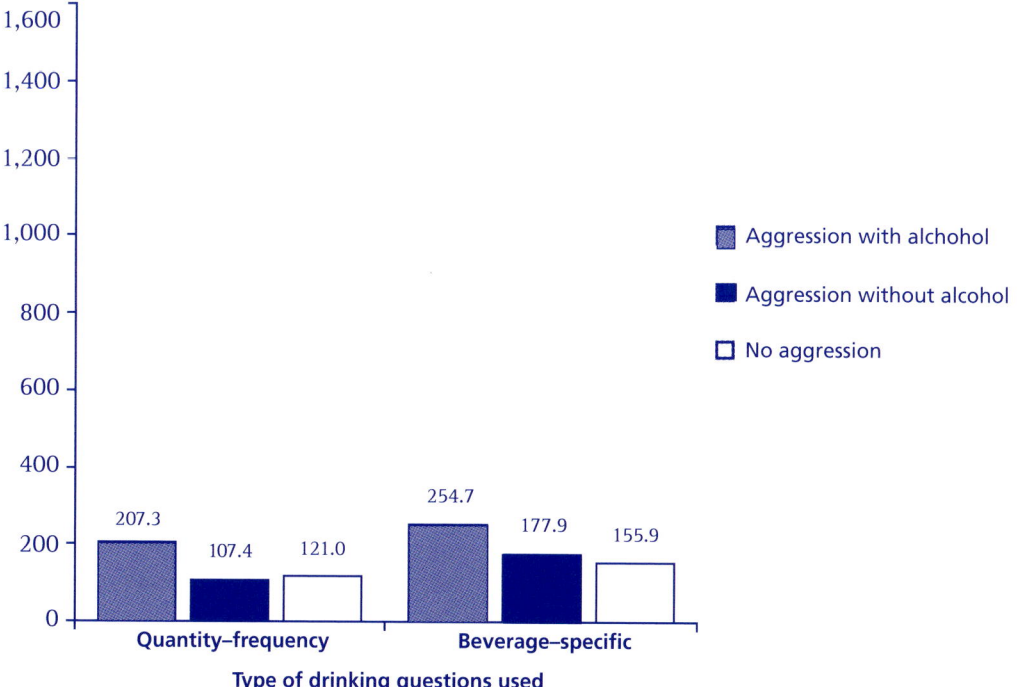

Type of drinking questions used	Aggression with alcohol	Aggression without alcohol	No aggression
Quantity–frequency	207.3	107.4	121.0
Beverage–specific	254.7	177.9	155.9

Discussion

The finding that 6.1% of women in the U.S. sample reported experiencing some form of partner physical aggression in the past two years falls within the range of prevalence rates reported in other recent U.S. surveys. On the one hand, the 6.1% rate is lower than the 18% of couples who reported partner physical violence in the past 12 months in surveys in 1992–1994 (Fox and Benson, 2006) and in 1995 (Schafer, Caetano, and Clark, 1998), probably reflecting in part the lack of information in the 2001 survey about aggression by women respondents toward their male partners. On the other hand, the 6.1% rate is higher than the 1.5% of women in the United States who reported physical assault by a partner in the past 12 months in a 1995–1996 survey (Tjaden and Thoennes, 2000a).

Alcohol and Partner Aggression

In 37.6% of occasions of partner physical aggression reported by women in the current sample, the male partner was drinking alcohol. This finding is quite similar to Thompson and Kingree's (2006) finding that 33.6% of the partner aggression events reported in the 1995–1996 National Violence against Women Survey involved drinking by the aggressive partner. Like most other country surveys reported in this book, we found that women who were current drinkers reported higher rates of partner physical aggression than abstainers, and that partner aggression involving alcohol was rated as more severe and life-threatening than aggression that did not involve alcohol. We also found consistent, although not statistically significant, associations between women's heavier drinking and higher rates of alcohol-related partner aggression.

Conclusions

The study reported in this chapter focused on drinking behavior and drinking-related problems of women. The survey did not include men and did not ask about women's aggression toward their male partners. Thus our results provide an incomplete picture of associations between alcohol use and partner aggression in the United States. Nonetheless, the findings do suggest that alcohol is involved in a sizable proportion of partner physical aggression events in the United States, and that partner aggression which involves alcohol is likely to be experienced as more severe and life-threatening than partner aggression not involving alcohol. Taken together with findings from other countries presented in this book, data from women in the United States underscore the need to take into account the role of alcohol in any attempts to understand, reduce, or prevent partner aggression.

The associations between alcohol use and partner physical aggression reported in this book may have implications for treating and preventing intimate partner violence. To deal with the effects of alcohol consumption on intimate partner violence, one possible strategy would be to make treatment for problems of alcohol abuse an integral part of treatment for intimate partner violence. There is evidence that men with substance use problems may have more negative outcomes than men without substance use problems from programs to reduce recurrent intimate partner violence (Jones and Gondolf, 2001;Gondolf, 2004). In the United States, there have been a few efforts to treat both intimate partner violence and substance abuse in the same program, such as the Dade County (Florida) Integrated Domestic Violence Model (Goldkamp, Weiland, Collins, and White, 1996) and Yale University's Substance Abuse Treatment Unit's Substance Abuse-Domestic Violence Program (Easton and Sinha, 2002). In general, however, U.S. programs for treating substance use problems and for treating violence against partners are separate and poorly linked (Fals-Stewart and Kennedy, 2005), with no guarantee that men who need treatment for both kinds of problems will get it. One hopes that publications like this one will encourage treatment programs in many countries to adopt a more inclusive treatment agenda.

Acknowledgments

The 2001 U.S. survey reported in this chapter was supported by Grant R01 AA004610 from the National Institute on Alcohol Abuse and Alcoholism (NIAAA), National Institutes of Health. Preparation of the chapter was supported by NIAAA Grants R21 AA012941 and R01 AA015775.

References

Aldarando E, Sugarman DB. (1996). Risk marker analysis of the cessation and persistence of wife assault. *Journal of Consulting and Clinical Psychology, 64,* 1010–1019.

Anderson KL. (2002). Perpetrator or victim? Relationships between intimate partner violence and well-being. *Journal of Marriage and the Family, 64,* 851–863.

Archer J. (2000). Sex differences in aggression between heterosexual partners: A meta-analytic review. *Psychological Bulletin, 126,* 651–680.

Austin JB, Dankwort J. (1999). Standards for batterer programs: A review and analysis. *Journal of Interpersonal Violence, 14,* 152–168.

Babcock JC, Green CE, Robie C. (2004). Does batterers' treatment work? A meta-analytic review of domestic violence treatment. *Clinical Psychology Review*, 23, 1023-1053.

Bell NS, Harford T, Fuchs CH, McCarroll JE, Schwartz CE. (2006). Spouse abuse and alcohol problems among white, African-American, and Hispanic U.S. Army soldiers. Alcoholism: *Clinical and Experimental Research*, 30, 1721-1733.

Bell NS, Harford T, McCarroll JE, Senier L. (2004). Drinking and spouse abuse among US Army soldiers. Alcoholism: *Clinical and Experimental Research*, 28, 1890-1897.

Brecklin L. (2002). The role of perpetrator alcohol use in the injury outcomes of intimate assaults. *Journal of Family Violence*, 17, 185-196.

Buzawa ES, Buzawa CG. (eds.) (1992). *Domestic Violence: The Changing Criminal Justice Response*. Westport, CT: Auburn House.

Caetano R, McGrath C, Ramisetty-Mikler S, Field CA. (2005). Drinking, alcohol problems and the five-year recurrence and incidence of male to female and female to male partner violence. *Alcohol: Clinical and Experimental Research*, 29, 98-106.

Cascardi M, Langhinrichsen J, Vivian D. (1992). Marital aggression: Impact, injury, and health correlates for husbands and wives. *Archives of Internal Medicine*, 152, 1178-1184.

Chen PH, White HR. (2004). Gender differences in adolescent and young adult predictors of later intimate partner violence: *A prospective study. Violence Against Women*, 10, 1283-1301.

Cunradi CB, Caetano R, Schafer J. (2002). Alcohol-related problems, drug use, and male intimate partner violence severity among U. S. couples. *Alcoholism: Clinical and Experimental Research*, 26, 493-500.

Danis FS. (2003). The criminalization of domestic violence: What social workers need to know. *Social Work*, 48, 237-246.

Dutton MA, Green BL, Kaltman SI, Roesch DM, Zeffiro TA, Krause ED. (2006). Intimate partner violence, PTSD, and adverse health outcomes. *Journal of Interpersonal Violence*, 21, 955-968.

Easton CJ, Sinha R. (2002). Treating the addicted male batterer: Promising directions for dual-focused programming. In C. Wekerle & A. Wall (eds.), *The Violence and Addiction Equation: Theoretical and Clinical Issues in Substance Abuse and Relationship Violence* (pp. 275-292). New York: Brunner-Routledge.

Fagan J. (1996). *The Criminalization of Domestic Violence: Promises and Limits*. Washington, DC: National Institute of Justice.

Fals-Stewart W. (2003). The occurrence of partner physical aggression on days of alcohol consumption: A longitudinal diary study. *Journal of Consulting and Clinical Psychology*, 71, 41-52.

Fals-Stewart W, Kennedy C. (2005). Addressing intimate partner violence in substance-abuse treatment. *Journal of Substance Abuse Treatment*, 29, 5-17.

Fals-Stewart W, Leonard KE, Birchler GR. (2005). The occurrence of male-to-female intimate partner violence on days of men's drinking: The moderating effects of antisocial personality disorder. *Journal of Consulting and Clinical Psychology*, 73, 239-248.

Feder L. and Wilson DB. (2005). A meta-analytic review of court-mandated batterer intervention programs: Can courts affect abusers' behavior? *Journal of Experimental Criminology*, 1, 239-262.

Fox GL. and Benson ML. (2006). Household and neighborhood contexts of intimate partner violence. *Public Health Reports*, 121, 419-427.

Fox JA, Zawitz MW. (2004). *Homicide Trends in the United States.* Washington, DC: U.S. Department of Justice, Bureau of Justice Statistics. At *www.ojp.usdoj.gov/bjs/homicide/homtrnd.htm*

Fryar CD, Hirsch R, Porter KS, Kottiri B, Brody DJ, Louis T. (2007). *Smoking and Alcohol Behaviors Reported by Adults: United States, 1999-2002. Advance data from Vital and Health Statistics 378* (29 November 2006; updated 27 March 2007). Centers for Disease Control and Prevention, U.S. Department of Health and Human Services. Published online at *www.cdc.gov/nchs/data/ad/ad378.pdf.*

Gerber MR, Ganz ML, Lichter E, Williams CM, McCloskey LA. (2005). Adverse health behaviors and the detection of partner violence by clinicians. *Archives of Internal Medicine, 165,* 1016-1021.

Golding JM. (1999). Intimate partner violence as a risk factor for mental disorders: A meta-analysis. *Journal of Family Violence, 14,* 99-132.

Goldkamp JS, Weiland D, Collins M, White M. (1996). *The Role of Drug and Alcohol Abuse in Domestic Violence and Its Treatment: Dade County's Domestic Violence Court Experiment.* Washington, DC: U.S. Department of Justice, National Institute of Justice, Crime and Justice Research Institute.

Gondolf EW. (2004). Evaluating batterer counseling programs: A difficult task showing some effects and implications. *Aggression and Violent Behavior, 9,* 605-631.

Goodman L, Bennett L, Dutton MA. (1999). Obstacles to victims' cooperation with the criminal justice prosecution of their abusers: The role of social support. *Violence and Victims, 14,* 427-443.

Greenfield LA, Rand MR, Craven D, Klaus PA, Perkins CA, Ringel C, et al. (1998). *Violence by Intimates.* Washington, DC: U.S. Department of Justice.

Hanna C. (1998). The paradox of hope: The crime and punishment of domestic violence. *William and Mary Law Review, 39,* 1505-1584.

Harrell A, Smith B. (1998). Effects of restraining orders on domestic violence victims. In American Bar Association & U.S. Department of Justice (eds.), *Legal Interventions in Family Violence: Research Findings and Policy Implications* (NCJ-171666) (pp. 49-51). Washington, DC: U.S. Government Printing Office.

Hotaling G, Sugarman D. (1986). An analysis of risk markers in husband to wife violence: The current state of knowledge. *Violence and Victims, 1,* 101-124.

Jones AS, Gondolf EW. (2001). Time-varying risk factors for reassault among batterer program participants. *Journal of Family Violence, 16,* 345-359.

Kaufman Kantor G, Asdigian NL. (1997a). Gender differences in alcohol-related spousal aggression. In R. W. Wilsnack & S. C. Wilsnack (eds.), Gender and Alcohol: Individual and Social Perspectives (pp. 312-334). New Brunswick, NJ: Rutgers Center of Alcohol Studies.

Kaufman Kantor G, Asdigian N. (1997b). When women are under the influence: Does drinking or drug use by women provoke beatings by men? In M. Galanter (ed.), *Recent Developments in Alcoholism, Volume 13: Alcoholism and Violence* (pp. 315-336). New York: Plenum Press.

Kilpatrick DG, Acierno R, Resnick HS, Saunders, BE, Best, CL. (1997). A two-year longitudinal analysis of the relationships between violent assault and substance use in women. *Journal of Consulting and Clinical Psychology, 65,* 834-847.

Kyriacou DN, Anglin D, Taliaferro E, Stone S, Tubb T, Linden JA, et al. (1999). Risk factors for injury to women from domestic violence. *New England Journal of Medicine, 341,* 1892-1898.

Lipsky S, Caetano R, Field CA, Larkin GL (2005). Psychosocial and substance-use risk factors for intimate partner violence. *Drug and Alcohol Dependence, 78*, 39–47.

Martino SC, Collins RL, Ellickson PL. (2005). Cross-lagged relationships between substance use and intimate partner violence among a sample of young adult women. *Journal of Studies on Alcohol, 66*, 139–148.

Muehlenhard CL, Kimes A. (1999). The social construction of violence: The case of sexual and domestic violence. *Personality and Social Psychology Review, 3*, 234–245.

Murphy CM, Winters J, O'Farrell TJ, Fals-Stewart W, Murphy M. (2005). Alcohol consumption and intimate partner violence by alcoholic men: Comparing violent and nonviolent conflicts. *Psychology of Addictive Behaviors, 19*, 35–42.

O'Leary KD, Schumacher JA. (2003). The association between alcohol use and intimate partner violence: Linear effect, threshold effect, or both? *Addictive Behaviors, 28*, 1575–1585.

Pan HS, Neidig PH, O'Leary KD. (1994). Predicting mild and severe husband-to-wife physical aggression. *Journal of Consulting and Clinical Psychology, 62*, 975–981.

Plichta SB. (2004). Intimate partner violence and physical health consequences. *Journal of Interpersonal Violence, 19*, 1296–1323.

Rebovich DJ. (1998). Prosecution response to domestic violence: Results of a survey of large jurisdictions. In American Bar Association & U.S. Department of Justice (eds.), *Legal Interventions in Family Violence: Research Findings and Policy Implications* (NCJ-171666) (pp. 59–61). Washington, DC: U.S. Government Printing Office.

Rennison CM. (2003). Intimate Partner Violence 1993-2001: Bureau of Crime Statistics Brief. Washington, DC: U.S. Department of Justice, Bureau of Justice Statistics, 2003.

Richardson DS. (2005). The myth of female passivity: Thirty years of revelations about female aggression. *Psychology of Women Quarterly, 29*, 238–247.

Rosenfeld BD. (1992). Court-ordered treatment of spouse abuse. *Clinical Psychology Review, 12*, 205–226.

Sartin RM, Hansen DJ, Huss MT. (2006). Domestic violence treatment response and recidivism: A review and implications for the study of family violence. *Aggression and Violent Behavior, 11*, 425–440.

Saunders DG. (1996). Feminist-cognitive-behavioral and process-psychodynamic treatments for men who batter: Interaction of abuser traits and treatment models. *Violence and Victims, 11*, 393–414.

Saunders DG. (2002). Are physical assaults by wives and girlfriends a major social problem? A review of the literature. *Violence Against Women, 8*, 1424–1448.

Schafer J, Caetano R, Clark C. (1998). Rates of intimate partner violence in the United States. *American Journal of Public Health, 88*, 1702–1704.

Schafer J, Caetano R, Cunradi CB. (2004). A path model of risk factors for intimate partner violence among couples in the United States. *Journal of Interpersonal Violence, 19*, 127–142.

Schmidt JD, Sherman LW. (1998). Does arrest deter domestic violence? In American Bar Association & U.S. Department of Justice (eds.), *Legal Interventions in Family Violence: Research Findings and Policy Implications* (NCJ-171666) (p. 54). Washington, DC: U.S. Government Printing Office.

Slade M, Daniel LJ, Heisler CJ. (1991). Application of forensic toxicology to the problem of domestic violence. *Journal of Forensic Science, 36*, 708–713.

Stith SM, Rosen KH, Middleton KA, Busch AL, Lundeberg K, Carlton RP. (2000). The intergenerational transmission of spouse abuse: A meta-analysis. *Journal of Marriage and the Family, 62*, 640-654.

Stith SM, Smith DB, Penn CE, Ward DB, Tritt D. (2004). Intimate partner physical abuse perpetration and victimization risk factors. *Aggression and Violent Behavior, 10*, 65-98.

Straus MA. (1995). Trends in cultural norms and rates of partner violence: An update to 1992. In S. M. Stith & M. A. Straus (eds.), *Understanding Partner Violence: Prevalence, Causes, Consequences, and Solutions* (pp. 30-33). Minneapolis, MN: National Council on Family Relations.

Straus MA. (2006). Future research on gender symmetry in physical assaults on partners. *Violence Against Women, 12*, 1086-1097.

Stuart GL, Meehan JC, Moore TM, Morean M, Hellmuth J, Folansbee K. (2006). Examining a conceptual framework of intimate partner violence in men and women arrested for domestic violence. *Journal of Studies on Alcohol, 67*, 102-112.

Stuart GL, Temple JR, Moore TM. (2007). Improving batterer intervention programs through theory-based research. *JAMA, 298*, 560-562.

Testa M, Livingston JA, Leonard KE. (2003). Women's substance use and experiences of intimate partner violence: A longitudinal investigation among a community sample. *Addictive Behaviors, 28*, 1649-1664.

Testa M, Quigley BM, Leonard KE. (2003). Does alcohol make a difference? Within participants comparison of incidents of partner violence. *Journal of Interpersonal Violence, 18*, 735-743.

Thompson MP, Kingree JB. (2006). The roles of victim and perpetrator alcohol use in intimate partner violence outcomes. *Journal of Interpersonal Violence, 21*, 163-177.

Tjaden P, Thoennes N. (2000a). *Extent, Nature, and Consequences of Intimate Partner Violence: Findings from the National Violence against Women Survey*. Washington, DC: U.S. Department of Justice, National Institute of Justice, NCJ 181867.

Tjaden P, Thoennes N. (2000b). Prevalence and consequences of male-to-female and female-to-male intimate partner violence as measured by the National Violence against Women Survey. *Violence Against Women, 6*, 142-161.

Tolman RM, Edleson JL. (1995). *Intervention for Men Who Batter: A Review of Research*. Minneapolis, MN: Minnesota Center Against Violence and Abuse.

United States, Department of Health and Human Services, Centers for Disease Control and Prevention, National Center for Injury Prevention and Control. (2003). *Costs of Intimate Partner Violence Against Women in the United States*. Atlanta, GA: Centers for Disease Control and Prevention.

United States, Department of Justice, Bureau of Justice Statistics (2000). Intimate partner violence against women declined from 1993 through 1998. Press release at *www.ojp.usdoj.gov/bjs/pub/press/intimate partner violence.pr*

United States Department of Justice (1998). *Violence by Intimates: Analysis of Data on Crimes by Current or Former Spouses, Boyfriends, and Girlfriends*. Washington, DC: U.S. Department of Justice, Bureau of Justice Statistics.

Weinsheimer RL, Schermer CR, Malcoe LH, Balduf LM, Bloomfield LA. (2005). Severe intimate partner violence and alcohol use among female trauma patients. *Journal of Trauma, Injury, Infection, and Critical Care, 58*, 22–29.

Williams SL, Frieze IH. (2005). Patterns of violent relationships, psychological distress, and marital satisfaction in a national sample of men and women. *Sex Roles, 52*, 771–784.

Wilsnack RW, Kristjanson AF, Wilsnack SC, Crosby RD. (2006). Are U.S. women drinking less (or more)?: Historical and aging trends, 1981 – 2001. *Journal of Studies on Alcohol, 67*, 341–348.

Wilsnack RW, Wilsnack SC, Klassen AD. (1984). Women's drinking and drinking problems: Patterns from a 1981 national survey. *American Journal of Public Health, 74*, 1231–1238.

Wilsnack SC, Klassen AD, Schur BE, Wilsnack RW. (1991). Predicting onset and chronicity of women's problem drinking: A five-year longitudinal analysis. *American Journal of Public Health, 81*, 305–318.

Wilsnack SC, Wilsnack RW, Kristjanson AF, Vogeltanz-Holm ND, Windle M. (2004). Alcohol use and suicidal behavior in women: Longitudinal patterns in a U.S. national sample. *Alcoholism: Clinical and Experimental Research, 28* (5) Suppl., 38S–47S.

Zorza J. (1992). The criminal law of misdemeanor domestic violence, 1970–1990. *Journal of Criminal Law and Criminology, 83*, 46–72.

Zorza J. (1998). Must we stop arresting batterers? Analysis and policy implications of new police domestic violence studies. In American Bar Association & U.S. Department of Justice (eds.), *Legal Interventions in Family Violence: Research Findings and Policy Implications* (NCJ-171666) (pp. 55–56). Washington, DC: U.S. Government Printing Office.

UNHAPPY HOURS:

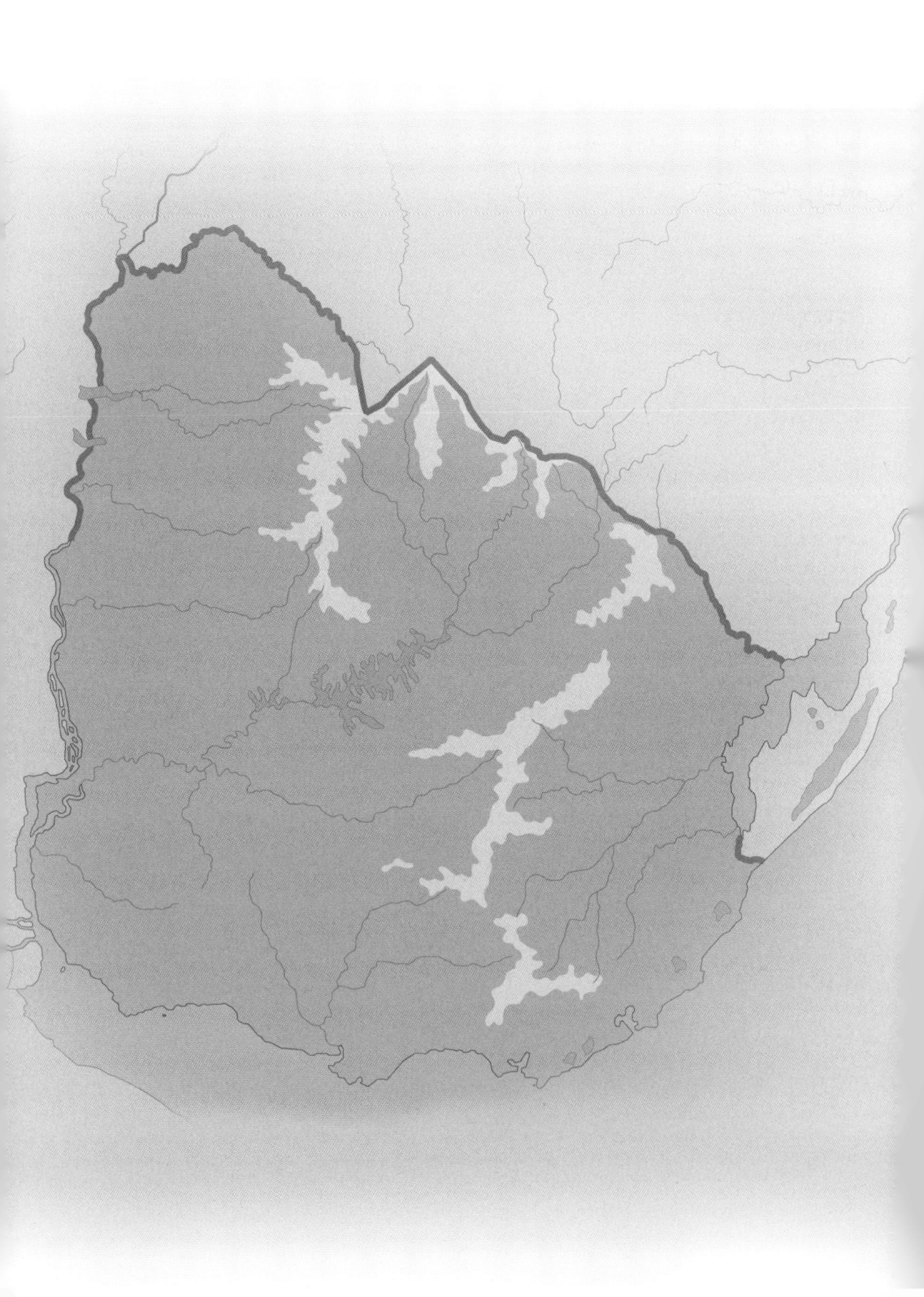

URUGUAY: Alcohol and Partner Physical Aggression in Various Cities

—*Raquel Magri, Hector Suárez, and Laurita Regueira*

Introduction

Despite its high human development index (HDI)[1] and a population that is highly engaged socially and politically, Uruguay also has gender-equity deficits in terms of income and political participation, including problems related to violence within intimate relationships (Traverso, 2007).

It is difficult to estimate the exact prevalence of intimate partner violence in Uruguay, despite the existence of mechanisms to gather information on this subject. In 2004, the National Consultation Council was established to enable the Ministry of the Interior and the judicial branch to compile statistics on domestic violence. Although the Council gathers information from all governmental and nongovernmental institutions working to deter family violence, only partial results have been obtained to date. The Observatory on Violence, which was created within the Ministry of Interior to monitor family violence, reported a 20% growth in one year. This increase is worrisome, although authorities think it might be the result of factors other than an actual increase in violence, such as greater awareness of this subject among the public, improvements in monitoring, and the application of new governmental policies.

In 2004, the National Consultation Council reported that 30% of deaths from family violence occurred in Montevideo, the capital, and 70% in the rest of the country. The deaths in the capital were among lower socioeconomic groups. Most occurred at home and more than half of the victims died during weekends and holidays. Deaths occurred more often from violence by a partner (one woman's death each 9 days and one man's death each 52 days) than from violence by another family member (CLADEM, 2002), with more women than men killed by their partner (44.6% of deaths for women vs. 10.7% for men) (Domínguez and Fernández, 2003).

Alcohol Consumption

Alcohol is the drug most frequently consumed in Uruguay. However, alcohol consumption patterns have changed in the last 20 years, shifting from daily drinking with meals (in the Mediterranean style that echoes Uruguay's Spanish and Italian ancestors' custom of drinking wine every day with meals, even diluting it with water to offer it to children) to a more pharmacological pattern of drinking for alcohol's

---

[1] The gender-related development index (GDI) was obtained through the human development index (HDI) prepared by UNDP. While the HDI measures the progress' average, the GDI adjusts the average of progress that reflects the inequalities between men and women under the following aspects: a long-lasting and healthy life, measured by life expectancy at birth; education, measured by adult literacy and the combined gross rate primary, secondary, and high school enrollment gross rate; and good living conditions, measured through the estimated income from work.

effects (Míguez, H. 2007). According to data collected by the Fourth National Census of Drug Consumption for the Total Population (November–December 2006) from a sample of 7,000 persons aged 12–65 years old living in cities of 10,000 population or more, almost 64.3% of adults had drunk alcohol in the 12 months prior to the census, 50.1% had consumed alcohol in the last 30 days, and 30% had consumed alcohol at problem levels in the last 30 days.

Men drink more than women; binge drinking is significantly more frequent among men than women, and it is more frequent outside of Montevideo than in the capital. About 5% of drinkers report signs of alcohol dependency, and the rate of dependency is six times greater for men. Those in the 19–25 age group report the highest rates of risky drinking (Uruguay, Junta National de Drogas, 2001). In 2004, 26.5% of recent detainees at police stations had been drinking prior to their offence (Magri, 2005); accidents that implied some type of crime, such as injuries to other parties, people, or property, were more related to alcohol consumption, while violent crimes were associated with the consumption of both alcohol and other drugs.

Legal and Educational Issues

Domestic violence was officially considered a violation in article 321 bis. of the Penal Code (art. 18). On July 12, 1995, Law No. 16.707 was approved, specifying domestic violence as follows:

"A person, who by any means of violence or threat at any time inflicts physical harm to persons with whom this person has or has had an affective or kinship relationship, regardless of legal connection, will be punished with between 6 and 24 months in prison. The penalty will be increased from a third and a half when the victim is a woman who fits the above requirements. The same law is applicable if the victim is under 16 years old or if a person has any physical or mental disability and is related to or cohabits with the offender."

Very few procedures were put in place when domestic violence was legally considered a crime, however, because the penalties required corroboration from persons with differing points of view. Nevertheless, the incorporation of this crime supported the perception that domestic violence is a social problem requiring sanctions. The Inter-American Convention on the Prevention, Punishment and Eradication of Violence against Women (Belém do Pará, Brazil, 1994) was ratified by Uruguay through Law No. 16.735, enacted on December 13, 1995. In May 18, 2001, Uruguay ratified the protocol of the United Nations' Convention on the Elimination of All Forms of Discrimination against Women with Law 17.338 (Uruguay had ratified the Convention in 1981). Law No. 17.514 on domestic violence was approved in july 2002. Article 2 states:

"Domestic violence is any direct or indirect act or failure to act which in any way impairs, by unlawfully limiting a person's free exercise or enjoyment of his or her human rights by another with whom the person is or has been betrothed or with whom he or she has or has had an affective relationship based on cohabitation and that has originated in kinship, marriage, or common law union."

The law stipulates an emergency jurisdiction within the family courts whereby third parties can report domestic violence to secure the victim's protection by the Judge in order to avoid secondary victimization (arts. 9 and 18), as well as the adoption of other protective measures. The law requires that the various jurisdictions coordinate their interventions through the National Consultative Council against Domestic Violence which oversees the prevention of violence and care of victims.

The law also activated an emergency process that allowed for preventive measures to be applied when someone reports a case of domestic violence. These measures, such as preventing the offender from entering the victim's home, must be applied immediately by the police (after the summary petition) and must be evaluated during the first ten days. At the same time, the National Consultative Council against Domestic Violence agreed to develop a national plan on domestic violence to, among other things, advise, coordinate actions, and seek the enforcement of the law. Law 17.707, enacted in 2003, grants the country's Supreme Court the ability to transform family courts into specialized domestic violence courts.

In practice, the family judge can adopt multiple protection measures, such as banning the aggressor from the household and issuing restraining orders; if these measures are not obeyed, the person then is penalized. However, these powers apply only to cases of domestic violence and sexual crimes; there are no specific sanctions for threats, hostility, or endangering women's lives, as these are considered to be already covered in the Penal Code under homicide, threats, damage, etc.

Despite the existence of legal avenues to address partner violence in Uruguay, the Organization of American States' Committee of Experts on Violence concluded in August 2005 that there were some failures in dealing with this matter in the country, given that there are no data on detentions or trials for violence against women, there are only 1% of officers from the Ministry of the Interior assigned to this issue, no one can provide victim protection, and there are no women's shelters.

Violence against women is not included as a subject within in the curricula of primary- or secondary-school teachers, physicians, psychologists, lawyers, or social workers. However, in 2001, post-graduate degrees on the study of violence against women were being developed at the university level, and several information courses have been given to judges, police, and others who deal with this subject.

Methods
Sample
During May 2004, face-to-face interviews were conducted with 376 men and 624 women between 18 to 65 years of age in some Uruguay cities, primarily in Montevideo (53.6% of interviews) and Canelones (11.6%). Based on a framework used in the 1996 National Census conducted by the Statistical and Census Institute, a geographic, multiple-phased method was used to randomly select individuals for this study from cities with a population of at least 10,000. The selection stages were: city; census tract; segment; street blocks; home; and individual. Interviewers were provided with guidelines for selecting an alternative person if the person who had been initially selected was unwilling to be interviewed or unavailable. Of the 7,271 households initially selected for the sample, 65.8% (4,781) were excluded because no one was home on either of the two visits made by the interviewer. Of the remaining households where a person was con-

tacted, 19.4% (484) were ineligible (e.g., only children were at home), 40.0% (996) refused to participate, 0.4% (10) did not complete the interview, and 40.2% (1,000) completed the interviews. Table 1 shows the characteristics of the persons participating in the survey. Of the 1,000 who participated 37.6% were men and 62.4% were women.

TABLE 1. Age, marital status, employment status and drinking pattern in the 12 months preceding the survey, for male and female respondents, Uruguay, 2004.

	Men (N=376)		Women (N=624)	
	Number	Percent or mean	Number	Percent or mean
Age		39.4 years		41.4 years
18–24 years	75	20.0%	103	16.5%
25–34 years	77	20.5%	120	19.2%
35–44 years	81	21.5%	118	18.9%
45–54 years	67	17.8%	139	22.3%
55 and older	76	20.2%	145	23.1%
Marital status				
Married	168	44.7%	277	44.4%
Cohabiting/living with partner	49	13.0%	79	12.7%
Divorced or separated	33	8.8%	99	15.9%
Never married	119	31.7%	126	20.2%
Widowed	7	1.9%	43	6.9%
Employment status				
In labor force (working, temporarily not working due to illness or parental leave)	263	70.0%	299	48.0%
Involuntarily unemployed	40	10.6%	55	8.8%
Voluntarily unemployed/homemaker	12	3.2%	169	27.1%
Student	29	7.7%	34	5.4%
Retired	32	8.5%	67	10.7%
Drinking pattern (past 12 months)				
Drank any alcohol past 12 months	305	81.1%	376	60.3%
Average number of drinking days (drinkers only)		86.1 days		51.1 days
Average number of drinks per occasion (drinkers only)		4.3 drinks		2.3 drinks
Average annual volume (drinkers only)		557.3 drinks		157.4 drinks
Drank five or more drinks on one or more occasions (drinkers only)	138	45.3%	46	12.2%

Measures that differed from the core questions:

Respondents to the Uruguay survey were not asked for information on the sex of their partner or sexual orientation; therefore, no cases were excluded based on the partner being the same sex. Whether the respondent drank five or more drinks on any occasion in the past year was based on the graduated frequency question described in the chapter "Common Survey Methods and Analyses Conducted for Each Country Chapter."

Results

There were no significant differences in the rates of partner aggression reported by male or female victims and aggressors (see Figure 1). As is evident in the figure, a higher percentage of female respondents reported being victims of physical aggression (6.6%) than male respondents reported being aggressive toward a partner (4.5%), although this difference did not reach statistical significance.

FIGURE 1. Percent of respondents who reported having been a victim or aggressor, by sex, GENACIS survey, Uruguay, 2004.

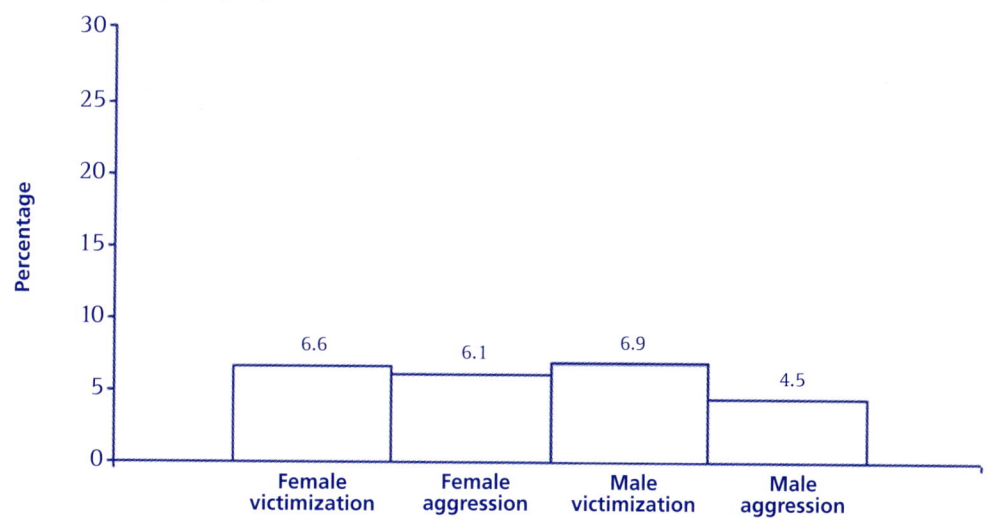

	Female victimization	Female aggression	Male victimization	Male aggression
Percentage	6.6	6.1	6.9	4.5

Some respondents reported having been both aggressive toward a partner and the victim of aggression by a partner. Of respondents who reported having been involved in any partner physical aggression, 34.5% (20) of women and 41.4% (12) of men had been victims only, 29.3% (17) of women and 10.3% (3) of men had been perpetrators only, and 36.2% (21) of women and 48.3% (14) of men reported having been both a victim and a perpetrator.

The average age of victims of partner physical aggression was 28.0 years for males and 32.7 years for females. Male respondents who reported aggression toward a partner were 25 years of age, on average, while female aggressors were 28.8 years old, on average. As shown in Figure 2, physical aggression by a partner and toward a partner tended to decrease with age for both men and women. The rates of partner physical aggression also varied by marital status (see Figure 3). Married respondents in all groups were the least likely to report partner physical aggression (significantly less than never-married respondents for all four groups and than cohabiting male and female aggressors and male victims at a significance level of $p < .01$). For male and female aggressors and male victims, those living with a partner were the most likely to report partner aggression (significant only compared to married respondents), followed by never married respondents (significant at $p < .01$ compared to married respondents).

FIGURE 2. Percent of respondents who reported having been a victim or aggressor, by age group and sex, GENACIS survey, Uruguay, 2004.

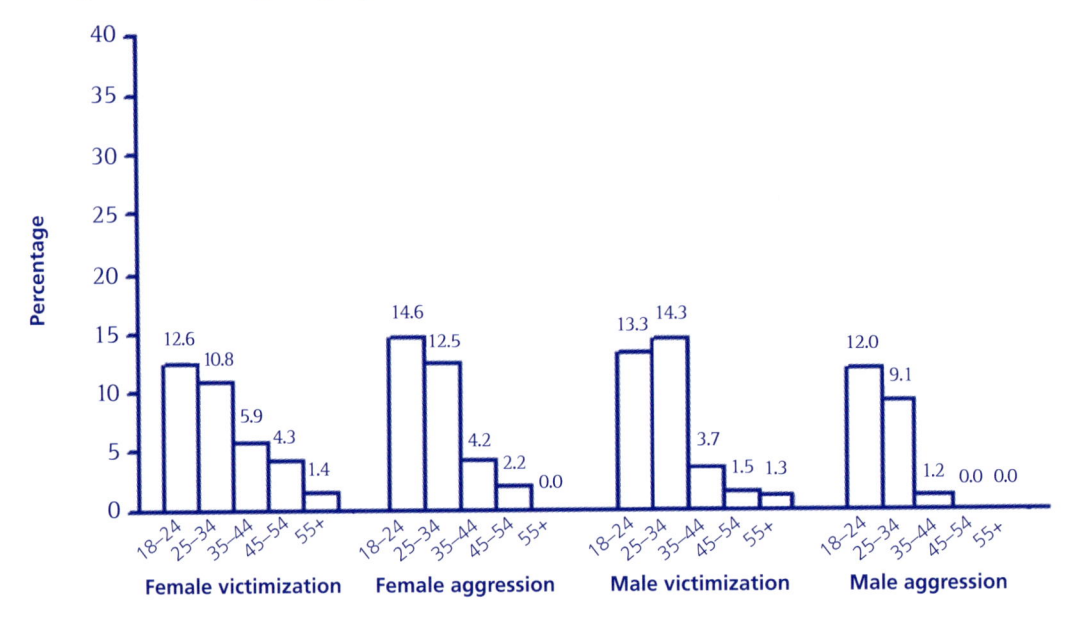

FIGURE 3. Percent of respondents who reported having been a victim or aggressor, by marital status and sex, GENACIS survey, Uruguay, 2004.

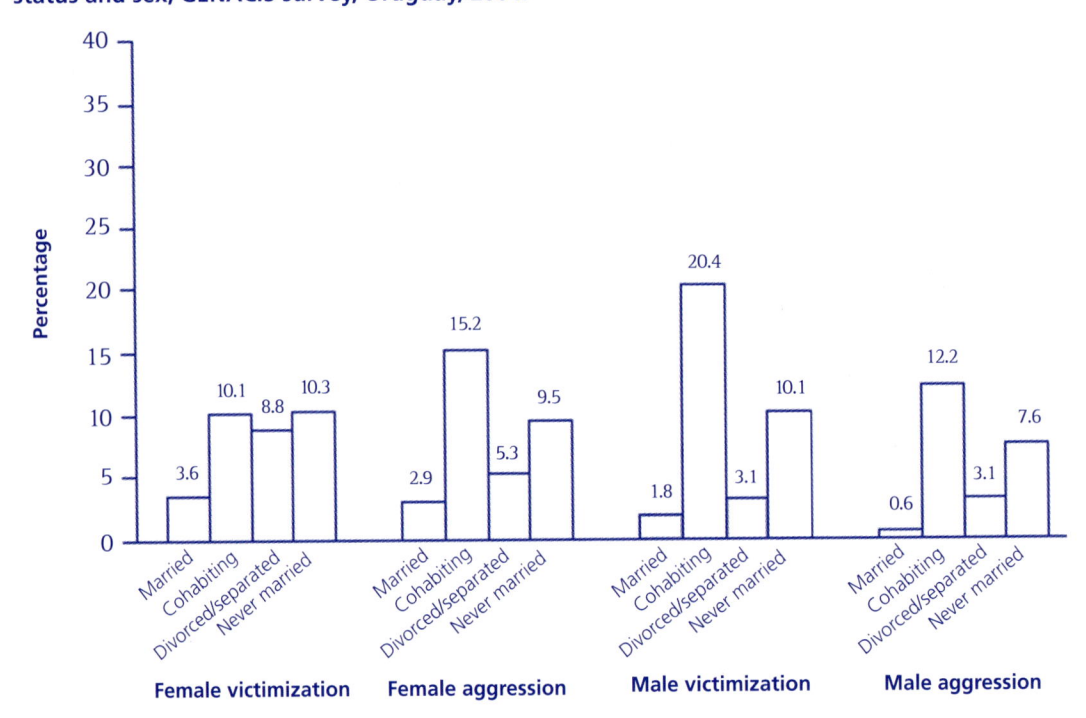

There were no significant differences in the type of aggressive act reported by male or female victims and aggressors, possibly because of the low numbers of participants who reported partner physical aggression. As shown in Figure 4, there was a trend for men (both among victims and aggressors) to report more pushing, shoving, and grabbing while female aggressors were more likely to report slapping and throwing something at the partner.

FIGURE 4. Type of aggressive act against females as reported by female victims and male aggressors and against males as reported by male victims and female aggressors, GENACIS survey, Uruguay, 2004.

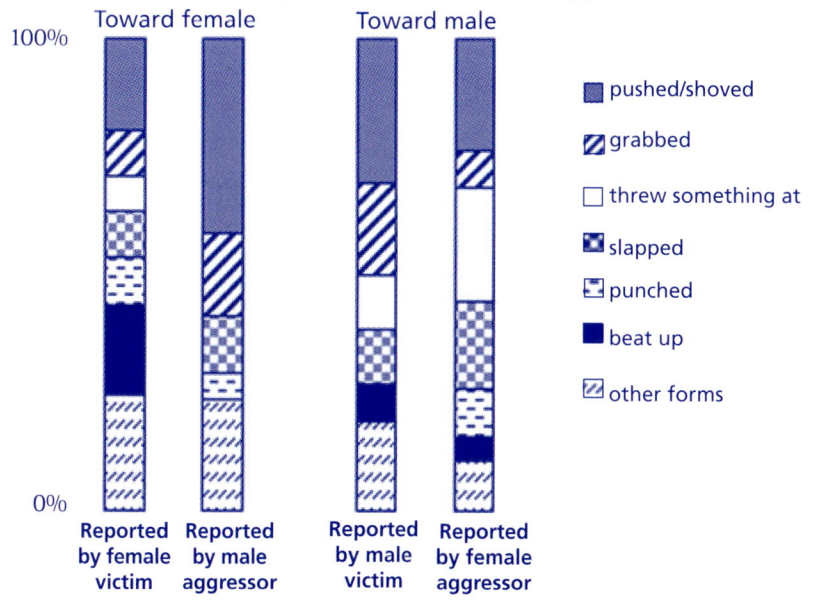

Figure 5 shows the mean ratings of severity of the physical aggression and how afraid, upset, and angry the respondent was at the time of the incident. Among respondents who reported having been victims of partner aggression, female victims rated the aggression as more severe than did male victims and they were more afraid, upset, and angry (all comparisons p < .001). Female aggressors rated the aggression as less severe and themselves as less afraid and upset than did male aggressors (significant only for upset p < .01). In comparing female victims to male aggressors, females rated the incident as more severe and themselves as more afraid, upset, and angry (significant only for level of fear at p < .05). Female aggressors rated the incident as more severe and themselves as more afraid, upset, and angry than did male victims (not significant for any rating). In addition to reporting higher severity ratings, a larger percentage of female victims (14.6%, 6 out of 41) than male victims (3.9%, 1 out of 26) reported having sought medical attention after the incident (although the difference did not meet the criterion of p < .05 for statistical significance).

As shown in Figure 6, male aggressors were more likely to report that they or their partner had been drinking at the time of the aggressive incident than was reported by female victims (85.4% of female victims said that no one had been drinking at the time of the aggressive incident, compared with 70.6% of male aggressors who said that no one had been drinking); however, no comparisons met the significance criterion of p < .05, and results should be interpreted with caution given the small numbers in each group. There were too few respondents who reported drinking at the time of aggression to permit further analyses comparing incidents with and without alcohol.

FIGURE 5. Mean ratings of severity of aggression, fear, upset, and anger, by male and female victims and aggressors, GENACIS survey, Uruguay, 2004.

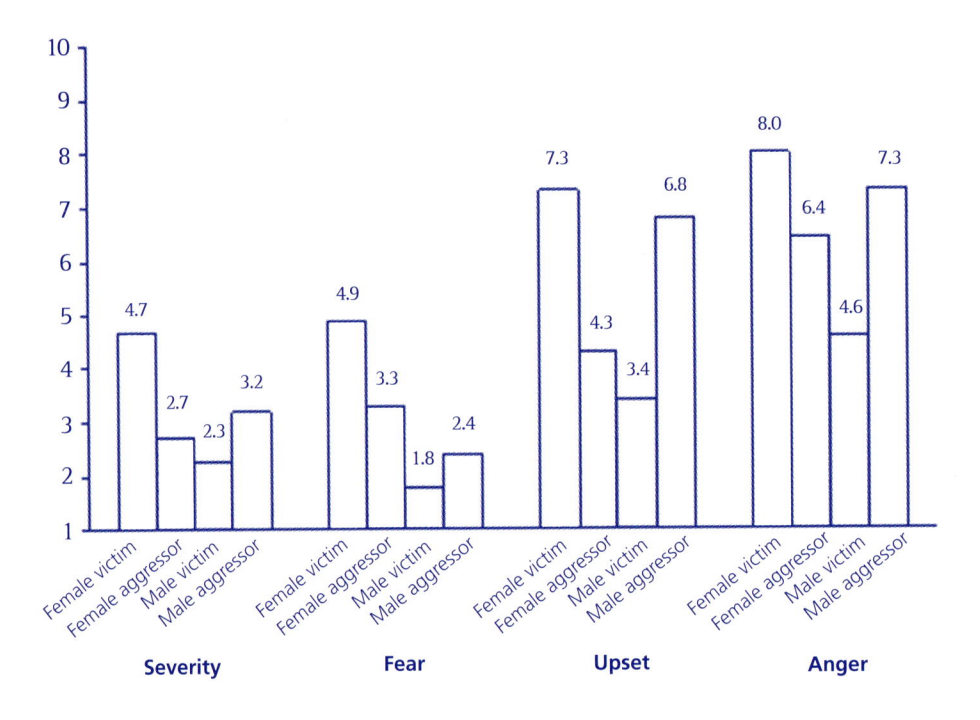

	Severity	Fear	Upset	Anger
Female victim	4.7	4.9	7.3	8.0
Female aggressor	2.7	3.3	4.3	6.4
Male victim	2.3	1.8	3.4	4.6
Male aggressor	3.2	2.4	6.8	7.3

FIGURE 6. Percent of incidents in which no partner had been drinking, both partners had been drinking, only the male partner had been drinking, or only the female partner had been drinking, as reported by male and female victims and aggressors, GENACIS survey, Uruguay, 2004.

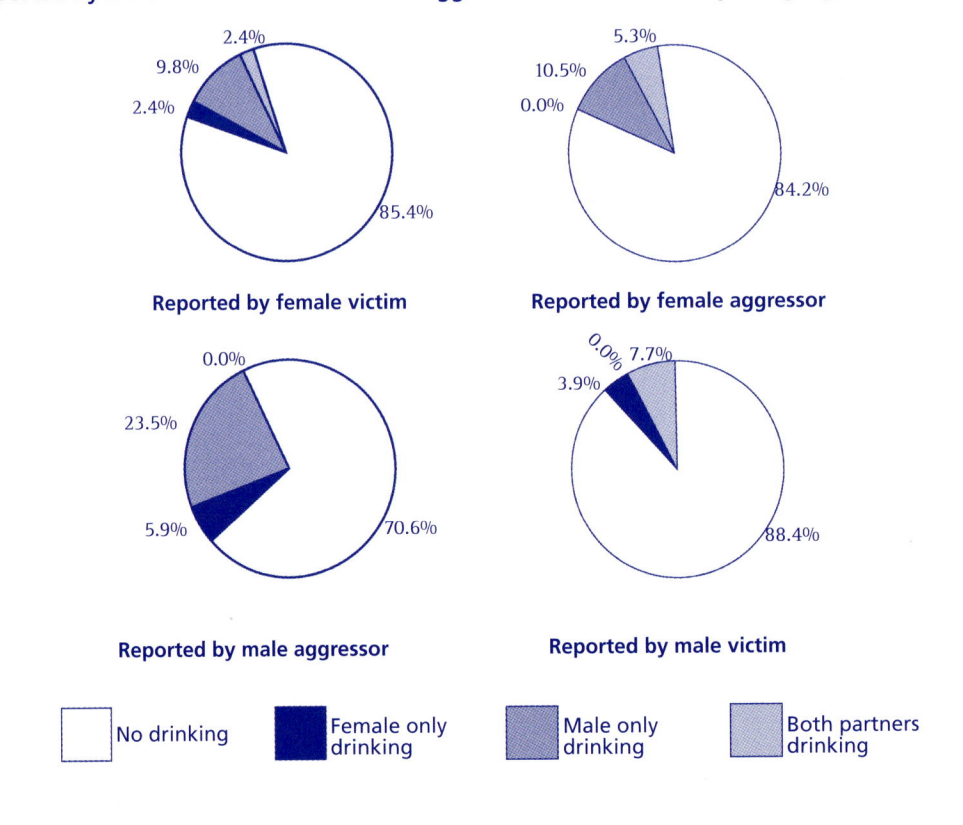

Reported by female victim: No drinking 85.4%, Female only drinking 2.4%, Male only drinking 9.8%, Both partners drinking 2.4%

Reported by female aggressor: No drinking 84.2%, Female only drinking 0.0%, Male only drinking 10.5%, Both partners drinking 5.3%

Reported by male aggressor: No drinking 70.6%, Female only drinking 5.9%, Male only drinking 23.5%, Both partners drinking 0.0%

Reported by male victim: No drinking 88.4%, Female only drinking 3.9%, Male only drinking 0.0%, Both partners drinking 7.7%

Relationship between Alcohol Consumption and Partner Aggression

Male and female respondents who drank any alcohol in the past year were more likely than past year abstainers to report aggression by a partner (8.2% of drinkers vs. 1.4% of abstainers for men; 7.2% of drinkers vs. 5.7% of abstainers for women) and aggression toward a partner (5.3% of drinkers vs. 1.4% of abstainers for men; 8.2% of drinkers vs. 2.8% of abstainers for women). However odds ratios predicting aggression by drinking status were not significantly greater than 1 after controlling for age.

Respondent's Drinking Pattern and Partner Aggression

As shown in Figure 7, the percent of female victims and aggressors and male victims and aggressors was higher among drinkers who consumed five or more drinks on at least one occasion in the year prior to the survey compared to those who never drank as much as five drinks on a single occasion (but odds ratios comparing those who drank five drinks or more with those who did not drink that much were not significantly greater than 1 for men or women victims or aggressors controlling for age).

FIGURE 7. Percent of respondents who reported victimization (aggression by a partner) or aggression (aggresion toward a partner) by whether the respondent had consumed five or more drinks on an occasion or never consumed five drinks on an occasion, by sex, GENACIS survey, Uruguay, 2004.

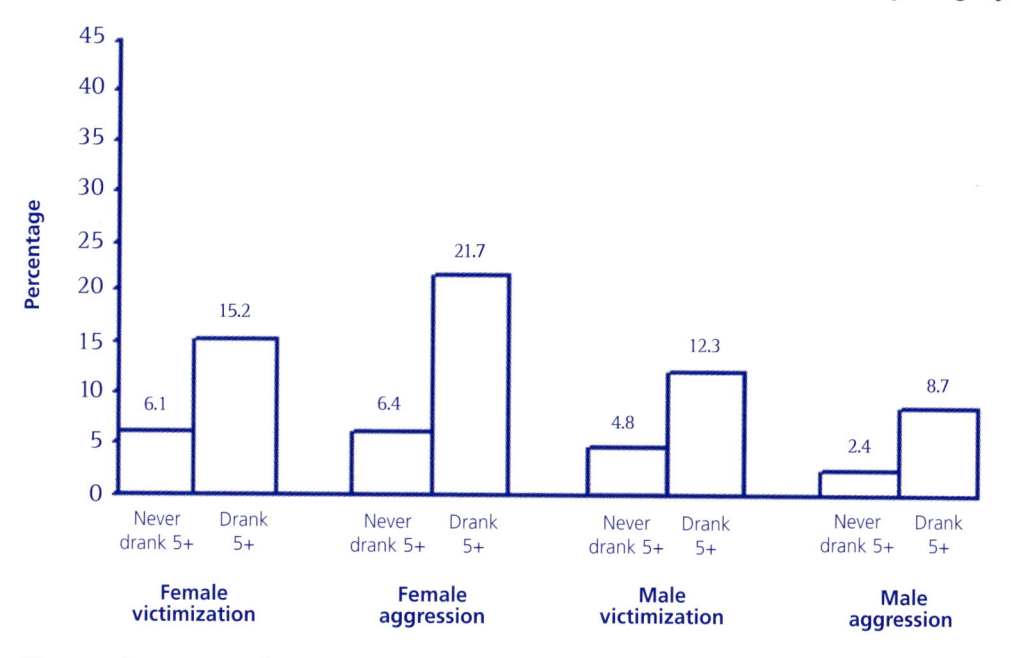

	Never drank 5+	Drank 5+
Female victimization	6.1	15.2
Female aggression	6.4	21.7
Male victimization	4.8	12.3
Male aggression	2.4	8.7

Those who reported aggression did not differ significantly in terms of frequency of drinking (Figure 8) or in terms of overall annual alcohol consumption (Figure 10) from those who reported no aggression; however, the tendency for higher overall annual consumption among those who reported aggression approached significance for female victimization (p = .073) and male aggression (p = .076). Usual number of drinks consumed per occasion (Figure 9) was significantly related to having been victimized (p< .001) and having been aggressive (p = .002) among females, with women who reported partner aggression consuming more alcoholic drinks per occasion than women who reported no aggression. The same pattern was evident for men, but it did not reach the p < .05 criterion for statistical significance. All analyses controlled for age of the respondent.

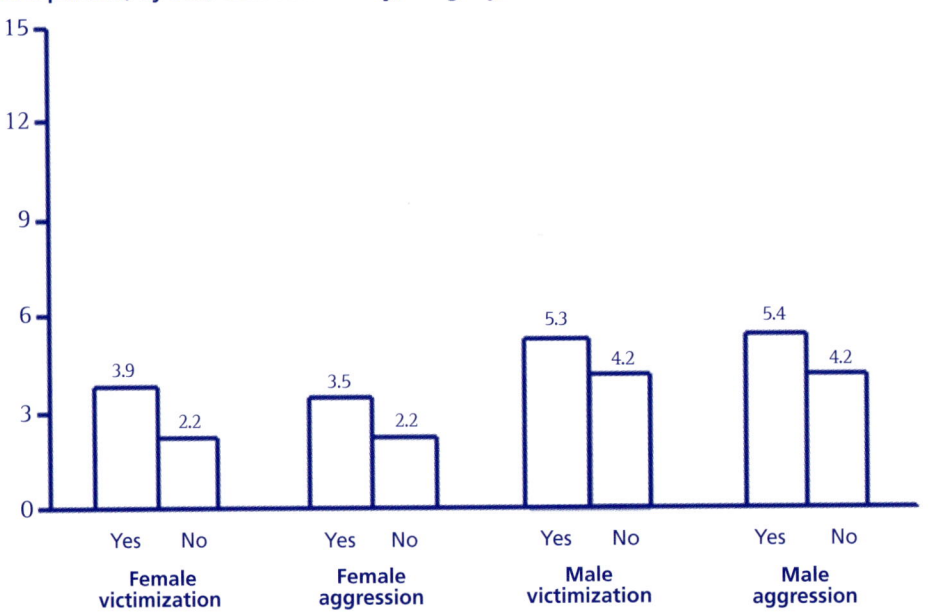

FIGURE 8. Mean number of drinking days in the year preceding the survey by whether the respondent had been a victim of partner aggression and whether the respondent had been aggressive toward a partner, by sex, GENACIS survey, Uruguay, 2004.

	Yes	No
Female victimization	4.8	51.3
Female aggression	31.4	52.8
Male victimization	67.6	87.7
Male aggression	78.6	86.5

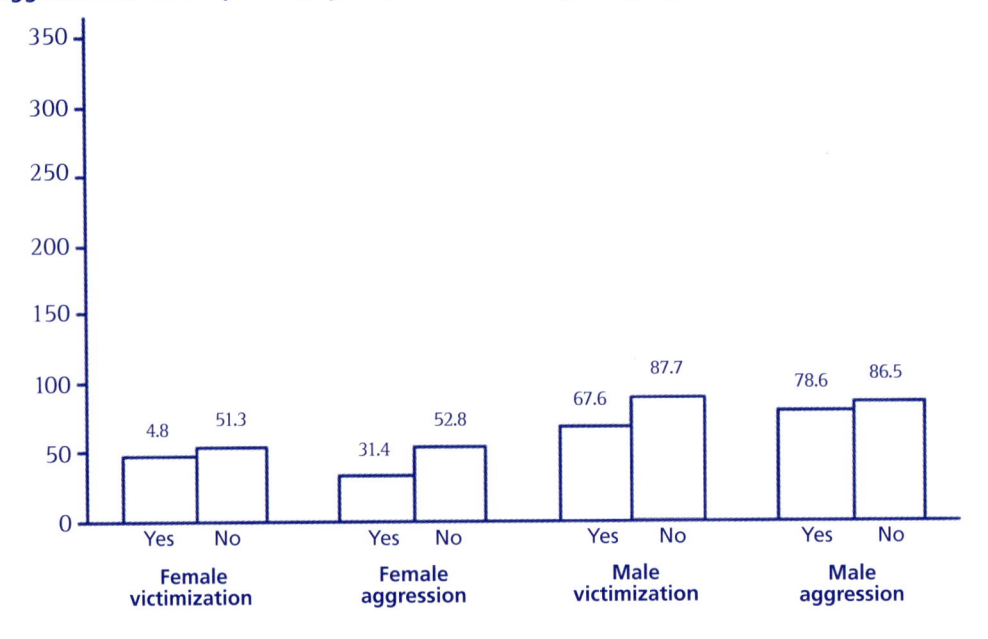

FIGURE 9. Mean number of drinks consumed on usual drinking occasions by whether the respondent had been a victim of partner aggression and whether the respondent had been aggressive toward a partner, by sex, GENACIS survey, Uruguay, 2004.

	Yes	No
Female victimization	3.9	2.2
Female aggression	3.5	2.2
Male victimization	5.3	4.2
Male aggression	5.4	4.2

FIGURE 10. Overall mean number of drinks consumed annually by whether the respondent had been a victim of partner aggression and whether the respondent had been aggressive toward a partner, by sex, GENACIS survey, Uruguay, 2004.

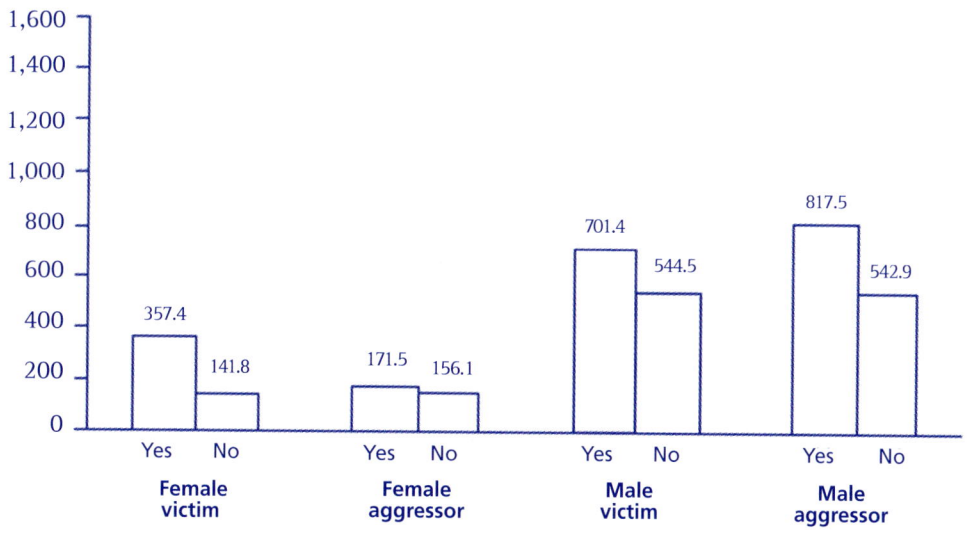

Discussion

Physical violence by a partner was reported by both men and women, but women experienced more severe aggression than did men. In this study, there was a non-significant trend for women to be more likely than men to report being beaten up or punched and to seek medical attention, as has been found by other studies (García-Moreno, 2002). In addition, female victims rated their own fear and the severity of the aggression higher than did male victims. Although this likely reflects greater strength on the part of male versus female aggressors, the less severe aggression reported by male victims might also relate to patriarchal culture, or it may be seen as a rationalization mechanism that men use for not seeing themselves as victims (Meiselman, 1990). While female victims reported the highest level of anger and upset, male aggressors were more angry and upset than were female aggressors.

The findings that no male victims reported drinking alcohol at the time of the aggressive incident and that the percentage of male aggressors who reported their own drinking during the aggression was higher than any other group of respondents suggests that male aggressors might have been using alcohol consumption as an excuse to diminish their responsibility and guilt about their aggressive acts. These findings must be treated with caution, however, given the low number of respondents who reported any drinking during the aggression.

There are factors that were associated with partner aggression for both men and women. In particular, higher rates of partner aggression were found for respondents who were under 35, and those who reported partner aggression were more likely to drink more drinks on occasions when they drank and to have higher overall annual consumption than those who reported no partner aggression. Such drinking patterns should be taken into account in developing prevention strategies. In particular, while more frequent drinking was not significantly related to partner aggression (and in fact, drinking was actually less frequent among those reporting aggression), the finding that aggression was associated with drinking more drinks per occasion suggests that it is not whether the person has been drinking but rather that he or she has consumed a large quantity of alcohol that increases the risk of partner aggression.

Despite the findings of a relationship between usual drinking habits and partner aggression, more than 70% of male aggressors and more than 80% of female aggressors and male and female victims reported that no one had been drinking alcohol before the incident. That is, the proportion of incidents of partner aggression involving alcohol was smaller than expected. A possible explanation is that certain types of alcoholic beverages are not recognized as alcohol by some people in a society where beverages such as wine are regularly ingested during the family's meals, and thus, respondents may not have considered such consumption as "drinking." It would be useful in future research to know the day and time in which partner aggression takes place, for example, how much aggression occurs after meals or on weekends, when drinking would have been likely.

The higher rate of partner aggression among younger adults suggests that prevention of violence (PAHO, 2005) as well as prevention of alcohol consumption and alcohol abuse must begin in the early stages of life. The current findings relating partner aggression with a pattern of consuming more drinks per occasion suggests that interventions focusing on both alcohol use and partner aggression would be useful.

Acknowledgments

Thanks to Sharon Bernards, Kate Graham, Sharon Wilsnack, Arlinda Kristjanson, Maristela Monteiro, Víctor H. González, and Hugo A. Míguez.

References

CLADEM (Comité de Latinoamérica y el Caribe para la Defensa de los Derechos de la Mujer (2002), http://www.cladem.org/espanol/nacionales/uruguay/uruguay7.asp

Corsi J. (2003). Maltrato y abuso en el ámbito doméstico, Ed. Paidos, Buenos Aires,

Domínguez C, Fernández M.(2003) Perfil de los Incidentes Familiares con Víctimas Fallecidas: Análisis estadístico y explicativo de la realidad uruguaya. Dirección Nacional de Prevención Social del Delito del Ministerio del Interior. http://www.dnpd.gub.uy
García-Moreno (2002). http://publications.paho.org/Spanish/capitulo_1_PO_12.pdf

Heise L, Ellsberg M, and Gottemoeller M.(1999). Ending Violence against Women. Population Reports. Series L. No. 11. Baltimore, Maryland: Population Information Program, Johns Hopkins University School of Public Health

Uruguay, Junta Nacional de Drogas (2006). 4a. EncuestaNacional de Prevalencia de Consumo de Drogas www.infodrogas.gub.uy

Magri R, et al. (2005) Legal and illegal drug consumption in recent detainees. Presented at Kettil-Bruun Society #1th Symposium. Riverside, Ca.

Magri R, Míguez H, Parodi V, Hutson J, Suárez H, Menéndez A, Koren G, Bustos R. (2007) Consumo de alcohol y otrasdrogas en embarazadas. *PediatrUrug* 78(2): 59-69.

Meiselman KC. (1990). Resolving the trauma of incest: Reintegration therapy with survivors. San Francisco: Jossey-Bass.

Miguez H. (2007) *http://www.hugomiguez.com.ar/Cambio.htm*

Organization of Amcerican States, Committtee of experts on Violence(CEVI) (2005). (MESECVI DOC.4/05/SER.L/II.7.10)

Pan American Health Organization (2005). Violencia de Genero, Salud y Derechos de la Americas. Accessed on 7 October 2001 *http://www.paho.org/Spanish/AD/GE/calltoactionsp.pdf*

Uruguay, Ministerio del Interior, National Consultation Council fighting against Domestic Violence for the National Plan 2004-2010 (2003) Ministerio del Interior

Traverso MT. (2000). Violencia en la Pareja: la cara oculta de la relación. New York BID

Comparison of Partner Physical Aggression Across Ten Countries

—Kathryn Graham and Sharon Bernards and (in alphabetical order by country) Myriam Munné, (Argentina), Claudina E. Cayetano (Belize), Florence Kerr–Corrêa and Maria Cristina Pereira Lima (Brazil), Julio Bejarano (Costa Rica), Martha Mendoza Romero, María Elena Medina–Mora and Jorge Velázquez Villatoro (Mexico), José Trinidad Caldera Aburto (Nicaragua), Marina Julia Piazza Ferrand (Peru), Sharon Wilsnack (United States), and Raquel Magri (Uruguay)

Introduction

Using the same questionnaire on alcohol consumption in several different countries has opened up a unique opportunity: it is now possible to identify the patterns of association between alcohol consumption and partner violence that are common across countries, instead of merely looking at patterns that occur only in certain cultures. This ability to identify common patterns is especially important when considering the role of alcohol consumption, because both the proportion of abstainers and the pattern of drinking among drinkers vary considerably from country to country. At one end of the continuum are countries where most people drink fairly often, but where drinking to intoxication is rare; at the other extreme are countries where only a small proportion of people drink, and those who drink consume alcohol only occasionally, but usually in large quantities.

This book includes the participation of ten countries in the Americas. Detailed results for each country were presented in the previous chapters. In this chapter, we evaluate the extent to which similar findings have emerged across countries. As a way to identify any patterns that may be characteristic of geographic location or region, the presentation of results is organized from south to north, beginning with Argentina and then ranging north to Canada.

Seven countries included questions on physical aggression both by a partner and toward a partner for both female and male respondents. Three countries (Belize, Mexico, and the United States of America) did not include questions on aggression toward a partner, and the United States sample included only women. Therefore, these three countries were excluded from some analyses. Peru included samples from two locations (the cities of Lima and Ayacucho) that were culturally quite different (Flake, 2005); therefore, these two samples were analyzed separately in the Peru chapter and in this comparative chapter.

In order to make patterns across countries visually apparent in the following tables, the highest numbers within each country are shown in dark blue and the lowest are left unshaded; values in between (where relevant) are shown in lighter shades of blue. Missing data, cells with fewer than 20 respondents, or cells where no gender comparisons were possible are shown using diagonal lines.

Gender Differences in Aggression By and Toward a Partner

Table 1a shows the percent of respondents who reported aggression in the ten participating countries, comparing the percent of female and male respondents who reported aggression by a partner (victims) and aggression toward a partner (aggressors). As shown in the table, a higher percent of female (shaded dark blue) than male (white) respondents reported being a victim of aggression by a partner in Brazil, Peru (both samples), Costa Rica, Belize, and Mexico; while a higher percent of male (shaded blue) than female (white) respondents reported being the victim of partner aggression in Argentina, Uruguay, Nicaragua, and Canada, suggesting no consistent gender difference across countries and no regional trends. The gender difference in reporting aggression by a partner was significant only for Argentina, Peru/Ayacucho, Belize, Mexico, and Canada. Gender differences in self-reported aggressors (the last two columns of Table 1a) showed a more consistent pattern across countries than was evident for victims, with a higher rate of perpetration reported by female than by male respondents in all countries, except in Peru/Ayacucho; however, this difference was small in many countries and significant only for Canada.[1]

TABLE 1a. Percent of respondents who reported aggression by a partner (victims) and aggression toward a partner (aggressors), by sex, ten participating countries.

Country	Female victimization	Male victimization	Female aggression	Male aggression
Argentina	9.4[a]	14.5[a]	8.4	8.2
Uruguay	6.6	6.9	6.1	4.5
Brazil	5.5	4.1	4.4	3.5
Peru (Lima)	8.4	7.5	8.8	6.5
Peru (Ayacucho)	19.8[a]	10[a]	12.6	12.9
Costa Rica	7.1	6.5	5.3	5.0
Nicaragua	6.0	6.1	6.4	6.1
Belize	4.4[a]	3.1[a]		
Mexico	7.6[a]	3.7[a]		
United States	6.1			
Canada	5.3[a]	7.2[a]	5.7[b]	3.4[b]

[a] significant difference (Chi-square p<.05) between female victims and male victims within country.
[b] significant difference (Chi-square p<.05) between female aggressors and male aggressors within country.

Table 1b shows the same results that were reported in Table 1a, but the results are organized so as to compare the percent of female respondents reporting victimization to the percent of male respondents reporting aggression toward a partner, and the percent of men reporting victimization to the percent of women reporting aggression toward a partner. As shown in this table, across all countries except Nicaragua, female respondents were more likely to report victimization than male respondents were to report aggression toward a partner (significant for Brazil and Canada). A comparison of male victims with female aggressors shows mixed results across countries (with significantly more males reporting victimization compared with females reporting aggression in Argentina and Canada).

---

[1] As noted elsewhere in this book, the use of the terms "victim" and "aggressor" reflects the operational definitions of physical aggression by and toward a partner and may not reflect the reality of the subjective experience. In addition, the questions excluded sexual aggression for most countries, as well as nonphysical aggression or abuse (as described in the chapter "Common Survey Methods and Analyses Conducted for Each Country Chapter.")

TABLE 1b. Percent of female respondents who reported aggression by a partner (victim) compared to male respondents who reported aggression toward a partner (aggressor); and percent of male respondents who reported aggression by a partner (victim) compared to female respondents who reported aggression toward a partner (aggressor), seven of the ten participating countries.

Country	Female victimization	Male aggression	Male victimization	Female aggression
Argentina	9.4	8.2	14.5[b]	8.4[b]
Uruguay	6.6	4.5	6.9	6.1
Brazil	5.5[a]	3.5[a]	4.1	4.4
Peru (Lima)	8.4	6.5	7.5	8.8
Peru (Ayacucho)	19.8	12.9	10.0	12.6
Costa Rica	7.1	5.0	6.5	5.3
Nicaragua	6.0	6.1	6.1	6.4
Canada	5.3[a]	3.4[a]	7.2[b]	5.7[b]

[a] Significant difference (Chi-square p<.05) between female victims and male aggressors within country.
[b] Significant difference (Chi-square p<.05) between male victims and female aggressors within country.

These comparisons involve independently sampled female and male respondents, not men and women who are part of a couple.[2] Therefore, discrepancies in reporting by victims and aggressors may be due to victim–aggressor biases in reporting, gender differences in reporting aggression, and/or gender differences in sampling. A possible explanation for the discrepancy between female victims and male aggressors shown in Table 1b is that victims are more willing to report aggression by their partner than aggressors are willing to report their aggression toward a partner. However, this does not account for the mixed results for male victims and female aggressors. It is possible that men may be underreporting their aggression in countries where there is a strong taboo against male-to-female aggression, while women may be less reluctant than men to report their own aggression in some countries if there is less of a taboo for female-to-male aggression. A second explanation relating to reporting bias is that men may be less likely than women to remember and report minor physical aggression, especially minor acts of aggression by the man toward the woman. Finally, gender differences in reporting aggression might be related to gender differences in sampling. For example, it may be that violent men are more reluctant than nonviolent men to participate in the surveys, while this may not be true for women. Whatever the explanation, it is worth noting the consistent pattern across countries that women are more likely to report victimization compared with the men reporting aggression, while the converse does not apply for male victims and female aggressors.

Relationship between Age and Partner Physical Aggression

Table 2 shows the percent of respondents in each of five age groups who reported aggression. As is clear from the shading, in all countries partner aggression decreased as people aged for both men and women and for both victimization and aggression. Except for female victims in Belize, the groups at highest risk were those aged 18–24 years or those aged 25–34 years; those at lowest risk in almost all countries were persons aged 55 and older, followed by those aged 45–54 years. This confirms previous research

---

[2] Although the Belize survey included more than one respondent from the same household, this analysis treats male and female respondents as independent samples, in order to allow the analyses to be comparable across countries.

(Bookwala, Sobin, and Zdaniuk, 2005; García-Moreno et al., 2005; Johnson, 2006; Orpinas, 1999; Rosales et al., 1999; Wilke and Vinton, 2005; Wilson, Johnson, and Daly, 1995) that, regardless of country, younger adults are more likely than older adults to be affected by partner aggression.

TABLE 2. Percent of respondents in each group who reported partner aggression, by sex and whether respondent was the victim or aggressor, ten participating countries.

Country	Sex	Role	Age Group 18–24	25–34	35–44	45–54	55+
Argentina							
	Female	Victim	19.3[d]	11.2	8.9	7.3	3.3[d]
		Aggressor	25.0[abcd]	9.5[a]	8.2[b]	1.6[c]	2.5[d]
	Male	Victim	25.3[cd]	23.7[fg]	11.6	4.4[cf]	1.7[dg]
		Aggressor	12.7	17.5[ef]	4.2[e]	2.9[f]	0.0
Uruguay							
	Female	Victim	12.6[d]	10.8[g]	5.9	4.3	1.4[dg]
		Aggressor	14.6[c]	12.5[f]	4.2	2.2[cf]	0.0
	Male	Victim	13.3	14.3	3.7	1.5	1.3
		Aggressor	12.0	9.1	1.2	0.0	0.0
Brazil							
	Female	Victim	6.2	8.6[g]	6.5	4.5	1.5[g]
		Aggressor	6.7	8.6[fg]	4.0	0.9[f]	1.1[g]
	Male	Victim	9.4	3.9	2.5	2.6	2.3
		Aggressor	8.4[d]	2.8	4.7[i]	1.1	0.7[dj]
Peru (Lima)							
	Female	Victim	12.4[c]	12.4[f]	8.2	2.1[cf]	3.8
		Aggressor	14.6[c]	12.4[f]	8.7	2.8[cf]	1.3
	Male	Victim	13.9	10.2	6.5	2.0	0.0
		Aggressor	10.1	11.1	3.9	2.0	0.0
Peru (Ayacucho)							
	Female	Victim	17.8	24.7	21.3	10.0	0.0
		Aggressor	24.7[b]	11.8	6.3[b]	5.0	0.0
	Male	Victim	17.7	7.3	5.9		0.0
		Aggressor	15.7	14.6	11.8		
Costa Rica							
	Female	Victim	10.4[d]	9.5[g]	5.5	8.4	1.4[dg]
		Aggressor	8.7[c]	8.9[f]	5.9	1.3[cf]	0.7
	Male	Victim	7.4	13.8	4.0	4.4	0.0
		Aggressor	9.5	5.3	6.6	1.5	0.0

TABLE 2. (continued)

Country	Sex	Role	Age Group 18–24	25–34	35–44	45–54	55+
Nicaragua							
	Female	Victim	8.7[c]	7.0	6.0	1.7[c]	0.8
		Aggressor	8.7	8.0	5.4	3.5	1.7
	Male	Victim	8.3	10.2	2.8	3.0	1.5
		Aggressor	9.5	8.2	3.7	3.0	1.5
Belize							
	Female	Victim	3.7	5.7[g]	7.4[hj]	1.9[h]	1.2[gj]
	Male	Victim	2.1[a]	6.3[ae]	3.4	3.0	0.3[e]
Mexico							
	Female	Victim	11.3	9.8	5.7	2.5	3.1
	Male	Victim	7.9	4.1	2.4	0.0	0.0
United States							
	Female	Victim	18.3[bc]	10.2[f]	5.8[b]	2.4[cf]	
Canada							
	Female	Victim	13.0[bcd]	9.8[efg]	5.2[bej]	4.9[cfk]	1.0[dgjk]
		Aggressor	18.2[abcd]	10.1[aefg]	6.1[behj]	2.9[cfhk]	0.9[dgjk]
	Male	Victim	17.0[abcd]	11.5[aefg]	8.0[behj]	5.0[cfhk]	1.6[dgjk]
		Aggressor	6.2[cd]	5.9[fg]	4.1[j]	2.9[cfk]	0.7[dgjk]

Note: Significant (p<.01) pairwise differences within country and within each respondent role using separate logistic regressionmodels for each age group as comparison category: [a]18–24 year olds vs. 25–34; [b]18–24 vs. 35–44; [c]18–24 vs 45–54; [d]18–24 vs 55+; [e]25–34 vs. 35–44; [f]25–34 vs. 45–54; [g]25–34 vs 55+; [h]35–44 vs 45–54; [j]35–44 vs 55+; [k]45–54 vs 55+.

Marital Status and Partner Aggression

Table 3a shows the percent of respondents reporting partner aggression by marital status. As shown in the table, a striking pattern in the association between marital status and partner aggression has emerged across many countries, with partner aggression most likely to be reported by respondents in a common–law relationship and least likely for respondents who were legally married. Because in many countries marital status is related to age (never married, cohabiting, and divorced/separated individuals are likely to be younger than married persons), it is important to control for age in assessing the relationship between partner aggression and marital status. To that end, Table 3b shows the odds of aggression for each marital status (compared to each other marital status) controlling for age. As is evident in this table, somewhat different results emerged from the pattern using raw percentages. Although being in a common–law relationship was still associated with an increased risk of aggression, being divorced/separated emerged as a more important risk factor compared with analyses that did not include age. In addition, controlling for age showed an increased risk for married respondents in some countries and reduced risk for respondents who had never been married.

TABLE 3a. Percent of respondents who reported partner aggression, by sex and marital status and whether respondent was the victim or aggressor, ten participating countries.

Country	Sex	Role	Married	Common–law union	Divorced/separated	Never married
Argentina						
	Female	Victim	5.5	17.7	14.5	10.3
		Aggressor	5.5	15.7	7.9	11.1
	Male	Victim	6.5	28.6	13.2	18.4
		Aggressor	5.8	21.4	0.0	8.2
Uruguay						
	Female	Victim	3.6	10.1	8.8	10.3
		Aggressor	2.9	15.2	5.3	9.5
	Male	Victim	1.8	20.4	3.1	10.1
		Aggressor	0.6	12.2	3.1	7.6
Brazil						
	Female	Victim	6.1	9.0	4.0	4.7
		Aggressor	3.9	8.0	2.9	5.0
	Male	Victim	1.9	8.9	5.0	5.1
		Aggressor	2.7	6.4	2.6	3.6
Peru (Lima)						
	Female	Victim	7.7	14.2	6.7	5.0
		Aggressor	5.8	15.8	6.7	7.5
	Male	Victim	4.3	7.1		10.6
		Aggressor	4.3	9.4		6.9
Peru (Ayacucho)						
	Female	Victim	23.0	32.8	21.6	7.3
		Aggressor	5.8	18.8	5.4	19.5
	Male	Victim	0.0	12.8		13.7
		Aggressor	5.1	19.2		11.8
Costa Rica						
	Female	Victim	5.8	18.9	8.4	4.4
		Aggressor	4.6	5.7	7.1	6.9
	Male	Victim	4.6	1.9	4.5	11.3
		Aggressor	3.5	7.4	0.0	7.0
Nicaragua						
	Female	Victim	5.7	9.4	6.6	3.8
		Aggressor	6.3	9.4	3.3	4.9
	Male	Victim	4.8	7.4		6.8
		Aggressor	3.7	9.3		6.4

TABLE 3a. (continued)

Country	Sex	Role	Marital Status			
			Married	Common–law union	Divorced/separated	Never married
Belize						
	Female	Victim	3.5	7.4	7.6	3.4
	Male	Victim	2.1	5.9	3.9	2.7
Mexico						
	Female	Victim	6.8	15.4	12.7	3.7
	Male	Victim	1.1	3.3	9.1	6.6
United States						
	Female	Victim	3.9	13.9	12.9	9.8
Canada						
	Female	Victim	2.7	6.7	9.1	9.8
		Aggressor	3.6	9.1	5.6	10.3
	Male	Victim	4.3	10.8	8.9	10.9
		Aggressor	2.5	5.2	3.7	4.7

TABLE 3b. Odds of respondents reporting partner aggression by sex, marital status, and whether respondent was the victim or aggressor, ten participating countries.

Country	Sex	Role	Marital Status			
			Married	Common–law union	Divorced/separated	Never married
Argentina						
	Female	Victim	C[b]	2.61 C	3.00[b] 1.15 C	1.02 .39 .34
		Aggressor	C	1.76 C	1.49 .85 C	.68 .39 .46
	Male	Victim	C	3.32 C[e]	2.32 .70 C	.91 .27[e] .39
		Aggressor	C	2.17 C[e]	(0)*	.30 .14[e]
Uruguay						
	Female	Victim	C	1.51 C	2.53 1.67 C	1.43 .95 .57
		Aggressor	C	2.06 C	2.08 1.67 C	1.00 .48 .48
	Male	Victim	C[a]	7.22[a] C[e]	2.05 .28 C	1.75 .24[e] .85
		Aggressor	C	7.54 C	7.04 .93 C	1.86 .25 .26

TABLE 3b. (continued)

			Marital Status			
Country	Sex	Role	Married	Common–law union	Divorced/separated	Never married
Brazil						
	Female	Victim	C	1.24 C	.72 .58 C	.55 .44 .76
		Aggressor	C	1.42 C	.95 .67 C	.65 .46 .68
	Male	Victim	C	4.04 C	2.69 .66 C	1.91 .47 .71
		Aggressor	C	1.54 C	.92 .60 C	.59 .38 .64
Peru (Lima)						
	Female	Victim	C[c] C[e]	1.11 C[e]	.94 .84 C	.26[c] .23[e] .28
		Aggressor	C	1.77 C[e]	1.29 .73 C	.58 .33[e] .45
	Male	Victim	C	.94 C		.78 .83
		Aggressor	C	1.13 C		.36 .32
Peru (Ayacucho)						
	Female	Victim	C[c]	.91 C[e]	.76 .84 C[f]	.10[c] .11[e] .13[f]
		Aggressor	C	2.24 C	.79 .35 C	1.70 .76 2.16
	Male	Victim	(0)*	C		.51
		Aggressor	C	2.75 C		1.07 .39
Costa Rica						
	Female	Victim	C[a]	2.93[a] C[e]	1.43 .49 C	.48 .16[e] .33
		Aggressor	C	.85 C	1.62 1.91 C	.81 .95 .50
	Male	Victim	C	.30 C	.88 2.99 C	1.38 4.65 1.56
		Aggressor	C	1.53 C	(0)*	.79 .52

TABLE 3b. (continued)

Country	Sex	Role	Married	Common–law union	Divorced/separated	Never married
Nicaragua						
	Female	Victim	C	1.44 C[e]	1.50 1.04 C	.52 .36[e] .35
		Aggressor	C	1.34 C[e]	.60 .45 C	.64 .48[e] 1.06
	Male	Victim	C	1.32 C		.75 .57
		Aggressor	C	2.20 C		.89 .41
Belize						
	Female	Victim	C	1.81 C[e]	2.57 1.42 C	.76 .42[e] .29
	Male	Victim	C	2.23 C[e]	2.28 1.02 C	.74 .33[e] .33
United States						
	Female	Victim	C	2.7 C	1.5 1.4 C[f]	1.1 0.9 0.3[f]
Canada						
	Female	Victim	C[bc]	1.57 C[d]	4.25[b] 2.71[d] C[f]	1.91[c] 1.22 .45[f]
		Aggressor	C[b]	1.41 C	1.88[b] 1.34 C	1.15 .82 .61
	Male	Victim	C[ab]	1.67[a] C	2.50[b] 1.50 C[f]	1.12 .67 .45[f]
		Aggressor	C	1.38 C	1.70 1.22 C	.86 .62 .51

Note: Shading indicates largest odds ratios (shades of blue) to smallest odds ratios (white), controlling for age. C denotes the comparison category. (*) cells with zero respondents were omitted from logistic regression.
Significant (p<.01) pairwise differences within country and within each respondent role using separate logistic regression models controlling for age for each marital status group as the comparison category: [a]married vs cohabiting; [b]married vs divorced/separated; [c]married vs never married; [d]cohabiting vs divorced/separated; [e]cohabiting vs never married; [f]divorced/separated vs never married

Results are consistent with previous research showing a higher risk of partner aggression among persons in common–law relationships versus legally married couples (see review in the chapter "General Issues in Research on Intimate Partner Violence: An Overview."). These findings suggest that being legally married may confer some protection; common–law relationships, on the other hand, may increase the risk for partner aggression, possibly because persons in common-law relationships have riskier lifestyles and/or because of the less secure nature or lower commitment of a common-law relationship (Stets and Straus, 1990), even though in many countries common-law relationships have the same legal status as formal marriages after a certain period of time. The higher risk for aggression among separated or divorced persons also is consistent with previous research (reviewed in the chapter "General Issues in Research on Intimate Partner Violence: An Overview"). The greater prominence of being divorced or separated as a risk factor when age is controlled for indicates a need for further research to identify the factors responsible for the higher risk of partner aggression among divorced/separated individuals.

Never-married persons were at higher risk than married persons in some countries and at lower risk in others. For example, even in analyses that controlled for age, single men in Costa Rica were the most likely of all marital status groups to report aggression by a partner, and single females in Canada were the second most likely. On the other hand, single women in Peru were the least likely of all marital status groups to report partner aggression. Thus, while being in a common-law relationship or being divorced/separated was associated with an increased risk in most countries, the results for married versus never married tended to vary by country and sex, especially when age was controlled for in the analyses (Table 3b). Further cross-cultural explorations are required in order to identify the reasons for these different patterns in different countries. Unfortunately, many previous surveys of violence against women have excluded women who have never been married or been in a cohabiting relationship (AuCoin, 2005; Bunge and Locke, 2000; Ellsberg, Peña, et al, 2000; Flake and Forste, 2006; García-Moreno, et al., 2006; Natera, et al., 1997; Stith et al., 2004), which has prevented further study of this important issue.

Gender Differences in Experiencing Aggression: Severity, Fear, Upset, and Anger Ratings

Table 4 presents the average ratings of severity of aggression by partner (for victims) and self (for aggressors), as well as respondents' ratings of fear, level of upset, and anger. Although the shading in Table 4 compares all four categories (male and female victims and aggressors), it was not possible to compare all four groups statistically within the same analysis because the groups were not mutually exclusive (i.e., some respondents were both victims and aggressors). Therefore, significance testing was done comparing female to male victims, female to male aggressors, female victims to male aggressors, and male victims to female aggressors (comparable to the groupings shown in Tables 1a and 1b) on ratings of severity, fear, upset, and anger. Significant differences are shown with superscripts.

A very clear pattern emerged when comparing male and female victims; namely, that severity of partner's aggression was rated as more severe and the respondent self-ratings of fear, upset, and angry were higher for female than for male victims (see Table 4). This difference was significant in almost all comparisons.

TABLE 4. Victims' and aggressors' ratings of severity of aggression and level of fear, upset, and anger at the time of the incident, by sex, nine of the ten participating countries.

	Country	Female victims	Male victims	Female aggressors	Male aggressors
Severity of aggression					
	Argentina	3.9[a]	2.8[ad]	3.6[d]	3.4
	Uruguay	4.7[a]	2.3[a]	2.7	3.2
	Brazil	5.8[a]	2.9[a]	4.5	4.2
	Peru (Lima)	4.7	3.8	3.3	3.8
	Peru (Ayacucho)	5.6		3.1	
	Costa Rica	5.6[ac]	2.1[ad]	3.8[d]	2.9[c]
	Nicaragua	5.4[a]	3.5[a]	3.7	4.3
	Belize	4.4[a]	2.5[a]		
	United States	4.0			
	Canada	3.7[ac]	2.8[a]	2.6	2.6[c]
Fear					
	Argentina	3.7[a]	1.9[a]	2.9	3.1
	Uruguay	4.9[ac]	1.8[a]	3.3	2.4[c]
	Brazil	5.6	4.1	4.6	5.1
	Peru (Lima)	5.7[a]	2.9[a]	3.2	4.1
	Peru (Ayacucho)	6.2		4.4	
	Costa Rica	7.4[a]	2.7[a]	3.5	4.0
	Nicaragua	6.2[ac]	3.5[a]	3.9	4.1[c]
	Belize	5.0[a]	2.0[a]		
	United States	5.6			
	Canada	4.7[ac]	1.9[ad]	2.7[d]	2.9[c]
Upset					
	Argentina	6.2[a]	4.6[a]	5.6	6.4
	Uruguay	7.3[a]	3.4[a]	4.3[b]	6.8[b]
	Brazil	8.9[ac]	6.8[a]	7.6	7.5[c]
	Peru (Lima)	8.1[ac]	4.1[a]	4.6	5.3[c]
	Peru (Ayacucho)	7.8		4.3	
	Costa Rica	9.2[ac]	4.7[a]	5.6	6.1[c]
	Nicaragua	7.0[ac]	4.1[a]	5.1	5.6[c]
	United States	7.6			
	Canada	6.9[ac]	4.4[ad]	6.0[bd]	5.5[bc]

TABLE 4. (continued)

	Country	Female victims	Male victims	Female aggressors	Male aggressors
Anger					
	Argentina	8.0[ac]	5.4[ad]	6.9[d]	5.8[c]
	Uruguay	8.0[a]	4.6[a]	6.4	7.3
	Brazil	8.7[ac]	5.6[ad]	7.8[d]	7.1[c]
	Peru (Lima)	8.3[ac]	5.0[a]	6.3	6.2[c]
	Peru (Ayacucho)	8.0		6.7	
	Costa Rica	8.1[ac]	5.9[ad]	8.7[bd]	7.0[bc]
	Nicaragua	7.8[ac]	5.7[ad]	7.4[d]	6.3[c]
	United States	7.8			
	Canada	6.5[ac]	4.3[ad]	6.2[bd]	5.4[bc]

Note: Significant mean differences (F-value $p<.05$) within country using 2-group ANOVA controlling for age for each pairwise comparison: [a]female victims vs. male victims; [b]female aggressors vs. male aggressors; [c]female victims vs. male aggressors; [d]male victims vs. female aggressors.

There were few significant differences between female and male aggressors (shown with [b]). There was, however, a pattern among male aggressors to rate themselves as more afraid and upset compared with female agressors, while female aggressors tended to rate themselves as more angry. While one might assume that fear expressed by female victims was fear of their partners, the same cannot be assumed for aggressors. In particular, because male aggressors consistently rated themselves as more afraid than did male victims, it is unlikely that male aggressors were afraid of their partners (to whom they were being aggressive) and more likely that they were expressing fear regarding the consequences of their aggression. This highlights the need for more research on how fear plays a role in partner aggression, including its contribution to both restraint (i.e., due to fear of consequences) and escalation of violence.

Female victims rated severity as significantly higher than did male aggressors, with sometimes quite large differences seen between the ratings (e.g., severity rating of 5.6 by female victims vs. 2.9 by male aggressors in Costa Rica), although these differences were not always statistically significant (see [c] in the note below Table 4). Female victims also rated themselves as more afraid, more upset, and more angry compared with male aggressors, although, again, not all comparisons were statistically significant. Because these ratings are made by independent samples of females and males, the reason for the higher rating of severity by female victims compared to male aggressors is unknown. A possible explanation for the pattern of findings is gender differences in perceived (but not necessarily actual) severity; that is, male aggressors may see their own behavior as less severe compared with the female victim's view of the same act. However, there is considerable literature to suggest that partner aggression is more likely to result in injuries for female than for male victims (Archer, 2000; Archer, 2002; Arias, Samios, and O'Leary, 1987; Bland and Orne, 1986; Cascardi, Langhinrichsena, and Vician, 1992; Mihorean, 2005; Straus, 1995; Tjaden and Thoennes, 2000), that more women than men are killed by their partner (Domínguez and Fernández, 2003; Fox and Zawitz, 2004; Johnson, 2006), and that women experience more fear from partner aggression than do men (Fergusson, Horwood, and Ridder, 2005). Moreover, all country surveys in the present analyses that measured whether the respondent sought medical attention following the incident found that female victims were more likely than male victims to have sought medical attention. Thus, the higher severity rating for female victims compared to male aggressors is not likely to be solely a difference in perception between the male aggressor and the female victim. This difference may relate to issues raised earlier such as social desirability or gender biases in sampling or participation in the survey. For example, men who engaged in more severe aggression may have been more likely to have refused to participate in the survey.

Interestingly, male victims in most countries rated the severity of their partners' aggression as less severe than female aggressors rated their own aggression, although the difference was often not large and significant in only a few comparisons (see [d] in the note at the end of the table). The lower rating by male victims compared to female aggressors could reflect gender differences in perceived severity, but may also reflect gender bias in sampling, such as a higher rate of nonparticipation among men in relationships in which more severe violence occurred.

Overall, it is clear across all countries that being the victim of partner aggression is very different for women than for men, with female victims perceiving aggression by their partner as more severe, more frightening, and more upsetting and female victims being more angry compared with male victims. Thus, even in countries where men and women are equally likely to report being the victim of partner aggression, severity of aggression and fear are especially important issues for female victims. Gender differences in ratings by those reporting aggression toward a partner (i.e., the aggressors) are more difficult to interpret. No clear pattern between male and female aggressors emerged across countries for severity ratings; however, for the other ratings, female aggressors tended to rate themselves as less afraid and upset and more angry compared with male aggressors.

Alcohol Consumption and Partner Physical Aggression

In the following sections, we examine the extent of alcohol consumption at the time of the incident of partner aggression, as well as gender and victim/aggressor differences in the relationship between the respondent's drinking pattern and aggression.

Gender Differences in Drinking at the Time of the Aggressive Incident

In all countries except Uruguay, female victims were more likely than male victims and male and female aggressors to report drinking at the time of the incident by one partner (usually the male partner) or both partners, as reported in the country chapters. Although in most countries the difference between female victims and other groups in the percent of incidents involving alcohol did not meet the $p < .05$ criterion for statistical significance (see Table 5), this consistent pattern across countries suggests that alcohol is more of an issue for female victimization than for other forms of partner aggression, at least as reported by females. This confirms previous studies of violence against women that have identified drinking by the male partner as an important aspect of partner aggression (see review in the chapter "General Issues in Research on Intimate Partner Violence: An Overview.").

TABLE 5. Percent of incidents in which one or both partners had been drinking, by whether respondent was the victim or aggressor and by sex, ten participating countries.

Country	Female victims	Male victims	Female aggressors	Male aggressors
Argentina	26.8	13.8	12.0	24.3
Uruguay	14.6	11.6	15.8	29.4
Brazil	57.1[ac]	27.6[a]	49.9[b]	27.3[bc]
Peru (Lima)	41.0	25.1	27.0	25.0
Peru (Ayacucho)	43.6		22.9	
Costa Rica	40.0	26.9	26.6	25.0
Nicaragua	35.7	36.1	30.3	33.3
Belize	52.8	41.0		
Mexico	39.0	26.0		
United States				
Canada	31.0[a]	17.6[ad]	25.6[d]	26.1

Significant differences (Chi-square $p<.05$) within country between genders and roles: [a]female victim vs. male victims; [b]female aggressors vs. male aggressors; [c]female victims vs. male aggressors; [d]male victims vs. female aggressors.

While female victims were most likely to report alcohol involvement (in all countries but one), male aggressors were least likely in three of the seven countries (significant for Brazil). This suggests gender differences in reporting alcohol involvement and/or possible sampling bias. However, the difference could also reflect the effects of alcohol. Some research suggests that people may underestimate the effects of alcohol on their behavior (Graham and Wells, 2001). This, combined with the possibility of forgetting incidents that occurred while drinking or underestimating their severity, could also account for the discrepancy in ratings of alcohol involvement for male aggressors versus ratings by female victims. That is, male aggressors may be less likely to remember incidents of their own aggression or underestimate its severity when drinking. The finding of gender differences in reporting of alcohol involvement in partner aggression has important implications for prevention and treatment. In particular, both prevention and treatment programs need to take into consideration that alcohol may affect the drinker's perception and memory of the aggressive incident, specifically, that aggressors who have been drinking may underestimate the severity of their own aggressiveness.

Drinking Pattern and Partner Physical Aggression

As shown in Table 6, there was a clear pattern for drinkers to be more likely than abstainers to report partner aggression, and for current drinkers who drank five or more drinks on at least one occasion in the past year to be more likely to report aggression than were current drinkers who never drank that much. Although this pattern did not always reach the criterion for statistical significance, and there were two instances where this pattern did not occur (both nonsignificant), the consistency of the pattern across countries suggests that drinkers, especially those who drink more per occasion, are especially at risk for partner aggression.

TABLE 6. Percent of respondents who reported partner aggression by whether the respondent was the victim and aggressor, whether respondent was a current drinker, and whether respondent drank five or more drinks in the past year, by sex, ten participating countries.

Country	Sex	Role	Current Drinker Yes	Current Drinker No	Drank five or more drinks[c] in the past year Yes	Drank five or more drinks[c] in the past year No
Argentina						
	Female	Victim	10.7	5.7	13.9	10.1
		Aggressor	8.8	7.0	13.9	8.0
	Male	Victim	15.5	2.9	19.8	9.4
		Aggressor	0.0	9.0	12.0	4.7
Uruguay						
	Female	Victim	7.2	5.7	15.2	6.1
		Aggressor	8.2	2.8	21.7	6.4
	Male	Victim	8.2	1.4	12.3	4.8
		Aggressor	5.3	1.4	8.7	2.4
Brazil						
	Female	Victim	8.4[a]	4.3[a]	18.2[b]	6.3[b]
		Aggressor	7.5[a]	3.1[a]	19.1[b]	5.0[b]
	Male	Victim	5.3	2.3	7.2	3.6
		Aggressor	4.9	1.4	4.3	5.5
Peru (Lima)						
	Female	Victim	10.3[a]	5.5[a]	11.2	9.3
		Aggressor	10.7[a]	5.8[a]	12.2	8.8
	Male	Victim	8.3	4.4	8.8	7.7
		Aggressor	7.6	1.5	9.1	3.9
Peru (Ayacucho)						
	Female	Victim	22.6	14.9	26.9[b]	9.5[b]
		Aggressor	13.6	10.9	14.9	9.5
	Male	Victim	11.9	0.0	11.4	
		Aggressor	14.4	4.6	15.2	
Costa Rica						
	Female	Victim	8.2	6.2	13.8	6.3
		Aggressor	8.2[a]	3.1[a]	14.9[b]	5.9[b]
	Male	Victim	8.4	2.3	11.3	4.8
		Aggressor	7.3	0.0	10.7[b]	3.2[b]

TABLE 6. (continued)

Country	Sex	Role	Current Drinker Yes	Current Drinker No	Drank five or more drinks[c] in the past year Yes	Drank five or more drinks[c] in the past year No
Nicaragua						
	Female	Victim	9.5	5.6	9.7	9.1
		Aggressor	7.4	6.3	8.6	5.5
	Male	Victim	10.3[a]	2.7[a]	10.7	
		Aggressor	10.7[a]	2.4[a]	10.7	
Belize						
	Female	Victim	8.5[a]	3.4[a]	10.7	6.8
	Male	Victim	5.6[a]	0.5[a]	6.1	4.6
Mexico						
	Female	Victim			15.1[b]	6.0[b]
	Male	Victim			4.5[b]	2.6[b]
United States						
	Female	Victim	8.3[a]	1.9[a]		
Canada						
	Female	Victim	5.8	4.0	9.8[b]	3.5[b]
		Aggressor	6.4[a]	3.4[a]	10.2[b]	4.0[b]
	Male	Victim	8.0[a]	3.6[a]	9.6	4.0
		Aggressor	3.8[a]	1.9[a]	4.8[b]	1.9[b]

[a] Significant difference ($p<.05$) within country and within each respondent role between drinkers and abstainers using logistic regression controlling for age.
[b] Significant difference ($p<.05$) within country and within each respondent role between those who drank five or more and those who never drank five drinks, using logistic regression controlling for age.
[c] Question in the U.S. survey asked whether respondent drank six or more drinks (not five or more) on any occasion in the past 12 months.

Frequency of Drinking

No consistent relationship between partner aggression and respondents' drinking frequency emerged across countries (see Table 7). The only differences that met the criterion for statistical significance were: in Peru/Ayacucho, where female aggressors drank more frequently than nonaggressors; in Costa Rica, where male aggressors drank more frequently than nonaggressors; and in Canada, where differences were fairly small but all were significant (more frequent drinking by female victims, male victims, and male aggressors, but less frequent drinking by female aggressors). It should be noted that the number of drinkers who reported partner aggression was too low for statistical comparison (based on a minimum cell size of 20) in some cases.

Usual Number of Drinks Consumed on Drinking Occasions

Table 8 shows that respondents who reported partner aggression consumed more drinks on their usual drinking occasions than did those who reported no aggression, although this difference did not always reach the significance criterion, and there were a few exceptions to this pattern. In general, however, the results are similar to those for ever consuming five or more drinks per occasion, namely that those who consume larger quantities per occasion are at higher risk for physical partner aggression.

TABLE 7. Average number of drinking days per year by whether respondent was a victim or aggressor, by sex, nine of the ten participating countries.

Country	Women				Men			
	Victim	Not a victim	Aggressor	Not an aggressor	Victim	Not a victim	Aggressor	Not an aggressor
Argentina	37.3	64.7	48.4	63.1	104.0	123.9	122.2	120.6
Uruguay	48.0	51.3	31.4	52.8	67.6	87.7		86.5
Brazil	47.9	32.4	42.6	33.0	100.5	85.5	55.5	87.9
Peru (Lima)	10.4	12.2	10.2	12.3	17.5	23.5	27.1	22.7
Peru (Ayacucho)	7.8	7.4	10.5[b]	7.1[b]		12.1		12.1
Costa Rica	39.0	26.9	27.6	27.9	54.5	54.0	82.1[d]	51.9[d]
Nicaragua		29.5		31.6	68.7	41.9	44.9	44.7
Belize	45.7	34.2			76.1	62.0		
United States	49.8	45.4						
Canada	72.6[a]	66.5[a]	63.8[b]	67.7[b]	108.8[c]	103.0[c]	109.1[d]	103.1[d]

Significant differences (F-value p<.05) within country between means using two-group ANOVA controlling for age for: [a]female victims vs. females who reported no victimization; [b]female aggressors vs. females who reported no aggression; [c]male victims vs. males who reported no victimization; [d]male aggressors vs. males who reported no aggression.

TABLE 8. Number of drinks consumed on usual drinking occasions by whether respondent was a victim or aggressor, by sex, ten participating countries.

Country	Women				Men			
	Victim	Not a victim	Aggressor	Not an aggressor	Victim	Not a victim	Aggressor	Not an aggressor
Argentina	2.0	1.7	1.7	1.7	4.2	3.6	3.9	3.6
Uruguay	3.9[a]	2.2[a]	3.5[b]	2.2[b]	5.3	4.2		4.2
Brazil	4.0[a]	2.4[a]	4.1[b]	2.4[b]	5.8	4.2	4.9	4.3
Peru (Lima)	4.6[a]	3.6[a]	4.9[b]	3.6[b]	6.9	7.0	7.1	7.0
Peru (Ayacucho)	4.9	4.1	4.5	4.3		7.2		6.9
Costa Rica	3.3	2.7	3.8[b]	2.6[b]	5.3	5.0	6.5	4.9
Nicaragua		6.9		6.7	13.7	12.1	13.7	12.1
Belize	3.7	3.5			6.7	7.5		
United States	2.3	2.1						
Canada	3.0[a]	2.0[a]	3.1[b]	2.1[b]	4.3[c]	3.1[c]	4.8[d]	3.2[d]

Significant differences (F-value p<.05) within country between means using ANOVA controlling for age for: [a]female victims vs. females who reported no victimization; [b]female aggressors vs. females who reported no aggression; [c]male victims vs. males who reported no victimization; [d]male aggressors vs. males who reported no aggression

Total Annual Consumption in Number of Drinks

The pattern for total annual consumption (see Table 9) was the same as that for the number of drinks per usual drinking occasion, with higher consumption associated with a higher risk of partner aggression, with a few exceptions and not all differences significant.

TABLE 9. Average annual consumption (total number of drinks per year) by whether respondent was a victim or aggressor, by sex, nine of the ten participating countries.

Country	Women				Men			
	Victim	Not a victim	Aggressor	Not an aggressor	Victim	Not a victim	Aggressor	Not an aggressor
Argentina	97.7	137.4	113.8	135.0	575.1	481.4	802.8[d]	466.4[d]
Uruguay	357.4	141.8	171.5	156.1	701.4	544.5		542.9
Brazil	321.9	98.6	350.2	98.5	764.2	579.7	335.1	602.8
Peru (Lima)	90.9	54.9	79.0	56.2	197.5	234.0	256.2	229.0
Peru (Ayacucho)	62.3	52.3	67.8	52.5		139.2		136.5
Costa Rica	132.8	91.6	120.0	92.8	384.8	343.8	692.5[d]	320.1[d]
Nicaragua		334.8		357.7	969.8	656.2	692.6	687.8
Belize	257.8	194.0			768.3	561.0		
United States	209.6	155.9						
Canada	282.1[a]	176.0[a]	269.3[b]	178.7[b]	699.4[c]	406.7[c]	720.2[d]	419.5[d]

Significant differences (F-value p<.05) within country between means using ANOVA controlling for age for: [a]female victims vs. females who reported no victimization; [b]female aggressors vs. females who reported no aggression; [c]male victims vs. males who reported no victimization; [d]male aggressors vs. males who reported no aggression.

These results are consistent with previous findings (see the chapter "General Issues in Research on Intimate Partner Violence: An Overview") of a relationship between heavier alcohol consumption and risk of partner aggression. However, the clear pattern of findings pertaining to the amount of alcohol consumed per usual occasion and of consuming five or more drinks on a single occasion, versus the mixed pattern for frequency of drinking, suggests that it may not be drinking per se that increases the risk of aggression, but primarily drinking large amounts on an occasion. This relationship between heavy drinking and partner aggression was evident across countries, despite variations in drinking patterns, proportions of heavy drinkers, and gender differences in drinking patterns seen from country to country. The importance of the amount consumed per occasion (versus frequency of drinking or total consumption) is consistent with previous research, suggesting that the quantity of alcohol consumed on a given occasion is more important than drinking frequency in predicting intimate partner aggression (Bondy, 1996; Wells, Graham, and West, 2000).

Analyses done within the chapters (where sufficient numbers were available to separate those who reported that one or both partners had been drinking at the time of the incident from those who reported that no one had been drinking) suggested that the relationship between aggression and the consumption of larger amounts of alcohol on a given occasion was stronger for respondents reporting alcohol-related aggression than for those who reported aggression that did not involve alcohol. Again, this is consistent with previous research showing that the link between drinking pattern and aggression applies mainly to aggression involving alcohol (Wells and Graham, 2003), rather than reflecting some common propensity to both drink and be aggressive.

The relationship between alcohol consumption and partner aggression may depend on whether the aggressor or the victim has consumed alcohol. For example, one explanation for the relationship between drinking and an increased risk of being aggressive toward a partner is that alcohol's effect on cognitive functioning, impulse control, problem solving, risk taking, and other functioning (Graham et al., 1998, 2000) may make it more likely that a person will behave aggressively and that aggression will be more severe when it does occur.

Establishing why drinking more drinks per occasion may also increase risk of victimization is more complex. One explanation, especially for female partners, is that drinking by females is highly correlated with drinking by their partners (Roberts and Leonard, 1997); therefore, the relationship between victimization and female drinking may be the result of female drinking serving as a proxy for male drinking, especially given the finding across countries that it was rare for only the female to be drinking at the time of the aggressive incident. A partner's heavy drinking might also put stress on the relationship, leading to conflicts that result in physical aggression (Dobash and Dobash, 1984).

Finally, alcohol's effects also could play a role for both nonaggressive and aggressive victims. For nonaggressive victims, alcohol could increase the extent to which they put themselves in risky situations, as well as affecting their problem-solving ability to avoid conflict situa-tions. For aggressive victims (i.e., persons who report both aggression by a partner and toward a partner), drinking may play a role in both partners' willingness to be aggressive, as well as in the escalation of aggression. It also is possible that victims and aggressors consume alcohol in large quantities as a way of coping with the effects of partner aggression. Finally, alcohol consumption and partner aggression might both be the results of other stresses in the relationship (Kantor and Straus, 1987).

Country Drinking Pattern and Alcohol Involvement in Partner Aggression

Alcohol might be expected to be more involved in partner aggression in those countries where most people drink and where people drink frequently, based on chance alone. That is, even if alcohol does not contribute to aggression, if people are generally more likely to be drinking, then it is also more likely that they will have been drinking when aggression occurred. However, cultures have been found to vary considerably in the extent to which people become aggressive when they drink (MacAndrew and Edgerton, 1969), and there is some evidence from Europe that alcohol-related aggression is more likely to occur in countries where drinking is infrequent (sometimes called "dry" countries) but where persons consume large amounts of alcohol when they do drink (Rossow, 2001) than in countries where persons drink frequently ("wet" countries). Therefore, it is useful to examine the relationship between drinking pattern and aggression for the countries included in the present analyses, in order to assess whether aggression is more strongly associated with drinking in countries with an infrequent but high-quantity drinking pattern versus countries where people drink more frequently but in lower quantities.

In figures 1, 3 and 5, we examine the relationship of whether the male respondent/partner was drinking at the time of the incident with percent of male respondents who were current drinkers and average frequency and quantity of drinking by male respondents from that country. In figures 2, 4, and 6, we examine the relationship of whether the female respondent/partner was drinking at the time of the incident with percent of female respondents who were current drinkers and average frequency and quantity of drinking by female respondents from that country. To illustrate the results visually in the figures, countries were ordered from highest to lowest for percent of current drinkers (Figures 1 and 2), average frequency of drinking in the country (Figures 3 and 4) and usual drinking quantity (Figures 5 and 6). In each figure, the bars show the percent of incidents of aggression in that country in which the male (Figures 1, 3, 5) or female (Figures 2, 4, and 6) respondent/partner had been drinking.

In Figure 1, the countries are ordered by the percent of male respondents who reported consuming alcohol in the year before the survey (i.e., current drinkers), from the highest percent (91.5% in Argentina) to the lowest (43.4% in Nicaragua). The bars show the percent of male partners who had been drinking at the time of the incident (combining the percentages for incidents in which only the male drank and those in which both

FIGURE 1. Percent of incidents in each country in which the male partner had been drinking (male only or both partners had been drinking), as reported by female victims and aggressors and male victims and aggressors, with countries shown in descending order by percent of men who were current drinkers, nine of the ten participating countries.

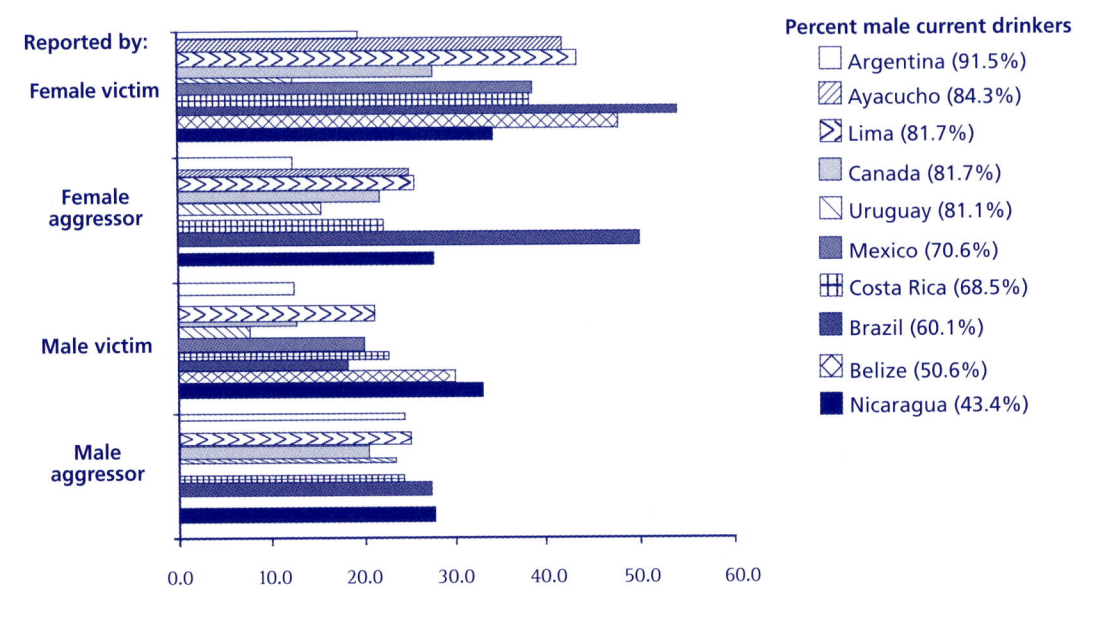

Note: Spearman rho rank order correlations between country rank on percent of current drinkers and percent of incidents involving drinking by the male partner: rho = −.32 (n = 10, p = .365) for female victims, rho = −.60 for female aggressors (n = 8, p = .120), rho = −.70 (n = 9, p = .036) for male victims, and rho = −.61 (n = 7, p = .148) for male aggressors.

partners drank) as reported by female victims, female aggressors, male victims, and male aggressors. Spearman rank order correlations (shown in a footnote to the table) were used as a simple way of quantifying the relationship between the country's ranking in terms of percent of male current drinkers and the percent of incidents in which the male partner had been drinking. Although most comparisons were not statistically significant (p < .05) due to the small number of countries in the analysis, Figure 1 shows a clear pattern in which drinking at the time of aggression was more likely to occur in countries with lower rates of current drinkers.

As shown in Figure 2, the relationship between percent of female drinkers in a country and the percent of incidents involving drinking by the female partner differed from the pattern seen for male drinkers. Overall, there was no apparent pattern in the relationship between percent of females who were current drinkers and whether the female was drinking at the time of the aggression.

FIGURE 2. Percent of incidents in each country in which the female partner had been drinking (female only or both partners had been drinking), as reported by female victims and aggressors and male victims and aggressors, with countries ordered by percent of women who were current drinkers (from highest to lowest), nine of the ten participating countries.

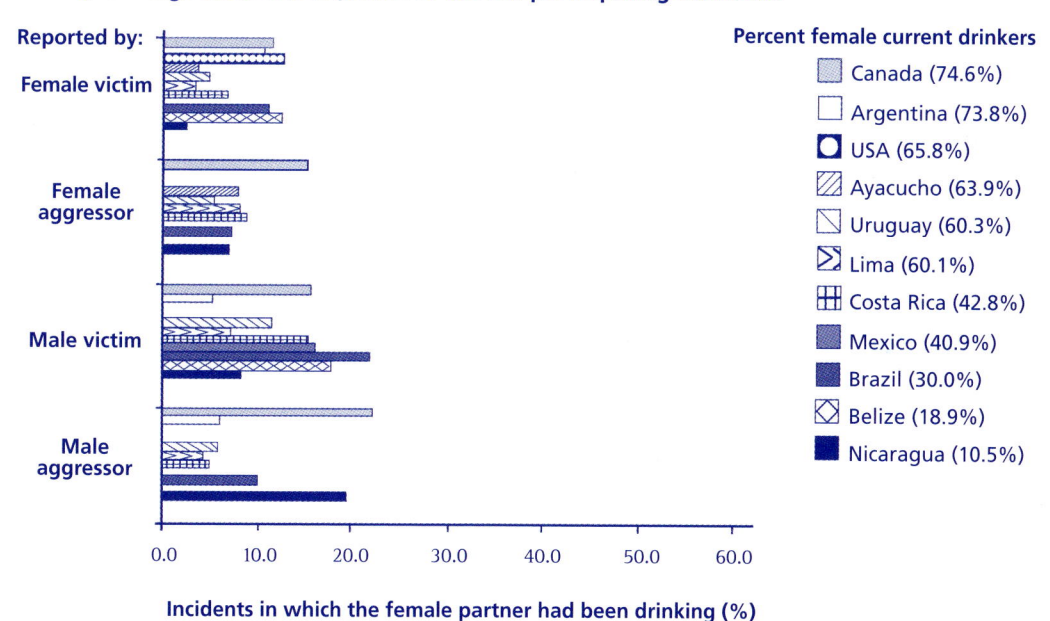

Percent female current drinkers
- Canada (74.6%)
- Argentina (73.8%)
- USA (65.8%)
- Ayacucho (63.9%)
- Uruguay (60.3%)
- Lima (60.1%)
- Costa Rica (42.8%)
- Mexico (40.9%)
- Brazil (30.0%)
- Belize (18.9%)
- Nicaragua (10.5%)

Incidents in which the female partner had been drinking (%)

Note: Spearman rho rank order correlations between country rank on percent of current drinkers and percent of incidents involving drinking by the female partner: rho = .34 (n = 11, p = .312) for female victims, rho = .12 for female aggressors (n = 8, p = .779), rho = −.40 (n = 9, p = .286) for male victims, and rho = .07 (n = 7, p = .879) for male aggressors.

Figures 3 and 4 show the percent of male (Figure 3) and female (Figure 4) partners who had been drinking during an aggressive incident, with countries ordered by frequency of drinking among current drinkers. Regarding the frequency of drinking among men in a given country, the pattern was the same as for the percent of current drinkers, with drinking by male partners at the time of aggression being more likely to occur in countries where men drank less frequently. The relationship between the frequency of females drinking and whether female partners had been drinking at the time of the aggressive incident showed the opposite pattern for female victims; that is, drinking by female victims was more likely to occur in countries where women drank at higher frequencies. There was no relationship between the frequency of females drinking at the country level and whether female partners had been drinking at the time of the incident for female aggressors.

FIGURE 3. Percent of incidents in each country in which the male partner had been drinking (male partner only or both partners had been drinking), as reported by female victims and aggressors and male victims and aggressors, with countries shown in descending order by average frequency of drinking by men who were current drinkers (from highest to lowest), nine of the ten participating countries.

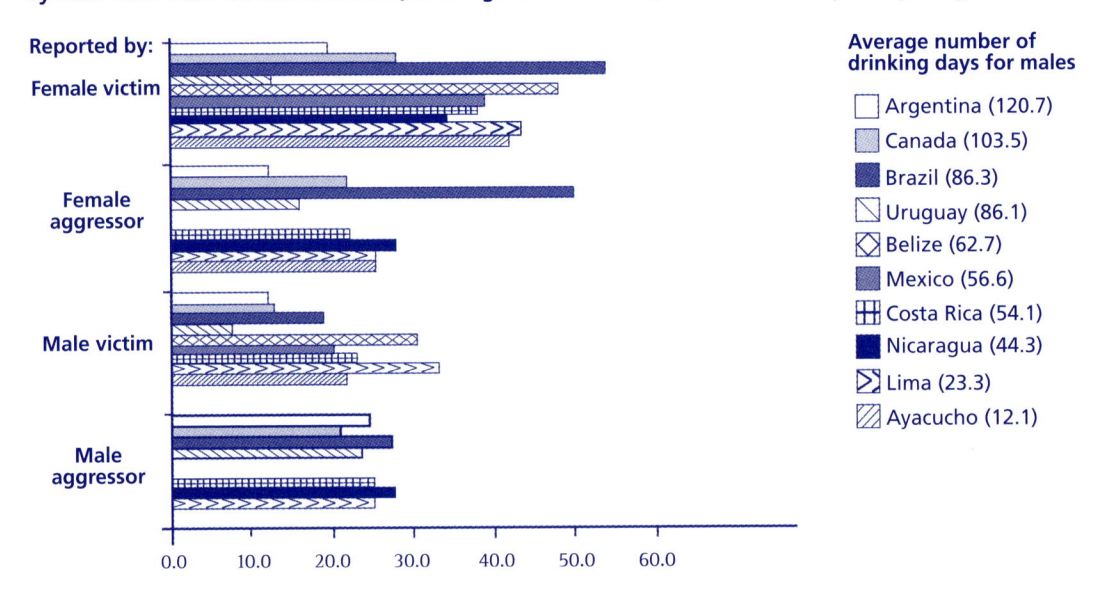

Average number of drinking days for males:
- Argentina (120.7)
- Canada (103.5)
- Brazil (86.3)
- Uruguay (86.1)
- Belize (62.7)
- Mexico (56.6)
- Costa Rica (54.1)
- Nicaragua (44.3)
- Lima (23.3)
- Ayacucho (12.1)

Incidents in which the male partner had been drinking (%)

Note: Spearman rho rank order correlations between country rank on frequency of drinking and percent of incidents involving drinking by the male partner: rho = –.36 (n = 10, p = .310) for female victims, rho = –.50 for female aggressors (n = 8, p = .207), rho = –.73 (n = 9, p = .025) for male victims, and rho = –.57 (n = 7, p = .180) for male aggressors.

Comparison of ten countries | 243

FIGURE 4. Percent of incidents in each country in which the female partner had been drinking (female partner only or both partners had been drinking), as reported by female victims and aggressors and male victims and aggressors in each country, with countries shown in descending order by average frequency of drinking by women who were current drinkers, ten participating countries

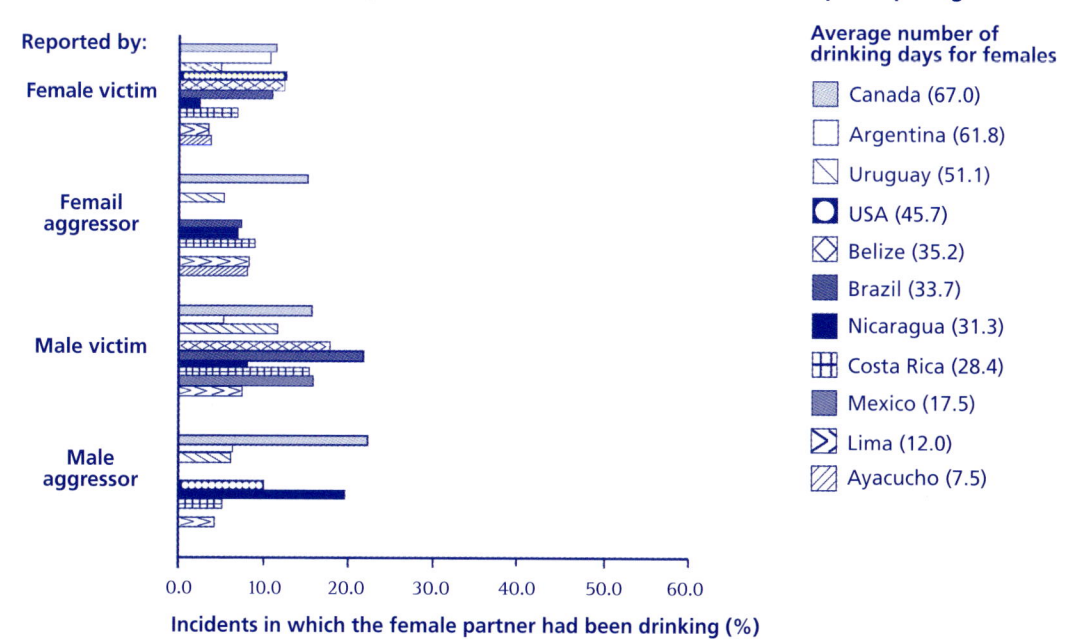

Average number of drinking days for females:
- Canada (67.0)
- Argentina (61.8)
- Uruguay (51.1)
- USA (45.7)
- Belize (35.2)
- Brazil (33.7)
- Nicaragua (31.3)
- Costa Rica (28.4)
- Mexico (17.5)
- Lima (12.0)
- Ayacucho (7.5)

Incidents in which the female partner had been drinking (%)

Note: Spearman rho rank order correlations between country rank on frequency of drinking and percent of incidents involving drinking by the female partner: rho = .68 (n = 11, p = .021) for female victims, rho = −.12 (n = 8, p = .779) for female aggressors, rho = .05 (n = 9, p = .898) for male victims; and rho = .54 (n = 7, p = .215) for male aggressors..

As shown in Figure 5, the percent of male partners who had been drinking at the time of the incident of partner aggression tended to be higher in countries where the usual quantity of alcohol consumed on drinking occasions by men in that country was higher. For female respondents who reported being the victim of partner aggression (see percents reported by female victims shown in Figure 6), on the other hand, the percent of women who reported drinking at the time of the aggressive incident tended to be lower in countries where the usual quantity consumed by women in the country was higher (rho = −.76, n = 11, p = .007); there was no relationship between whether the female partner had been drinking and usual amount consumed by women in that country found for incidents reported by female aggressors or for male aggressors or male victims.

FIGURE 5. Percent of incidents in each country in which the male partner had been drinking (male partner only or both partners had been drinking), as reported by female victims and aggressors, and male victims and aggressors, with countries shown in descending order by average number of drinks per occasion by men who were current drinkers, nine of the ten participating countries.

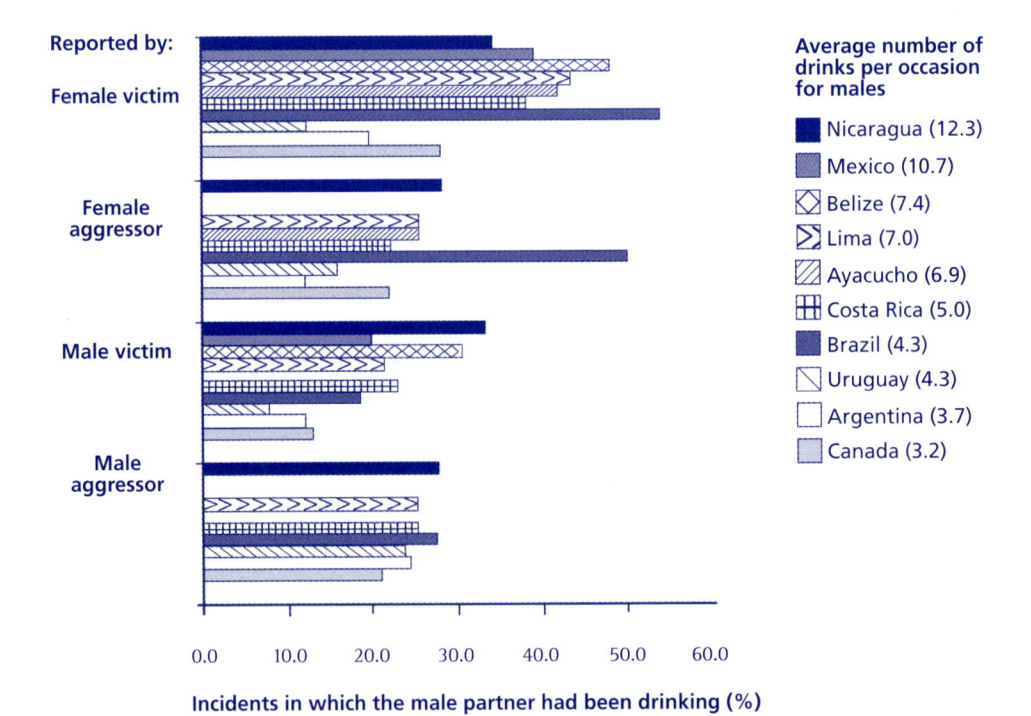

Average number of drinks per occasion for males:
- Nicaragua (12.3)
- Mexico (10.7)
- Belize (7.4)
- Lima (7.0)
- Ayacucho (6.9)
- Costa Rica (5.0)
- Brazil (4.3)
- Uruguay (4.3)
- Argentina (3.7)
- Canada (3.2)

Incidents in which the male partner had been drinking (%)

Note: Spearman rho rank order correlations between country rank on usual quantity per occasion and percent of incidents involving drinking by the male partner: rho = .44 (n = 10, p = .200) for female victims, rho = .69 (n = 8, p = .058) for female aggressors, rho = .82 (n = 9, p = .007) for male victims, and rho = .86 (n = 7, p = .014) for male aggressors.

As the results for Figures 1 through 6 indicate, the relationship between the drinking pattern in a given country and whether there was drinking at the time of aggression differed for men and women. The pattern among men is consistent with the hypothesis that men are more likely to have been drinking at the time of an aggressive incident in those countries where drinking is relatively infrequent and where those who drink consume larger amounts per occasion. This was especially true when partner aggression was reported by male respondents, both as victims and aggressors. These findings provide additional evidence that it is the quantity of alcohol consumed per occasion not just whether the person is a drinker that accounts for the relationship between drinking and partner aggression. Findings are also consistent with research suggesting that problem behavior from drinking may be more likely to occur in "dry" countries (i.e., countries where drinking is not the norm) than in "wet" countries where drinking is more routinely done (see Room, 2001).

FIGURE 6. Percent of incidents in each country in which the female partner had been drinking (female partner only or both partners had been drinking), as reported by female victims and aggressors, and male victims and aggressors, with countries shown in descending order by average number of drinks per occasion by women who were current drinkers, ten participating countries.

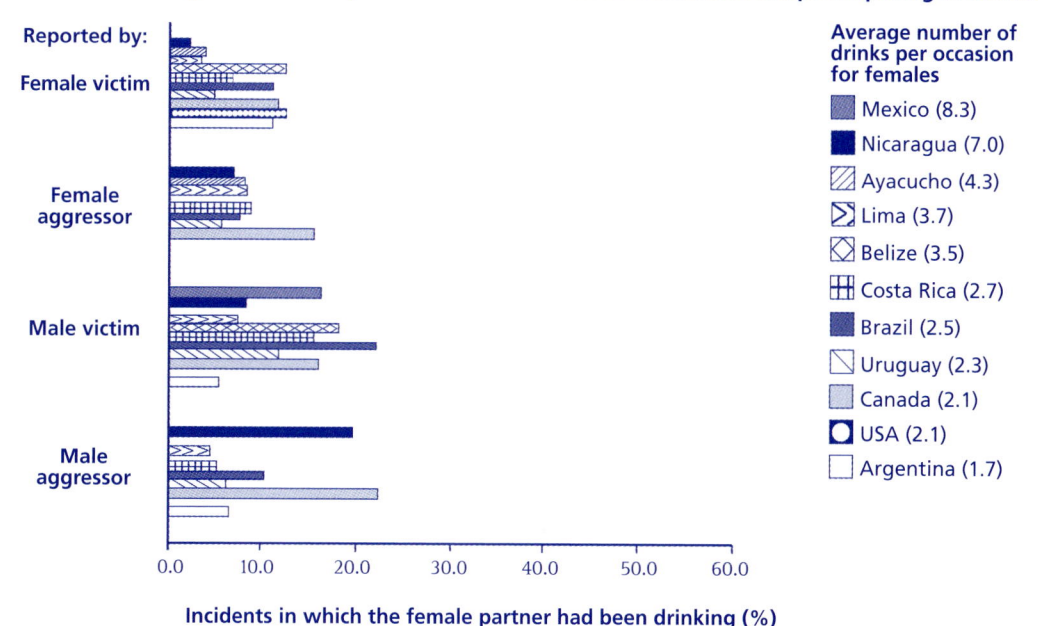

Reported by:

Female victim

Female aggressor

Male victim

Male aggressor

Incidents in which the female partner had been drinking (%)

Average number of drinks per occasion for females
- Mexico (8.3)
- Nicaragua (7.0)
- Ayacucho (4.3)
- Lima (3.7)
- Belize (3.5)
- Costa Rica (2.7)
- Brazil (2.5)
- Uruguay (2.3)
- Canada (2.1)
- USA (2.1)
- Argentina (1.7)

Note: Spearman rho rank order correlations between country rank on usual quantity per occasion and percent of incidents involving drinking by the female partner: rho = −.76, n = 11, p = .007 for female victims, rho = .17 (n = 8, p = .693) for female aggressors, rho = .17 (n = 9, p = .668) for male victims, and rho = −.25 (n = 7, p = .589) for male aggressors).

For women, the only patterns that emerged were that female victims (as reported by female victims and male aggressors) were more likely to have been drinking at the time of aggression in those countries where drinking by women was more frequent, and less likely (as reported by female victims but not by male aggressors) in those countries where women consumed larger quantities of alcohol on drinking occasions. It would be premature to speculate on the reasons for the particular pattern found for women, because the sample of female drinkers and the proportion of women drinking at the time of the aggressive incident were both quite small in some countries. However, it is important to note that there is no evidence that the consistent relationship between drinking pattern and drinking at the time of aggression found for men also applies to women. Thus, additional research is needed to better understand the cultural and pharmacological factors in women's drinking and how these relate to women's involvement in partner aggression.

Conclusions

Many of these findings are surprisingly consistent across the ten countries, despite differences in language, culture, economic prosperity, and other factors. For example, partner aggression appears to decrease with age in all the countries. Married persons are least likely to report partner aggression and those in a common-law relationship are most likely to do so across most countries. In addition to identifying high-risk subpopulations, these findings point to a need for research to better understand how young age and common-law marital status increase the risk of partner violence.

Ratings of aggression severity, fear, upset, and anger confirm that, although both men and women engage in partner aggression, the experience is more severe for female than for male victims; thus, these findings reinforce the priority given to stopping violence against women. In almost all countries, gender differences also were found in the percent of respondents who reported having been drinking at the time of the incident, with female victims being especially likely to report that the male partner or both partners had been drinking. Thus, alcohol use seems to be particularly important in terms of violence against women.

In terms of the relationship between drinking pattern and partner aggression, the results showed that current drinkers were more likely than abstainers to report partner aggression (both as victims and as aggressors), and that those who drank more per occasion were more likely to be involved in aggression than those who drank less; however, no clear pattern emerged linking partner aggression to drinking frequency. Thus, the evidence is mounting across countries with different drinking patterns and cultures that the link between drinking and partner aggression is primarily related to the quantity of alcohol consumed, at least at the individual level, adding insight into previously observed relationships between male-to-female partner physical aggression and alcohol use and problems (Stith et al., 2004).

At the country level, the relationship between drinking pattern and whether alcohol was consumed at the time of partner aggression differed for male versus female drinkers. For men, there was a greater likelihood that the male partner would have been drinking at the time of the aggressive incident in those countries where there was a high abstinence rate among men, less frequent drinking and more alcohol consumed per occasion on average by men in that country. When a relationship was found related to female drinking, on the other hand, it was found only for female victims and was in the opposite direction from that found for male drinking. These puzzling findings related to female drinking indicate a need for further research on gender differences in the link between partner aggression and alcohol consumption.

Finally, despite differences in countries and cultures, consistent gender differences in reporting partner aggression raised common methodological concerns. In particular, the consistency in the finding that female respondents were more likely than male respondents to report aggression toward the female partner raised the possibility of response or sampling bias, especially for male respondents. More research, including qualitative research, on female versus male perspectives on aggressive acts between partners would be useful in trying to sort out not only the discrepancy between reports of female victims and male aggressors, but also findings that male aggressors reported feeling more afraid at the time of the incident than did male victims, and that country-level relationships between drinking patterns and drinking at the time of aggression were different for men and women.

References

Archer J. (2000). Sex differences in aggression between heterosexual partners: A meta-analytic review. *Psychological Bulletin*, 126, 651-680.

Archer J. (2002). Sex differences in physically aggressive acts between heterosexual partners: A meta-analytic review. *Aggression and Violent Behavior*, 7, 213-351.

Archer J. (2006). Cross-cultural differences in physical aggression between partners: A social role analysis. *Personality and Social Psychology Review*, 10, 133-153.

Arias I, Samios M, O'Leary, K. (1987). Prevalence and correlates of physical aggression during courtship. *Journal of Interpersonal Violence*. 2, 82-90.

AuCoin K. (Ed.) (2005). *Family violence in Canada: A statistical profile*. Ottawa, Canada: Canadian Centre for Justice Statistics, Statistics Canada. www.statcan.ca. Catalogue no. 85-224-XIE

Bland R, Orne H. (1986). Family violence and psychiatric disorder. *Canadian Journal of Psychiatry*. 31, 129-137.

Bondy S. (1996). Overview of studies on drinking patterns and consequences. *Addiction*. 91, 1663-1674.

Bookwala J, Sobin J, Zdaniuk, B. (2005). Gender and aggression in marital relationships: A life-span perspective. *Sex Roles*, 52(11/12), 797-806.

Bunge VP, Locke D. (Eds.) (2002). *Family violence in Canada: A statistical profile*. Ottawa, Canada: Canadian Centre for Justice Statistics, Statistics Canada. www.statcan.ca. Catalogue no. 85-224-XIE

Cascardi M, Langhinrichsen J, Vivian, D. (1992). Marital aggression: Impact, injury, and health correlates for husbands and wives. *Archives of Internal Medicine*, 152, 1178-1184.

Dobash R, Dobash R. (1984). The nature and antecedents of violent events. *British Journal of Criminology*, 24, 269-288.

Domínguez C, Fernández M. (2003). *Perfil de los Incidentes Familiares con Víctimas Fallecidas: Análisis Estadístico y Explicativo de la Realidad Uruguaya*. Dirección Nacional de Prevención Social del Delito del Ministerio del Interior.

Ellsberg M, Peña R, Herrera A, Liljestrand J, Winkvist A. (2000). Candies in hell: women's experiences of violence in Nicaragua. *Social Science and Medicine*, 51, 1595-1610.

Fergusson D, Horwood L, Ridder, E. (2005). Partner violence and mental health outcomes in a New Zealand birth cohort. *Journal of Marriage and Family*, 67, 1103-1119.

Flake D. (2005). Individual, family, and community risk markers for domestic violence in Peru. *Violence Against Women*, 11, 353-373.

Flake DF, Forste R. (2006). Fighting families: Family characteristics associated with domestic violence in five Latin American countries. *Journal of Family Violence*, 21, 19-29.

Fox JA, Zawitz, MW. (2004). Homicide trends in the United States. Washington, DC: U.S. Department of Justice, Bureau of Justice Statistics. At www.ojp.usdoj.gov/bjs/homicide/homtrnd.htm

García-Moreno C, Jansen HAFM, Ellsberg M, Heise L, Watts, C. (2006). Prevalence of intimate partner violence: findings from the WHO multi-country study on women's health and domestic violence. *Lancet*, 368, 1260-1269.

Graham K, Leonard KE, Room R, Wild TC, Pihl RO, Bois C, Single, E. (1998). Current directions in research on understanding and preventing intoxicated aggression. *Addiction*, 9, 659-676.

Graham K, Wells S. (2001). "I'm okay. You're drunk!" Self-other differences in the perceived effects of alcohol in real-life incidents of aggression. *Contemporary Drug Problems*, 28, 441-462.

Graham K, West P, Wells S. (2000). Evaluating theories of alcohol-related aggression using observations of young adults in bars. *Addiction*, 95(6), 847-863.

Johnson H. (2006) Measuring violence against women. Statistical trends 2006. Ottawa, Canada: Canadian Centre for Justice Statistics, Statistics, Canada.

Kantor G, Straus, M. (1987). The "drunken bum" theory of wife beating. *Social Problems*, 34, 213-230.

MacAndrew C, Edgerton, RB. (1969). *Drunken comportment. A social explanation*. Chicago: Aldine.

Mihorean K. (2005). Trends in self-reported spousal violence. In K. AuCoin (Ed.) *Family violence in Canada: A statistical profile*. Ottawa, Canada: Canadian Centre for Justice Statistics, Statistics Canada. www.statcan.ca. Catalogue no. 85-224-XIE.

Natera G, Tiburcio M, Villatoro J. (1997) Marital violence and its relationship to excessive drinking in Mexico. *Contemporary Drug Problems*, 24, 787-804.

Orpinas P. (1999). Who is violent? Factors associated with aggressive behaviors in Latin America and Spain. *Rev Panam Salud Publica*. Vol 5, Washington, D.C.

Roberts LJ, Leonard KE. (1997). Gender differences and similarities in the alcohol and marriage relationship (pp. 289-311). In S. Wilsnack and R. Wilsnack (Eds.), *Gender and alcohol*. Piscataway, NJ: Rutgers Center of Alcohol Studies.

Room R. (2001). Intoxication and bad behaviour: Understanding cultural differences in the link. *Social Science and Medicine*, 53, 189-198.

Rosales J, Loaiza E, Primante D, Barberena A, Blandon L, Ellsberg M. (1999). Encuesta Nicaraguense de Demografia y Salud, 1998. Managua, Nicaragua: Instituto Nacional De Estadisticas y Censos, INEC and Macro International, Inc.

Rossow I. (2001). Alcohol and homicide: A cross-cultural comparison of the relationship in 14 European countries. *Addiction*, 96(Supplement 1), S77-S92.

Stets JE, Straus MA. (1990). The marriage license as a hitting license: A comparison of assaults in dating, cohabiting and married couples. In M. A. Straus & R. J. Gelles & C. Smith (Eds.), *Physical violence in American families: Risk factors and adaptations to violence in 8,145 families* (pp. 227-244). New Brunswick, New Jersey: Transaction Publishers.

Stith SM, Smith DB, Penn CE, Ward DB, Tritt D. (2004). Intimate partner physical abuse perpetration and victimization risk factors: A meta-analytic review. *Aggression and Violent Behavior*, 10, 65-98.

Straus MA. (1995). Trends in cultural norms and rates of partner violence: An update to 1992. In S. M. Stith & M. A. Straus (eds.), Understanding partner violence: prevalence, causes, consequences, and solutions (pp. 30-33). Minneapolis, MN: National Council on Family Relations.

Tjaden P, Thoennes N. (2000). Prevalence and consequences of male-to-female and female-to-male intimate partner violence as measured by the National Violence Against Women Survey. *Violence Against Women*, 6, 142-161.

Wells S, Graham K. (2003). Aggression involving alcohol: Relationship to drinking patterns and social context, *Addiction*, 98, 33-42.

Wells S, Graham K, West, P. (2000). Alcohol-related aggression in the general population. *Journal of Studies on Alcohol*, 61, 626-632.

Wilke D, Vinton L. (2005). The nature and impact of domestic violence across age cohorts. *AFFILIA*, 20, 316-328.

Wilson M, Johnson H, Daly M. (1995). Lethal and nonlethal violence against wives. *Canadian Journal of Criminology*, 37, 331-361.

Acknowledgments

This book is part of the project, Gender, Alcohol and Culture: An International Study (GENACIS). GENACIS is a collaborative international project affiliated with the Kettil Bruun Society for Social and Epidemiological Research on Alcohol, and coordinated by GENACIS partners from the University of North Dakota, the University of Southern Denmark, the Charité-University Medicine Berlin, the Pan American Health Organization, and the Swiss Institute for the Prevention of Alcohol and Drug Problems. Support for aspects of the project comes from the World Health Organization, the Quality of Life and Management of Living Resources Programme of the European Commission (Concerted Action QLG4-CT-2001-0196), the United States National Institute on Alcohol Abuse and Alcoholism (part of the National Institutes of Health) (Grant Numbers R21 AA012941 and R01 AA015775), Canadian Institutes of Health Research (CIHR) (No. 108626), the German Federal Ministry of Health, the Pan American Health Organization, and national funds from Switzerland. Data from some countries were collected as part of the PAHO Multicentric Study led by Maristela G. Monteiro (PI), Jürgen Rehm (PI), and Ben Taylor (Project Coordinator).

The following authors and co-authors contributed chapters to this book. Also sources of funding for the surveys in each country are gratefully acknowledged.

Chapter
Funding Source(s) of survey
Author(s) (Affiliation(s))

Preface
Dr. Mirta Roses Periago (Director, Pan American Health Organization)

Foreword
Lori Heise (Research Fellow, Gender Violence and Health Centre, London School of Hygiene and Tropical Medicine; Core Research Team Member, WHO Multi-Country Study on Women's Health and Domestic Violence against Women; Director, Global Campaign for Microbicides, PATH)

Introduction
Maristela Monteiro (Senior Advisor on Tobacco Control, Alcohol, and Substance Abuse, Pan American Health Organization)

Marijke Velzeboer-Salcedo (Senior Advisor, Gender, Ethnicity and Health, Pan American Health Organization)

Gender, Alcohol, and Culture: An International Study (GENACIS): A brief history, present work, and future initiatives
Benjamin Taylor (Centre for Addiction and Mental Health, Ontario, Canada)

Sharon Wilsnack (Department of Clinical Neuroscience, University of North Dakota School of Medicine and Health Sciences, Grand Forks, North Dakota, USA)

Jürgen Rehm (Centre for Addiction and Mental Health, Ontario, Canada)

General issues in research on intimate partner violence: an overview
Sharon Wilsnack (Department of Clinical Neuroscience, University of North Dakota School of Medicine and Health Sciences, Grand Forks, North Dakota, USA)

Richard Wilsnack (Department of Clinical Neuroscience, University of North Dakota School of Medicine and Health Sciences, Grand Forks, North Dakota, USA)

Common survey methods and analyses conducted for each country chapter
Sharon Bernards (Centre for Addiction and Mental Health, Ontario, Canada)

Kathryn Graham (Centre for Addiction and Mental Health, Ontario, Canada; Department of Psychology, University of Western Ontario, Canada; National Drug Research Institute, Curtin University of Technology, Australia)

Chapter
Funding Source(s) of survey
Author(s) (Affiliation(s))

Argentina: Alcohol and partner physical aggression in Buenos Aires province and city
World Health Organization and conducted as part of GENACIS
Myriam Munné (Research Institute of University of Buenos Aires)

Belize: Alcohol and partner physical aggression
Pan American Health Organization and completed as part of the PAHO Multicentric Study and affiliated with GENACIS

Claudina Ellington Cayetano (Mental Health Program, Ministry of Health, Belize)

Kathryn Graham (Centre for Addiction and Mental Health, Ontario, Canada; Department of Psychology, University of Western Ontario, Canada; National Drug Research Institute, Curtin University of Technology, Australia)

Brazil: Alcohol and partner physical aggression in Metropolitan São Paulo
São Paulo State Research Support Foundation – Fundação de Apoio à Pesquisa do Estado de Saõ Paulo (FAPESP 04/11729–2) also conducted in affiliation with the PAHO Multicentric Study and GENACIS

Florence Kerr–Corrêa (Department of Neurology, Psychology, and Psychiatry, Botucatu Medical School, São Paulo State University, UNESP, Botucatu, São Paulo)

Janaina Barbosa de Oliveira (Ph D student–Mental Health Post graduation, São Paulo University Medical School, USP–RibeirãoPreto, São Paulo)

Maria Cristina Pereira Lima (Department of Neurology, Psychology, and Psychiatry, Botucatu Medical School, São Paulo State University, UNESP, Botucatu, São Paulo; CAPES post–doctoral fellowship)

Adriana Marcassa Tucci (Department of Health Sciences, São Paulo Federal University–UNIFESP–Santos, São Paulo)

Maria Odete Simão (Department of Neurology, Psychology and Psychiatry, Botucatu Medical School, São Paulo State University, UNESP, Botucatu, São Paulo)

Mariana Braga Cavariani (MSc student–Department of Public Health, Botucatu Medical School, São Paulo State University, UNESP, Botucatu, São Paulo and FAPESP Fellowship)

Miriam Malacize Fantazia (Department of Neurology Psychology, and Psychiatry, Botucatu Medical School, São Paulo State University, UNESP, Botucatu, São Paulo and FAPESP fellowship)

Canada: Alcohol and partner physical aggression in the 10 provinces
Canadian Institutes of Health Research (CIHR) (No. 108626), Kathryn Graham (PI) and Andree Demers (Co–PI) and also conducted as part of GENACIS

Kathryn Graham (Centre for Addiction and Mental Health, Ontario, Canada; Department of Psychology, University of Western Ontario, Canada; National Drug Research Institute, Curtin University of Technology, Australia)

Sharon Bernards (Centre for Addiction and Mental Health, Ontario, Canada)

Costa Rica: Alcohol and partner physical aggression in the Greater Metropolitan Area
World Health Organization and conducted as part of GENACIS
Julio Bejarano (Instituto sobre Alcoholismo y Farmacodependencia)

Chapter
Funding Source(s) of survey
Author(s) (Affiliation(s))

Mexico: Alcohol and partner physical aggression in Ciudad Juárez, Monterrey, Querétaro, and Tijuana
CONADIC (National Council against Addictions), the State Councils against Addictions of the states of Baja California, Chihuahua, Monterrey, and Quéretaro, and the National Institute of Psychiatry (INP) and also conducted in affiliation with the PAHO Multicentric Study and GENACIS
Martha Romero Mendoza (National Institute of Psychiatry)
María Elena Medina–Mora (National Institute of Psychiatry)
Jorge Velázquez Villatoro (National Institute of Psychiatry)
Clara Fleiz (National Institute of Psychiatry)
Leticia Casanova (National Institute of Psychiatry)
Francisco Juárez (National Institute of Psychiatry)

Nicaragua: Alcohol and partner physical aggression in Bluefields, Estelí, Juigalpa, León, and Rivas
Pan American Health Organization and completed as part of the PAHO Multicentric Study and affiliated with GENACIS

José Trinidad Caldera Aburto (Professor, University of Colonia, León, Nicaragua)
Sharon Bernards (Centre for Addiction and Mental Health, Ontario, Canada)
Myriam Munné (Research Institute of University of Buenos Aires)

Peru: Alcohol and partner physical aggression in Lima and Ayacucho
Pan American Health Organization and completed as part of the PAHO Multicentric Study and affiliated with GENACIS

Marina Piazza (Professor, School of Public Health and Administration, Universidad Peruana Cayetano Heredia, Lima, Peru)

United States: Alcohol and partner physical aggression—Findings from a national sample of women
National Institute on Alcohol Abuse and Alcoholism, National Institutes of Health (Grants R01 AA004610, R01 AA015775, and R21 AA012941) and also conducted as part of GENACIS

Sharon Wilsnack (Department of Clinical Neuroscience, University of North Dakota School of Medicine and Health Sciences, Grand Forks, North Dakota, USA)

Richard Wilsnack (Department of Clinical Neuroscience, University of North Dakota School of Medicine and Health Sciences, Grand Forks, North Dakota, USA)

Arlinda Kristjanson (Department of Clinical Neuroscience, University of North Dakota School of Medicine and Health Sciences, Grand Forks, North Dakota, USA)

Uruguay: Alcohol and partner physical aggression in various cities
World Health Organization and conducted as part of GENACIS
Raquel Magri (Former National Secretary on Drugs, Montevideo)
Héctor Suárez (Observatory on Drugs (Junta Nacional de Drogas)
Laurita Regueira (Observatory on Drugs (Junta Nacional de Drogas)

Comparison of partner physical aggression across ten countries
Kathryn Graham (Centre for Addiction and Mental Health, Ontario, Canada; Department of Psychology, University of Western Ontario, Canada; National Drug Research Institute, Curtin University of Technology, Australia)

Sharon Bernards (Centre for Addiction and Mental Health, Ontario, Canada)

UNHAPPY HOURS: